Serono Symposia, USA
Norwell, Massachusetts

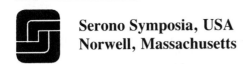

Serono Symposia, USA
Norwell, Massachusetts

William F. Crowley, Jr.   P. Michael Conn
Editors

Modes of Action of GnRH and GnRH Analogs

With 117 Figures

Springer-Verlag
New York Berlin Heidelberg London Paris
Tokyo Hong Kong Barcelona Budapest

William F. Crowley, Jr., M.D.
Reproductive Endocrine Unit
Department of Medicine
Massachusetts General Hospital
Boston, MA 02114
USA

P. Michael Conn, Ph.D.
Department of Pharmacology
University of Iowa College of
 Medicine
Iowa City, IA 52242-1109
USA

Proceedings of the Symposium on Modes of Action of GnRH and GnRH Analogs, sponsored by Serono Symposia, USA, held February 26 to March 2, 1991, in Scottsdale, Arizona.

For information on previous volumes, please contact Serono Symposia, USA.

Library of Congress Cataloging-in-Publication Data
Modes of action of GnRH and GnRH analogs/William F. Crowley, Jr., P.
  Michael Conn, editors.
     p. cm.
    "Proceedings of the Symposium on Modes of Action of GnRH and GnRH
  Analogs, sponsored by Serono Symposia, USA, held February 26 to
  March 2, 1991, in Scottsdale, Arizona."—T.p. verso.
    Includes bibliographical references and indexes.
    ISBN 0-387-97802-X (alk. paper).—ISBN 3-540-97802-X (alk. paper)
    1. Luteinizing hormone releasing hormone—Mechanism of action—
  Congresses.   2. Luteinizing hormone releasing hormone—Derivatives—
  Mechanism of action—Congresses.   I. Crowley, William F. (William
  Francis)   II. Conn, P. Michael.   III. Serono Symposia, USA.
  IV. Symposium on Modes of Action of GnRH and GnRH Analogs (1991:
  Scottsdale, Ariz.)
    [DNLM: 1. Gonadorelin—analogs & derivatives—congresses.
  2. Gonadorelin—physiology—congresses.   3. Gonadorelin—therapeutic
  use—congresses.   WK 515 M691 1991]
  QP572.L85M63   1992
  612.6—dc20
  DNLM/DLC   92-2157

Printed on acid-free paper.

Production coordinated by Technical Texts and managed by Francine Sikorski; manufacturing supervised by Jacqui Ashri.
Typeset by Best-set Typesetter Ltd., Hong Kong.
Printed and bound by Edwards Brothers, Inc., Ann Arbor, MI.

Printed in the United States of America.

9 8 7 6 5 4 3 2 1

ISBN 0-387-97802-X Springer-Verlag New York Berlin Heidelberg
ISBN 3-540-97802-X Springer-Verlag Berlin Heidelberg New York

SYMPOSIUM ON MODES OF ACTION OF GnRH AND GnRH ANALOGS

Scientific Committee

P. Michael Conn, Ph.D., Cochairman
University of Iowa College of Medicine

William F. Crowley, Jr., M.D., Cochairman
Massachusetts General Hospital
and Harvard Medical School

Organizing Secretary

L. Lisa Kern, Ph.D.
Serono Symposia, USA
100 Longwater Circle
Norwell, Massachusetts

Preface

Since the awarding of the Nobel Prize to Drs. Guillemin and Schally in 1971 for isolation and chemical characterization of gonadotropin releasing hormone, we have experienced a remarkable period of growth of interest in this hormone. The last 20 years have been characterized by a swift translation of basic science discovery into clinical utility. Approval of GnRH and its analogs for treatment of prostate cancer, endometriosis, and precocious puberty and for induction of ovulation indicate the range of usefulness of these agents.

In order to bring together the leaders in the basic and clinical science of GnRH, a conference was organized on "Modes of Action of GnRH and GnRH Analogs" and held in Scottsdale, Arizona, February 26 to March 2, 1991. The presentations, given as chapters in this volume, show both the advances in the body of information in this discipline and the efforts underway to reduce basic science to clinical practice. The audience was a combination of representatives from universities, government, industry, and physicians in practice. The lively discussions and insightful questions indicated the interest in the topics discussed and frequently served to catalyze planned interactions of the meeting participants.

The organizers are grateful to the speakers and poster presenters for their contributions and for the timely preparations of the manuscripts included in the present volume. We are also thankful to the staff of Serono Symposia, USA, for the organizational skills and support that allowed the meeting organizers to focus on the science and medicine presented.

WILLIAM F. CROWLEY, JR.
P. MICHAEL CONN

Contents

Part III.   GnRH Physiology: Animal Models

Part IV. GnRH Antagonists

Contributors

J.P. ADELMAN, Vollum Institute, Oregon Health Sciences University, Portland, Oregon, USA.

CARRIE J. BAGATELL, Medical Service, Veterans Affairs Medical Center, Department of Medicine, Population Center for Research in Reproduction, and the Regional Primate Research Center, University of Washington, Seattle, Washington, USA.

ANGELA C. BAUER-DANTOIN, Department of Neurobiology and Physiology, Northwestern University, Evanston, Illinois, USA.

MICHEL R. BLANC, Station de Physiologie de la Reproduction, Institut National de la Recherche Agronomique, 37380 Nouzilly, France.

C.T. BOND, Vollum Institute, Oregon Health Sciences University, Portland, Oregon, USA.

PHILIPPE BOUCHARD, Service d'Endocrinologie, Hôpital de Bicêtre, 94270 Le Kremlin Bicêtre, France.

TIM D. BRADEN, Department of Pharmacology, University of Iowa College of Medicine, Iowa City, Iowa, USA.

WILLIAM J. BREMNER, Medical Service, Veterans Affairs Medical Center, Department of Medicine, Population Center for Research in Reproduction, and the Regional Primate Research Center, University of Washington, Seattle, Washington, USA.

ALAIN CARATY, Station de Physiologie de la Reproduction, Institut National de la Recherche Agronomique, 37380 Nouzilly, France.

MELVIN CHING, Laboratory of Molecular and Integrative Neurosciences, National Institute of Environmental Health Sciences, National Institutes of Health, Research Triangle Park, North Carolina, USA.

I.J. Clarke, Prince Henry's Institute of Medical Research, South Melbourne, Victoria, Australia.

P. Michael Conn, Department of Pharmacology, University of Iowa College of Medicine, Iowa City, Iowa, USA.

William F. Crowley, Jr., Reproductive Endocrine Unit, Department of Medicine, Massachusetts General Hospital, Boston, Massachusetts, USA.

Gordon B. Cutler, Jr., National Institutes of Health, Bethesda, Maryland, USA.

Alan C. Dalkin, Divisions of Endocrinology and Metabolism, Department of Internal Medicine, University of Virginia, Charlottesville, Virginia, USA.

Douglas R. Danforth, The Jones Institute for Reproductive Medicine, Department of Obstetrics and Gynecology, Eastern Virginia Medical School, Norfolk, Virginia, USA.

R. Fernald, Department of Biology, Stanford University, Stanford, California, USA.

R. Francis, Department of Biology, Stanford University, Stanford, California, USA.

Marie J. Gibson, Department of Medicine, Mount Sinai School of Medicine, New York, New York, USA.

David F. Gordon, Department of Medicine, University of Colorado Health Sciences Center and Veterans Affairs Medical Center, Section of Endocrinology (111H), Denver, Colorado, USA.

Keith Gordon, The Jones Institute for Reproductive Medicine, Department of Obstetrics and Gynecology, Eastern Virginia Medical School, Norfolk, Virginia, USA.

Andrea C. Gore, Wisconsin Regional Primate Research Center, University of Wisconsin, Madison, Wisconsin, USA.

Kenneth G. Gould, Yerkes Regional Primate Research Center, Atlanta, Georgia, USA.

Sajiv Gugneja, Department of Biochemistry, Molecular Biology, and Cell Biology, Northwestern University, Evanston, Illinois, USA.

DANIEL J. HAISENLEDER, Divisions of Endocrinology and Metabolism, Department of Internal Medicine, University of Virginia, Charlottesville, Virginia, USA.

JANET E. HALL, Reproductive Endocrine Unit, Massachusetts General Hospital, Boston, Massachusetts, USA.

GARY D. HODGEN, The Jones Institute for Reproductive Medicine, Department of Obstetrics and Gynecology, Eastern Virginia Medical School, Norfolk, Virginia, USA.

FRED J. KARSCH, Reproductive Sciences Program and Department of Physiology, University of Michigan, Ann Arbor, Michigan, USA.

MARVIN J. KARTEN, Contraceptive Development Branch, Center for Population Research, National Institute of Child Health and Human Development, National Institutes of Health, Bethesda, Maryland, USA.

J.C. KING, Department of Anatomy and Cellular Biology, Tufts University Health Sciences Campus, Boston, Massachusetts, USA.

ERIC LEE, National Institutes of Health, Bethesda, Maryland, USA.

JON E. LEVINE, Department of Neurobiology and Physiology, Northwestern University, Evanston, Illinois, USA.

ZSOLT LIPOSITS, Laboratory of Molecular and Integrative Neurosciences, National Institute of Environmental Health Sciences, National Institutes of Health, Research Triangle Park, North Carolina, USA.

FRANCISCO LÓPEZ, Laboratory of Molecular and Integrative Neurosciences, National Institute of Environmental Health Sciences, National Institutes of Health, Research Triangle Park, North Carolina, USA.

DAVID R. MANN, Department of Physiology, Morehouse School of Medicine, Atlanta, Georgia, USA.

JOHN C. MARSHALL, Divisions of Endocrinology and Metabolism, Department of Internal Medicine, University of Virginia, Charlottesville, Virginia, USA.

KELLY E. MAYO, Department of Biochemistry, Molecular Biology, and Cell Biology, Northwestern University, Evanston, Illinois, USA.

PAMELA MELLON, Regulatory Biology Laboratory, Salk Institute, La Jolla, California, USA.

ISTVAN MERCHENTHALER, Laboratory of Molecular and Integrative Neurosciences, National Institute of Environmental Health Sciences, National Institutes of Health, Research Triangle Park, North Carolina, USA.

JOHN M. MEREDITH, Department of Neurobiology and Physiology, Northwestern University, Evanston, Illinois, USA.

GREGORY M. MILLER, Department of Medicine, Mount Sinai School of Medicine, New York, New York, USA.

SUZANNE M. MOENTER, Reproductive Sciences Program and Department of Physiology, University of Michigan, Ann Arbor, Michigan, USA.

YUKO NAKAYAMA, National Institutes of Health, Bethesda, Maryland, USA.

ANDRÉS NEGRO-VILAR, Laboratory of Molecular and Integrative Neurosciences, National Institute of Environmental Health Sciences, National Institutes of Health, Research Triangle Park, North Carolina, USA.

OK-KYONG PARK, Department of Biochemistry, Molecular Biology, and Cell Biology, Northwestern University, Evanston, Illinois, USA.

SPYROS N. PAVLOU, Department of Medicine, Division of Endocrinology, Vanderbilt University School of Medicine, Nashville, Tennessee, USA.

DONALD W. PFAFF, Laboratory of Neurobiology and Behavior, The Rockefeller University, New York, New York, USA.

SALLY RADOVICK, Case Western Reserve University, School of Medicine, Division of Endocrinology and Hypertension, Cleveland, Ohio, USA.

B.S. RUBIN, Department of Anatomy and Cellular Biology, Tufts University Health Sciences Campus, Boston, Massachusetts, USA.

YOUICHI SAITOH, Department of Medicine, Mount Sinai School of Medicine, New York, New York, USA.

MARLENE SCHWANZEL-FUKUDA, Laboratory of Neurobiology and Behavior, The Rockefeller University, New York, New York, USA.

R. SEAL, Vollum Institute, Oregon Health Sciences University, Portland, Oregon, USA.

ANN-JUDITH SILVERMAN, Department of Cell Biology and Anatomy, Columbia College of Physicians and Surgeons, New York, New York, USA.

R. SIMERLY, Oregon Regional Primate Research Center, Beaverton, Oregon, USA.

ROBERT A. STEINER, Departments of Obstetrics and Gynecology, Physiology and Biophysics, Population Center for Research in Reproduction, and the Regional Primate Research Center, University of Washington, Seattle, Washington, USA.

FRANK J. STROBL, Department of Neurobiology and Physiology, Northwestern University, Evanston, Illinois, USA.

WEI SUN, Department of Medicine, University of Colorado Health Sciences Center and Veterans Affairs Medical Center, Section of Endocrinology (111H), Denver, Colorado, USA.

EI TERASAWA, Wisconsin Regional Primate Research Center, University of Wisconsin, Madison, Wisconsin, USA.

CHRISTINE TICKNOR, Case Western Reserve University, School of Medicine, Division of Endocrinology and Hypertension, Cleveland, Ohio, USA.

JANICE H. URBAN, Department of Neurobiology and Physiology, Northwestern University, Evanston, Illinois, USA.

MARCELO VALENÇA, Laboratory of Molecular and Integrative Neurosciences, National Institute of Environmental Health Sciences, National Institutes of Health, Research Triangle Park, North Carolina, USA.

KIM WALLEN, Department of Psychology, Emory University, Atlanta, Georgia, USA.

CHUN WANG, Department of Medicine, University of Colorado Health Sciences Center and Veterans Affairs Medical Center, Section of Endocrinology (111H), Denver, Colorado, USA.

RICHARD WEINER, Reproductive Endocrinology Center, University of California, San Francisco, California, USA.

BRUCE D. WEINTRAUB, National Institutes of Health, Bethesda, Maryland, USA.

HEINER WESTPHAL, National Institutes of Health, Bethesda, Maryland, USA.

WILLIAM WETSEL, Laboratory of Molecular and Integrative Neurosciences, National Institute of Environmental Health Sciences, National Institutes of Health, Research Triangle Park, North Carolina, USA.

RANDALL W. WHITCOMB, Reproductive Endocrine Unit, Department of Medicine, Massachusetts General Hospital, Boston, Massachusetts, USA.

MARGARET E. WIERMAN, Department of Medicine, University of Colorado Health Sciences Center and Veterans Affairs Medical Center, Section of Endocrinology (111H), Denver, Colorado, USA.

ROBERT F. WILLIAMS, The Jones Institute for Reproductive Medicine, Department of Obstetrics and Gynecology, Eastern Virginia Medical School, Norfolk, Virginia, USA.

FREDRIC E. WONDISFORD, Case Western Reserve University, School of Medicine, Division of Endocrinology and Hypertension, Cleveland, Ohio, USA.

WILLIAM W. WOOD, Department of Medicine, University of Colorado Health Sciences Center and Veterans Affairs Medical Center, Section of Endocrinology (111H), Denver, Colorado, USA.

SUSAN WRAY, National Institutes of Health, Bethesda, Maryland, USA.

Part I

Overview of GnRH Secretion and Mechanism of Action

1

Critical Determinants of GnRH-Gonadotrope Interactions in the Human

RANDALL W. WHITCOMB AND WILLIAM F. CROWLEY, JR.

The study of GnRH physiology in the human has proven to be complex, with both technical and practical obstacles. Specifically, the rapid metabolism of GnRH continues to make its direct measurement in the peripheral circulation limited in utility in defining the neuroendocrine control of reproduction in the human (1, 2). The inaccessibility of the hypophyseal-portal blood supply to direct sampling also means that a series of indirect approaches must be undertaken, using several strategies to piece together a complete story of the hypothalamic control of gonadotropin function. Thus, we have chosen to use complementary approaches involving the tandem study of GnRH-deficient men as well as of normal men with intact hypothalamic pituitary axes (3).

The role of LH an alternative marker of hypothalamic secretion has been dramatically improved by two advances. The first is the widespread agreement that increasing the intensity of sampling of peripheral blood for LH levels to 10-min intervals has harvested considerably more precise information about patterns of LH release, permitted a sharper discernment of each individual LH pulse, and consequently allowed more precise estimates of LH, and therefore of GnRH, pulse frequency (4). Secondly, a growing body of experimental evidence in several species has now confirmed the concordancy of GnRH secretion from the hypothalamus with subsequent bursts of pulsatile LH release from the anterior pituitary (5–8). Taken together, these advances have yielded considerably more information as well as enhancing the certitude of this information.

An additional advance has been the recognition that the free alpha subunit (FAS) of glycoprotein hormones is also released in a pulsatile fashion with nearly 100% concordance with LH (9, 10). The utility of FAS as a surrogate marker of GnRH secretion in physiologic states in which rapid pulse frequency is evident (i.e., the midcycle surge) may in fact prove superior to that of LH, as a result of the more rapid half-life of FAS and of the consequently improved visualization of pulsatile secretory activity. FAS may also be the earliest marker of GnRH secretory activity during early GnRH exposure—i.e., FAS demonstrates pulsatility prior to LH or FSH. Thus, additional and complementary information may be obtained using measurements of both LH and FAS as markers of GnRH secretion.

Models for the Study of GnRH Physiology

Each of the various models chosen for the study of GnRH physiology has its unique strength; however, this strength is invariably combined with a limitation such that interpretations of GnRH physiology on the basis of any single model is flawed in some fundamental way.

The first model is that of the normal male (Figs. 1.1 and 1.2). Its advantages are numerous, including the relative abundance of subjects and their ease of study. They also permit a visualization of the intact hypothalamic-pituitary-gonadal axis. Such studies afford an understanding of the interindividual variability in the normal male reproductive system. Thus, when they are studied in sufficient numbers to overcome this variance, examination of normal men permits assembly of a robust normative data base. This precision of normative information can then be used to establish statistical limits of confidence that can be used to define clinical abnormalities of the reproductive system. The study of the normal

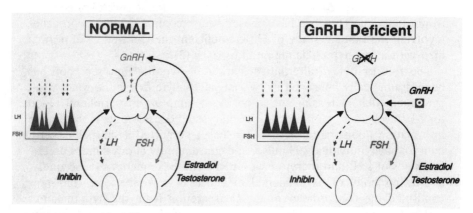

FIGURE 1.1. Hypothalamic-pituitary-gonadal axes in normal (left panel) and GnRH-deficient (right panel) men. The free-running nature of the normal male GnRH secretory system results in GnRH-induced LH pulses of differing amplitudes and frequencies, with evidence of feedback of gonadal steroids and/or inhibin potentially occurring at the hypothalamus and/or the pituitary. In contrast, GnRH-deficient men receiving an experimentally definable regimen of exogenous GnRH have gonadotropin pulse amplitudes and frequencies that can be fixed. Hence they are capable of responding to gonadal feedback only at the level of the pituitary.

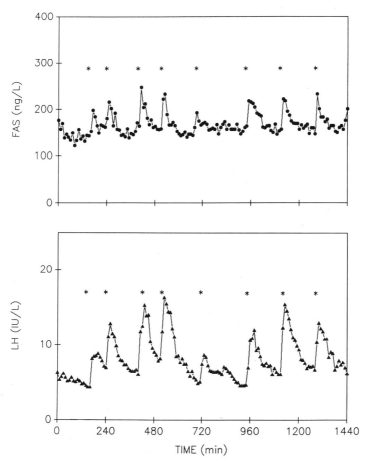

FIGURE 1.2. Normal man sampled at 10-min intervals for 24 h for FAS (upper panel) and LH (lower panel). Note the excellent correlation in pulsatile secretion between these two glycoproteins.

male possesses certain limitations. The variance inherent in this model demands the study of large numbers of patients. In addition, since their hypothalamic-pituitary axes are fully integrated, they may have compensatory adaptations that occur in response to any experimental manipulation of this system that might be attempted. Consequently, the normal male, when studied alone, does not permit a dissection of the hypothalamic from the pituitary components of the reproductive system and thus requires the parallel study of a complementary model.

GnRH-deficient men represent a unique "experiment of nature" that in many ways is invaluable to study in parallel with the intact male (Figs. 1.1 and 1.3). Since these patients completely lack functional secretion of GnRH (11), their reproductive competency can be totally restored with the proper regimen of pulsatile GnRH (12–14). When competency

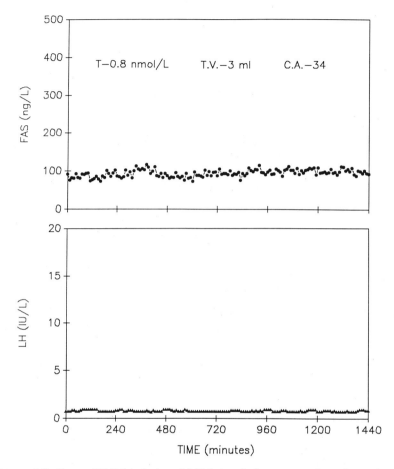

FIGURE 1.3. Serum FAS (circles) and LH (triangles) concentrations determined at 10-min intervals in a representative man with complete GnRH deficiency. The patient had testicular volumes (T.V.) of 3 ml, anosmia, and no history of spontaneous puberty. Note the complete absence of pulsatility of both LH and FAS. (C.A. = chronological age, T = serum testosterone levels in ng/dl.)

of their pituitary-gonadal axes has been restored to normal with a physiologic program of exogenous GnRH administration, these men permit a separation of the hypothalamic from the pituitary component of this system's responsiveness, since any physiologic manipulation must occur at the level of the anterior pituitary (Fig. 1.1). There are, however, significant limitations in the use of this rare human disease state as a investigational model. It is, for example, critical to define individually the "physiologic nature" of the exogenous GnRH regimen used in terms of GnRH dose, frequency, etc. In addition, longitudinal studies are required, since the administration of exogenous GnRH to these patients for the first 2–3 months elicits priming of the pituitary responsiveness with a changing pattern of pituitary responsiveness during this period (13).

The Role of the Bolus Dose of GnRH in Gonadotrope Secretion

A review of the 24-h pattern of pulsatile LH release in the normal male as outlined in Figure 1.2 reveals a striking variability of the LH and FAS pulse amplitude over a 24-h period. The question thus arises, is this variation in LH pulse amplitude due to (a) varying bolus doses of endogenous GnRH secretion, (b) varying intervals of pituitary stimulation by a fixed dose of GnRH, (c) feedback effects of gonadal steroids and/or proteins at the anterior pituitary, or (d) a combination of these factors?

Of course, it is not possible to examine this issue further in an intact male other than to document its presence. This problem can, however, be approached by using GnRH-deficient men in whom the dose and frequency of GnRH stimulation can be experimentally controlled. In vivo, this frequency of GnRH stimulation was set to the mean frequency documented to occur in normal males (approximately 2 h), a frequency deduced from sampling a large series of normal adult males at 10-min intervals for 24 h (15). Prior to exogenous GnRH administration, all GnRH-deficient men exhibited a complete absence of endogenous GnRH activity as attested to by their apulsatile LH and FAS secretion during baseline studies (Fig. 1.3). Each man subsequently received exogenous GnRH administered at 2-h intervals until normalization of his pituitary-gonadal axis had been documented for at least 3 months. Subsequently, the men were admitted to the General Clinic Research Center of the Massachusetts General Hospital, where the frequency of their GnRH regimen was held constant at 2-h intervals, their gonadal steroid levels were determined to be within the physiologic range for normal adult males, and the intravenously administered doses of GnRH were varied to span two log orders (2.5–250 ng/kg/bolus). As can be seen in Figure 1.4, a linear relationship exists between the LH and FAS amplitude (or area under the curve) and the log of the GnRH dose. This dose-response relationship is tenfold higher for LH than for FSH (Fig. 1.5) and exists for both biologically and immunologically active LH (16).

These studies confirm a quantitative relationship between the amount of GnRH administered exogenously (or presumably secreted endogenously), and all 3 of the ensuing gonadotrope glycoprotein secretory responses. Moreover, these dose-response relationships can now be quantitated in relation to the data obtained from extensive sampling

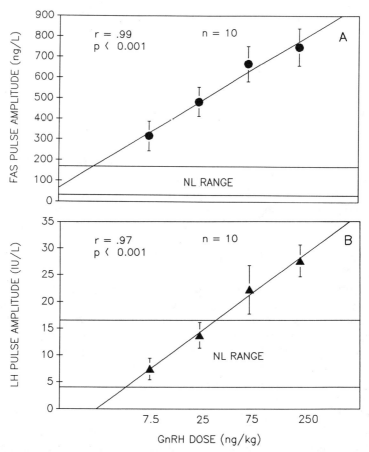

FIGURE 1.4. Dose-response relationships between GnRH and FAS (A) and between GnRH and LH (B) in 10 GnRH-deficient men compared with the normal adult range. Both panels exhibit a log linear response between the dose of GnRH and the resultant pulse amplitude. Doses of 7.5 and 25 ng/kg resulted in LH pulse amplitudes within the normal range, whereas the FAS responses to these 2 doses of GnRH were 88% and 187% higher, respectively, than the upper 95% confidence limits of the normal (NL) male range for FAS pulse amplitudes. Reprinted by permission from Ref. 10, © by The Endocrine Society, 1990.

of our normal population (Fig. 1.4), such that an individual dose of exogenous GnRH can be selected in each GnRH-deficient subject that will predictably evoke an LH secretory response whose amplitude is within the midnormal range, when applied at a physiologic frequency and in a physiologic gonadal hormonal milieu.

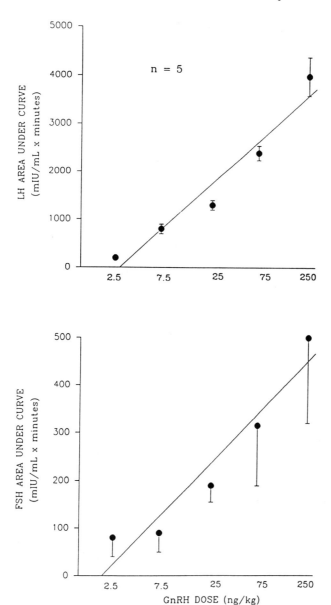

FIGURE 1.5. Mean (±SEM) immunoactive dose-response curves for LH and FSH constructed from area under the secretory curve of pulses after varying doses of GnRH in 5 men with GnRH deficiency. Note that this relationship is 10-fold higher for LH than for FSH in these men with intact gonads.

The Role of Frequency of GnRH Stimulation in Gonadotrope Secretion

Although there is a clearcut linear dose-response relationship between the dose of exogenous GnRH and the subsequent pituitary response, this information is not sufficient to answer the question first posited regarding the LH amplitudes that occur in the normal male—i.e., whether all their variability is attributable to individual differences of endogenous GnRH doses secreted by the hypothalamus. Thus, the next series of experiments examined the role of increasing and decreasing the frequency of a fixed and "physiologic" bolus of GnRH input. These studies were designed to examine the alternative hypothesis that variations in frequency of stimulation by a fixed (and "physiologic") dose of GnRH could also result in varied pituitary responsiveness per se. This is a particularly important hypothesis to examine, since the hypothalamus is known to vary greatly the frequency of endogenous GnRH secretion and hence of gonadotroph stimulation during puberty (17, 18) and the menstrual cycle (19) and after removal of gonadal influences (20).

Increasing Frequency of GnRH Stimulation

An individualized GnRH dosage was administered intravenously at the mean normal adult male frequency of every 2 h to a series of GnRH-deficient patients (21). After an 8-h period of baseline monitoring (i.e., four individual pulses), the frequency of this fixed GnRH dose was progressively increased at weekly intervals from 120- to 60- to 30- to 15-min frequencies. The patients were admitted every 7 days for an equivalent 8-h period of monitoring of these intravenous GnRH doses. The increase to the next frequency was then made in the middle of each admission. As shown in representative subjects in Figure 1.6, a progressive rise of the mean LH level occurred with increasing frequencies of GnRH stimulation, whereas FSH levels did not change significantly. This increase in mean LH levels was, however, accompanied by a decreasing amplitude of individual LH responses at each level of increased frequency, a phenomenon that is considerably more apparent for FSH than for LH, since the mean FSH level did not increase in spite of the progressive shortening of the interpulse interval of GnRH stimulation (Fig. 1.7). This failure, of LH and especially of FSH, to rise in parallel with the expectations that had been established by the earlier dose-response relationships represents the earliest example of "desensitization" of pituitary gonadotropin secretion induced by frequency changes. This term signifies the shortfall in pituitary gonadotropin responsiveness from that which would be expected to accompany increasing GnRH stimulation. Moreover, this earliest form of desensitization associated

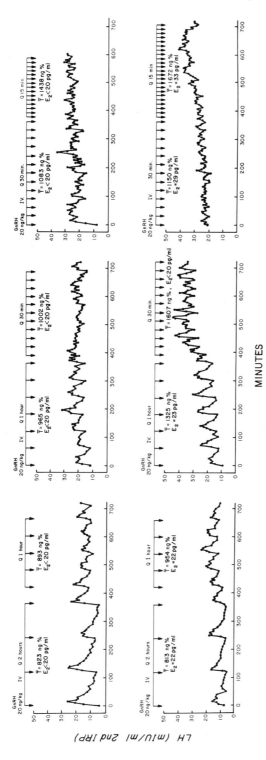

MINUTES

LH (mIU/ml 2nd IRP)

FIGURE 1.6. Serum LH concentrations determined at 5- and 10-min intervals during 3 sequential admissions of 2 GnRH-deficient subjects as the GnRH frequencies were progressively increased in the middle of each 12-h study from 2h to 1h to 0.5h. Testosterone concentrations (T) were determined in serum pools formed from samples from each 6-h period and expressed in ng/dl. Note that at higher frequencies, GnRH injections were not uniformly followed by LH pulses. Reprinted by permission from Ref. 21, © by The Endocrine Society, 1987.

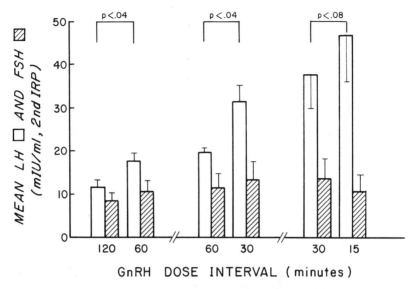

FIGURE 1.7. Mean (±SEM) serum LH and FSH concentrations during the 3 weekly 12-h admissions described in Figure 1.6, while the frequency of GnRH administration of a physiologic dose of GnRH was progressively increased to 5 GnRH-deficient men as shown in Figures 1.6 and 1.8. Mean LH concentrations increased progressively as GnRH frequency increased, whereas no significant change in FSH levels occurred. Thus, LH was preferentially secreted at higher frequencies of GnRH, whereas FSH secretion was preferentially desensitized by increasing GnRH frequency. Reprinted by permission from Ref. 21, © by The Endocrine Society, 1987.

with increasing the frequency of GnRH stimulation appears to be an unstable process—as can be seen in Figure 1.8, wherein both striking rises and falls in gonadotrope response to fixed doses and intervals of frequent GnRH stimulation occur as the mean frequency is increased. The resemblance of these rises and falls to those occurring during both the onset and the termination of the LH surge in the normal menstrual cycle is quite striking. This observation then raises the question of whether this frequency-mediated form of desensitization of gonadotropin secretion might play a role in these other physiologic states. Additionally, this progressive rise in mean LH levels with a fixed FSH level results in a high LH:FSH ratio associated with these rapid GnRH pulse frequencies (Fig. 1.6). This high ratio of LH to FSH is analogous to those gonadotropin ratios which have been documented to occur in the clinical entity of polycystic ovarian disease (22). Subsequently, other studies from our group have demonstrated that patients with polycystic ovarian disease do exhibit a similarly high, relatively fixed frequency of GnRH secretion (23).

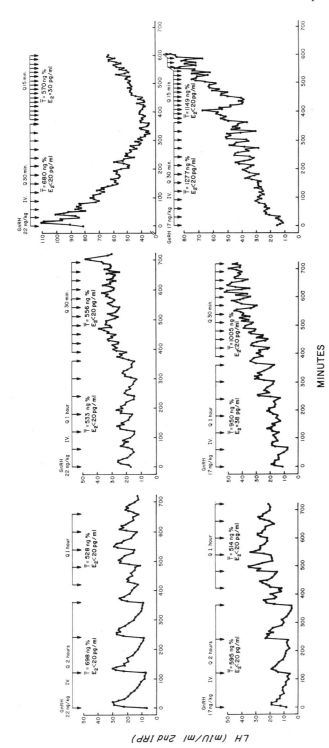

FIGURE 1.8. Serial serum LH concentrations determined in 2 additional GnRH-deficient subjects as described in Figure 1.6, as GnRH frequency of a midphysiologic dose was progressively increased from q 2h to q 30min. The instability of LH responses to these fixed and midphysiologic doses of GnRH administered at q 30-min frequencies seen in the panels at the far right demonstrates the unstable nature of the desensitization process. The rise in LH levels in response to a fixed dose and rapid frequency (q 30-min) GnRH frequency shown in the right panels is strikingly similar to that which occurs in normal women at the midcycle LH surge. Reprinted by permission from Ref. 21, © by The Endocrine Society, 1987.

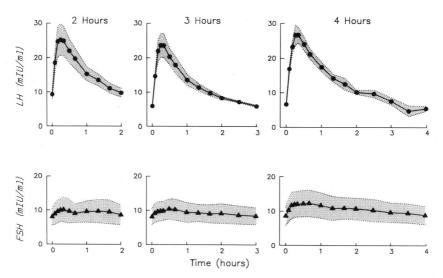

FIGURE 1.9. Mean (±SEM) serum LH and FSH concentrations of 4 GnRH-induced pulses in 4 men with GnRH deficiency when the frequency of IV GnRH administration was progressively decreased at weekly intervals from 2 h to 3 h to 4 h. Reprinted by permission from Ref. 24. Copyright by the American Society of Clinical Investigation, 1988.

Decreasing Frequency of GnRH Stimulation

After examination of the ability of increasing frequencies of fixed GnRH doses to alter the quantity and ratios of gonadotropins secreted, the effects of decreasing the frequency of the "ED$_{50}$" or physiologic dosage of GnRH progressively were determined. As can be seen in Figure 1.9, mild decreases in the frequency of GnRH stimulation from 2 to 3 to 4 h—i.e., in line with those intervals that can occur in normal adult males (15)—are associated with a relatively fixed peak of the LH pulse; but progressive increases in LH amplitudes and area under the secretory curve are associated with a more prolonged interval between pulses of GnRH stimulation. These longer intervals permit mean gonadotropin levels to fall to a lower baseline level by allowing increased time for metabolic clearance to occur (24). This phenomenon is apparent as the frequency of GnRH stimulation is decreased form 2 h to 8 h, at which point the interval between the episodes of GnRH stimulation is so long that the pretreatment apulsatile baseline state of the patient's GnRH deficiency can be observed (Fig. 1.10). When groups of patients with GnRH deficiency are pooled during decreases of GnRH stimulation from 2 h to 8 h, it is clear once again that the LH amplitude and area under the secretory curve increase even more strikingly, primarily due to further fall in the baseline before each pulse.

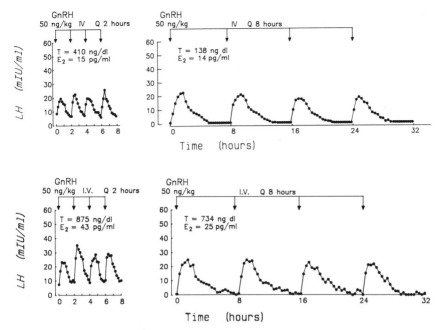

FIGURE 1.10. Serum LH concentrations determined at frequent intervals in 2 men with isolated GnRH deficiency as the frequency of GnRH administration was decreased from every 2 h to every 8 h at weekly intervals without testosterone (T) replacement (upper panels) or with T replacement (lower panels). Note that the increase in pituitary responsiveness to the slower GnRH administration was independent of changes in ambient gonadal steroid levels. Reprinted by permission from Ref. 24. Copyright by the American Society of Clinical Investigation, 1988.

However, as the pulse frequencies are reduced to 8 h, serum testosterone levels fall as a result of the long absence of LH stimulation from the Leydig cells (Fig. 1.11). Consequently, the increased amplitude and area under the LH secretory curve observed during these declining GnRH frequencies might well have been due to the decreasing negative feedback of testosterone on the pituitary. To control for this variable, a companion series of patients received exogenous testosterone as their GnRH frequency was decreased to 8 h; they showed identical changes in gonadotropin secretory dynamics. This finding indicates that the increasing responsiveness of LH secretion observed during decreasing frequencies of GnRH stimulation is unrelated to any changes in ambient serum testosterone levels. Somewhat in contrast to previous findings (25), the serum FSH levels failed to demonstrate any changes in these subjects with intact gonads over a wide range of increasing and decreasing GnRH frequencies. These results indicate that the overriding control of circulat-

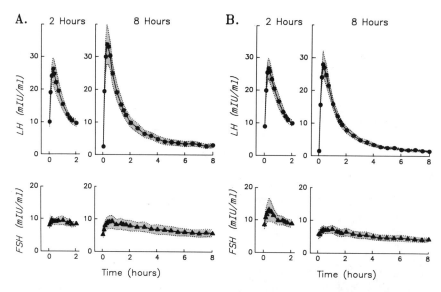

FIGURE 1.11. Mean (±SEM) serum LH and FSH concentrations of 4 GnRH-induced pulses in 4 GnRH-deficient men when GnRH was administered every 2 h or 8 h (A) without T replacement or (B) with T replacement. Reprinted by permission from Ref. 24. Copyright by the American Society of Clinical Investigation, 1988.

ing FSH levels in the adult male may well not be GnRH dosage, frequency, or ambient sex steroid levels. Rather, gonadal peptides such as inhibin and activin may be the dominant influence on FSH.

The Role of Sex Steroid Modulation in GnRH-Induced Gonadotropin Secretion

To define the site of action of sex steroid feedback in the human male, the models of the intact and GnRH-deficient man were again studied in tandem. By infusing sex steroids into normal men with intact hypothalamic-pituitary axes, the net effect of sex steroids upon both the hypothalamus and the anterior pituitary can be examined. By combining these studies with those of the GnRH-deficient men who can only experience sex steroid feedback at the level of the anterior pituitary, the hypothalamic component of sex steroid feedback can be dissected from that of the pituitary. The responses of the GnRH-deficient men represent the isolated pituitary component that can then be "subtracted" from that of normal men to deduce the role of the hypothalamus in steroid hormone feedback.

Estradiol

Estradiol was infused intravenously at a dose of 90 µg/24 h for a period of 96 h. This dose of estradiol represents twice the endogenous production rate of the normal male (26) and had been used by previous investigators in similar studies (27). The normal men were sampled at 10-min intervals for 12 h prior to and during the last day of the estradiol infusion. The GnRH-deficient men were sampled similarly, during which period 3 intravenous doses of the "ED_{50}" physiologic dose of GnRH were administered, followed by a GnRH dose-response curve spanning from 7.5 to 250 ng/kg. All blood sampling was performed prior to and during the last day of the estradiol infusion in both normal and GnRH-deficient men.

As can be seen in Figure 1.12, estradiol suppressed LH pulse amplitude in both normal and GnRH-deficient men (28). The data revealed that there was equivalent suppression of gonadotropins in both normal and GnRH-deficient men in terms of both mean LH levels and amplitudes of response (Fig. 1.12). Additionally, there was a slight decrease in the apparent frequency of LH pulses in the normal men; however, most of this change in frequency was due to the difficulty of visualizing low-amplitude LH pulses in some of the normal men and thus was largely artifactual. Thus, the percentages of decrease in mean LH and FSH levels in both normal and GnRH-deficient men were identical (Fig. 1.13). Consequently, it is apparent that the majority, if not all, of the effects of estradiol are exerted at the level of the anterior pituitary.

Testosterone

Unlike estradiol, testosterone, administered at a dose of 15 mg/24 h (i.e., at similar twice-production-rate levels) (29), exhibited marked differences between the GnRH-deficient and normal men, thus indicating that testosterone has a dual site of action. In the normal men (Fig. 1.14), the predominant effect of testosterone was to reduce the endogenous GnRH pulse frequency dramatically (30). In some cases, it virtually eradicated all evidence of GnRH secretion. In contrast, in the GnRH-deficient men in whom the frequency of GnRH stimulation was fixed, there was a mild but discernible effect of testosterone at the level of the anterior pituitary, with decreases in mean LH levels and LH pulse amplitudes following its administration. When these men are viewed as a group, the advantages of being able to control the GnRH pulse frequency and dosage in the GnRH-deficient men become readily apparent (Fig. 1.14). Since these patients can exhibit no decrease in mean GnRH pulse frequency, all decreases in their mean levels must be solely attributable to the isolated impact of testosterone on the amplitude of the pituitary LH response to GnRH. It is also noteworthy that the majority of this blunting effect of testosterone on the anterior pituitary was manifest in response to those

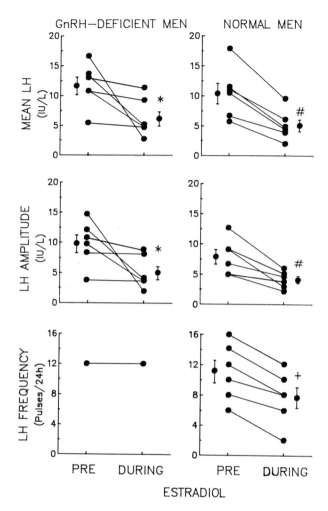

FIGURE 1.12. Individual mean LH levels, LH amplitude, and LH frequency in 6 GnRH-deficient (left-hand panels) and 6 normal (right-hand panels) men before and during 96-h IV infusion of estradiol (90 μg/24 h). Group means ± SE for each parameter are indicated to the side of each graph. (∗ = P < 0.01.) Reprinted by permission from Ref. 28, © by The Endocrine Society, 1991.

doses of GnRH which produced LH pulse amplitudes within the normal adult male range. In contrast, the testosterone infusions had no significant effect on the LH pulse amplitudes that occurred after GnRH doses of 250 ng/kg—i.e., a dose of GnRH that routinely produces LH pulse amplitudes above the normal range and hence represents a pharmacologic dose of GnRH. This finding may well explain previous studies that have demonstrated that the responsiveness to a dose of exogenous GnRH in

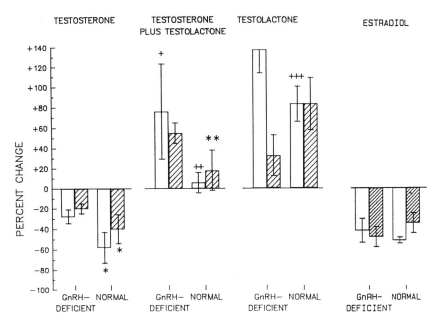

FIGURE 1.13. Percent age of change in mean LH (open bars) and FSH (hatched bars) levels in GnRH-deficient and normal men during administration of testosterone (T), testosterone plus testolactone (TL), TL alone, or estradiol. (* = P < 0.01 for mean LH and FSH levels in GnRH-deficient men receiving T alone. ** = P < 0.02 vs. mean FSH levels in GnRH-deficient men receiving T plus TL. + = P < 0.05 vs. mean LH levels in GnRH-deficient men receiving T alone. ++ = P < 0.01 vs. mean LH levels in normal men receiving TL alone. +++ = P < 0.05 for mean LH levels in normal men receiving T plus TL.) Reprinted by permission from Refs. 28 and 30, © by The Endocrine Society, 1991.

the pharmacologic range used for GnRH testing is unaffected by testosterone infusion. The final point of interest during the testosterone studies is that, given that testosterone induces striking decreases in the endogenous GnRH pulse frequency in normal men and that in our previous studies controlled decreases in GnRH frequency demonstrated an increased amplitude in the ensuing LH pulse, the fact that the normal men did not exhibit accompanying rises in LH pulse amplitude associated with their decreased endogenous GnRH frequency can now be discerned to represent the direct pituitary effect of testosterone feedback in the normal men.

Testosterone plus Testolactone

To determine the degree to which the effects of testosterone on the hypothalamic-pituitary axis of the normal male and on the pituitary

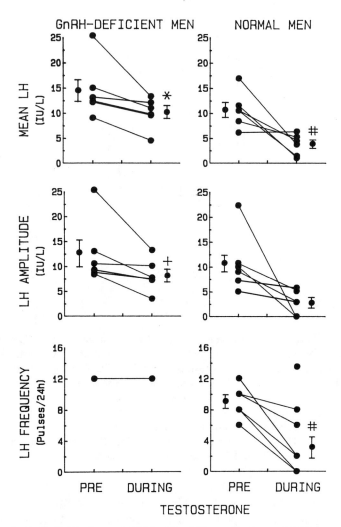

FIGURE 1.14. Individual mean LH levels, LH amplitude, and LH frequency in 6 GnRH-deficient (left-hand panels) and 6 normal (right-hand panels) men before and during 96-h IV testosterone infusion (15 mg/24 h). Group means ± SE for each parameter are indicated to the side of each graph. (∗ = P < 0.02, + = P < 0.05, # = P < 0.01.) Reprinted by permission from Ref. 30, © by The Endocrine Society, 1991.

responses of GnRH-deficient males might be related to aromatization, a parallel series of studies were undertaken in which the testosterone infusions were repeated with the addition of 2 g/day of testolactone administered orally in both normal and GnRH-deficient men (30). A companion series of steroid production rate studies, performed in col-

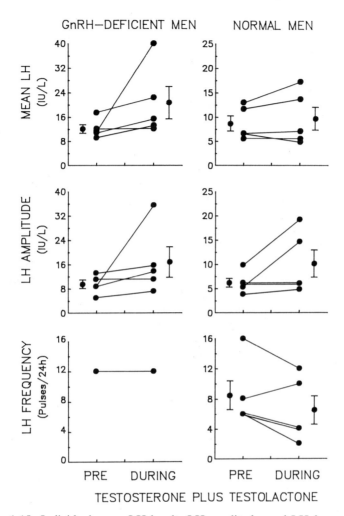

FIGURE 1.15. Individual mean LH levels, LH amplitude, and LH frequency in 5 GnRH-deficient (left-hand panels) and 5 normal (right-hand panels) men before and during testosterone plus testolactone administration. Group means ± SE for each parameter are indicated to the side of each graph. Reprinted by permission from Ref. 30, © by The Endocrine Society, 1991.

laboration with Dr. Chris Longcope, confirmed that aromatization had been inhibited by 67% to 80% in the two sets of subjects as studied with blood and urinary steroid production rates. The results of blockade of aromatization produced strikingly different results in both normal and GnRH-deficient (Fig. 1.15) men. In the normal males, inhibition of aromatization completely blocked the effect of testosterone on GnRH pulse frequency as well as mean LH levels and amplitude. Thus, blockade of aromatase activity rendered normal men virtually immune to the effects of exogenous testosterone infusion (Figs. 1.13 and 1.15). In contrast, GnRH-deficient men exhibited a striking increase in both LH pulse amplitude and mean LH level in view of their controlled frequency of GnRH administration. This "overshoot" of the GnRH-deficient men during aromatase blockade was taken to signify the liberation of the pituitary from estradiol feedback (previously documented in the above studies) combined with the fact that the frequency of GnRH stimulation was controlled. Consequently, the fact that the normal men did not exhibit this overshoot seen in the GnRH-deficient men suggests that testosterone itself, independently of its aromatization to estradiol, has an additional effect on the hypothalamus in normal men to slow GnRH frequency and/or to reduce its dosage of secretion, and thus to prevent the overshoot seen in GnRH-deficient men whose dose and frequency of GnRH stimulation remained unchanged.

When the mean LH and FSH levels are compared for all these studies (Fig. 1.13), one can see that the differences between estradiol's ability to suppress FSH and LH in normal and GnRH-deficient men are quite small, indicating that the predominant effect of this steroid is at the level of the anterior pituitary (Figs. 1.12 and 1.13). On the other hand, testosterone suppresses gonadotropins to a greater degree in the normal than in the GnRH-deficient men, indicating that it has both a pituitary and a hypothalamic effect. Quantitating these effects would indicate that approximately half of testosterone's effect is due to its anterior pituitary site of action, and half appears due to its hypothalamic effect on GnRH frequency as judged by suppression of mean LH levels (Fig. 1.13). Finally, the effects of testosterone plus testolactone represent merely a restoration of the gonadotropins to pretreatment levels in normals, whereas the GnRH-deficient subjects exhibit the above-mentioned overshoot, suggesting that freedom from inhibition of the anterior pituitary by blockade of aromatase as seen in the GnRH-deficient subjects is somehow further restrained in the normal men, thus targeting an additional hypothalamic site to testosterone's direct action.

Summary and Conclusion

The traditional difficulty in studying the neuroendocrine control of reproduction in the human male has been the inability to tease out the hypothalamic from the pituitary component of this neuroendocrine system. The use of multiple models, each with its own strength and weakness, represents an overlapping approach that has permitted further insights to be gained into the hypothalamic control of the neuroendocrine regulation of gonadotropin secretion in the human. Such an insight is an important prerequisite to the understanding of the pathophysiology of various disease states, the unraveling of the control of FSH secretion by GnRH versus other modulators, and the subsequent design of rational therapies for male reproductive disorders.

Acknowledgments. We acknowledge the key contributions of D.I. Spratt, J.S. Finkelstein, L.St.L. O'Dea, J.P. Butler, and D.M. Musket to this work. This work was supported by NIH Grant HD15788 and FDA Grant FD-U-000523-01.

References

1. Handelsman DJ, Swerdloff RS. Pharmacokineteics of gonadotropin-releasing hormone and its analogs. Endocr Rev 1986;7:95–105.
2. Spratt DI, Crowley WF, Butler JP, Hoffman AR, Conn PM, Badger TM. Pituitary luteinizing hormone responses to intravenous and subcutaneous administration of gonadotropin-releasing hormone in men. J Clin Endocrinol Metab 1985;61:890–5.
3. Crowley WF, Filicori M, Spratt DI, Santoro N. The physiology of gonadotropin-releasing hormone (GnRH) in men and women. Recent Prog Horm Res 1985;41:473–531.
4. Filicori M, Flamigni C, Crowley WF. The critical role of blood sampling frequency in the estimation of episodic LH secretion in normal women. In: Crowley WF, Hoefler JG, eds. The episodic secretion of hormones. New York: Churchill Livingstone, 1987:5–13.
5. Levine JE, Pau K-YF, Ramirez VD, Jackson GL. Simultaneous measurement of luteinizing hormone-releasing hormone and luteinizing hormone release in unanesthetized, ovariectomized sheep. Endocrinology 1982;111:1449–55.
6. Caraty A, Orgeur P, Thiery JC. Demonstration of the pulsatile secretion of LH-RH into hypophyseal portal blood of ewes using an original technique for multiple samples. C R Seances Acad Sci 1982;295:103–6.
7. Clarke IJ, Cummins JT. The temporal relationship between gonadotropin releasing hormone (GnRH) and luteinizing hormone (LH) secretion in ovariectomized ewes. Endocrinology 1982;111:1737–9.
8. Karsch FJ, Bittman EL, Foster DL, Goodman RL, Legan SJ, Robinson JE. Neuroendocrine basis of seasonal reproduction. Recent Prog Horm Res 1984;40:185–232.
9. Winters SJ, Troen P. Pulsatile secretion of immunoreactive alpha-subunit in man. J Clin Endocrinol Metab 1985;60:344–8.
10. Whitcomb RW, O'Dea LStL, Finkelstein JS, Heavern DM, Crowley WF. Utility of free alpha subunit (FAS) as an alternative neuroendocrine marker of gonadotropin-releasing hormone (GnRH) stimulation of the gonadotroph in the human: evidence from normal and GnRH-deficient men. J Clin Endocrinol Metab 1990;70:1654–61.
11. Spratt DI, Carr DB, Merriam GR, Scully RE, Rao PN, Crowley WF. The spectrum of abnormal patterns of gonadotropin-releasing hormone (GnRH) secretion in men with idiopathic hypogonadotropic hypogonadism: clinical and laboratory correlations. J Clin Endocrinol Metab 1987;64:283–91.

12. Valk TW, Corley KP, Kelch RP, Marshall JC. Hypogonadotropic hypogonadism: hormonal responses to low dose pulsatile administration of gonadotropin-releasing hormone. J Clin Endocrinol Metab 1980;51:730–8.
13. Hoffman AR, Crowley WF. Induction of puberty in men by long-term pulsatile administration of low-dose gonadotropin-releasing hormone. N Engl J Med 1982;307:1237–41.
14. Whitcomb RW, Crowley WF. Diagnosis and treatment of isolated gonadotropin-releasing hormone deficiency in men. J Clin Endocrinol Metab 1990;70:3–7.
15. Spratt DI, O'Dea LStL, Schoenfeld DA, Butler JP, Rao PN, Crowley WF. Neuroendocrine-gonadal axis in men: frequent sampling of LH, FSH, and testosterone. Am J Physiol 1988;254:E658–66.
16. Spratt DI, Finkelstein JS, Badger TM, Butler JP, Crowley WF. Bio- and immunoactive luteinzing hormone responses to low doses of gonadotropin-releasing hormone (GnRH): dose-response curves in GnRH-deficient men. J Clin Endocrinol Metab 1986;63:143–50.
17. Boyar R, Finkelstein J, Roffwarg H, Kapen S, Weitzman E, Hellman L. Synchronization of augmented luteinizing hormone secretory pattern in puberty. N Engl J Med 1972;287:582–6.
18. Jackacki RI, Kelch RP, Sauder SE, Lloyd JS, Hopwood NJ, Marshall JC. Pulsatile secretion of luteinizing hormone in children: J Clin Endocrinol Metab 1982;55:453–8.
19. Filicori M, Santoro NF, Merriam GR, Crowley WF. Characterization of the physiological pattern of episodic gonadotropin secretion throughout the human menstrual cycle. J Clin Endocrinol Metab 1986;62:1136–44.
20. Yen SSC, Tsai CC, Naftolin F, Vandenberg G, Ajabor L. Pulsatile patterns of gonadotropin release in subjects with and without ovarian function. J Clin Endocrinol Metab 1972;34:671–5.
21. Spratt DI, Finkelstein JS, Butler JP, Badger TM, Crowley WF. Effects of increasing the frequency of low doses of gonadotropin-releasing hormone (GnRH) on gonadotropin secretion in GnRH-deficient men. J Clin Endocrinol Metab 1987;64:1179–86.
22. Rebar R, Judd HL, Yen SSC, Rakoff J, Vandenberg G, Naftolin F. Characterization of the inappropriate gonadotropin secretion in polycystic ovary syndrome. J Clin Invest 1976;57:1320–5.
23. Waldstreicher J, Santoro NF, Hall JE, Filicori M, Crowley WF. Hyperfunction of the hypothalamic-pituitary axis in women with polycystic ovarian disease: indirect evidence for partial gonadotroph desensitization. J Clin Endocrinol Metab 1988;66:165–72.
24. Finkelstein JS, Badger TM, O'Dea LStL, Spratt DI, Crowley WF. Effects of decreasing the frequency of gonadotropin-releasing hormone stimulation on gonadotropin secretion in gonadotropin-releasing hormone-deficient men and perifused rat pituitary cells. J Clin Invest 1988;81:1725–33.
25. Gross KM, Matsumoto AM, Bremner WJ. Differential control of luteinizing hormone and follicle-stimulating hormone secretion by luteinizing hormone-releasing hormone pulse frequency in man. J Clin Endocrinol Metab 1987;64:675–80.
26. Baird DT, Horton R, Longcope C, Tait JF. Steroid dynamics under steady-state conditions. Recent Prog Horm Res 1965;25:611–64.

27. Sherins RJ, Loriaux DL. Studies on the role of sex steroids in the feedback control of FSH concentrations in men. J Clin Endocrinol Metab 1973;36:886–93.
28. Finkelstein JS, O'Dea LStL, Whitcomb RW, Crowley WF. Sex steroid control of gonadotropin secretion in the human male: II. Effects of estradiol administration in normal and GnRH-deficient men. J Clin Endocrinol Metab 1991;73:621–9.
29. Horton R, Shinsako J, Forsham PH. Testosterone production and metabolic clearance rates with volumes of distribution in normal adult men and women. Acta Endocrinol 1965;48:446–58.
30. Finkelstein JS, Whitcomb RW, O'Dea LStL, Longcope C, Schoenfeld DA, Crowley WF. Sex steroid control of gonadotropin secretion in the human male: I. Effects of testosterone administration in normal and GnRH-deficient men. J Clin Endocrinol Metab 1991;73:609–20.

2

Gonadotropin Releasing Hormone and Its Actions*

Tim D. Braden and P. Michael Conn

Gonadotropin releasing hormone plays a central role in regulating the reproductive process. Since isolation of this decapeptide and identification of its structure almost twenty years ago, our understanding of the neural control of reproduction and neuroendocrinology as a whole has experienced tremendous growth. Analogs of GnRH are now being used clinically to treat precocious puberty in children, endometriosis, polycystic ovarian disease, and two of the most prevalent steroid-dependent neoplasia, prostate cancer and breast cancer. In addition, GnRH and its analogs have proven useful in enhancing the reproductive efficiency of animals produced for both food and fiber. Clearly, basic research into the physiology and pharmacology of GnRH can be regarded as particularly successful in light of the relatively short time-span from basic studies to practical utility. In addition to the direct clinical applications of GnRH, the study of this hormone has contributed to our understanding of the mechanisms and pattern of hormone release, as well as the mechanisms by which responsiveness of target glands are regulated. Therefore, studies on GnRH have spanned the many areas of physiology, pharmacology, endocrinology, reproductive biology, cellular biology, and molecular biology.

Hypothalamic GnRH is synthesized primarily in the arcuate nucleus region, and is transported to and released from the median eminence into the hypothalamic-hypophyseal portal system. The release of GnRH occurs in a pulsatile fashion that can be regulated by various external signals (i.e., steroid hormones). GnRH has its effects at the pituitary gonadotrope and stimulates the release of the gonadotropins, luteinizing hormone and follicle stimulating hormone, into the peripheral circulation.

*Adapted, with permission, from The Stevenson Lecture (Can J Physiol Pharmacol 1991). Supported by NIH Grant HD19899. Dr. Braden is supported by a Carver Fellowship of the University of Iowa College of Medicine.

The pulsatile nature of GnRH release results in the pulsatile release of LH and FSH. In addition to gonadotropin release, GnRH evokes several other cellular responses of gonadotropes such as desensitization, up- and down-regulation of GnRH receptors, and biosynthesis of gonadotropins and GnRH receptors.

Structure/Binding/Function Relationships of GnRH and Its Analogs

Structure of the GnRH Gene

The gene encoding for GnRH is a single gene in rat, mouse, and man and is located on the short arm of chromosome 8 in the human (1). Information obtained from cloned cDNAs of hypothalamic and placental origins indicates 4 exons (2, 3). The coding sequence translates for a 92 amino acid precursor protein for GnRH and a 56 amino acid peptide termed GAP (GnRH-associated peptide). The first exon consists of a 5'-untranslated region that differs between cDNAs from hypothalamic and placental tissues. The second exon codes for the signal peptide, GnRH, and the first 11 amino acid residues of GAP. The third exon codes for GAP residues 12–43. The fourth exon codes for the 13 terminal amino acids residues of GAP and the remaining 3'-untranslated mRNA (review, 4). Identification of the gene for GnRH has led to the isolation and reversal of a defect in a strain of hypogonadal mice (*hpg*) that do not normally progress through puberty. The GnRH gene in *hpg* mice was found to have a large deletion that omits the third and fourth exons. By using transgenic animals carrying a wild-type GnRH gene and crosses with heterozygous *hpg* mice, animals that were homozygous for the *hpg* mutation and yet carried the wild-type GnRH transgene were produced. These homozygous *hpg* mice underwent normal puberty and were fertile (4, 5). Alleviation of the *hpg* phenotype through gene incorporation suggests the possibility that similar human deficiencies may also be corrected through the use of gene therapy.

Amino Acid Structure

Since publication of the amino acid sequence of native mammalian GnRH (6–8), over 3500 different analogs of GnRH have been synthesized. The linear sequence of mammalian GnRH is:

$$\text{pyroGlu}^1\text{-His}^2\text{-Trp}^3\text{-Ser}^4\text{-Tyr}^5\text{-Gly}^6\text{-Leu}^7\text{-Arg}^8\text{-Pro}^9\text{-Gly}^{10} \text{ amide}$$

GnRH from virtually all mammals has the same structure. Distinct variant forms in the primary structure of GnRH have been identified in the chicken (2 variants; 9–11), salmon (12), and lamprey (13). Generally, the structure of GnRH has been conserved throughout evolution; however, significant variations are observed at positions 7 and 8 (reviews, 14, 15). Amino acid substitution analysis has led to identification of the structural requirements for binding to the GnRH receptor and activation of the target cell (16). The native GnRH molecule can undergo major conformational changes from a fully extended form to a highly folded form. The formation of a type II β turn at Gly^6-Leu^7 results in a configuration that has a high affinity for GnRH receptors (17). This least-energy configuration is apparently stabilized by the formation of hydrogen bonds between the pyrrolidone carbonyl residue (position 1) and the glycineamide group (position 10; 18, 19). Therefore, the close opposition of amino acids in positions 1 and 10 is involved in binding of GnRH to its receptor (20). Substitution at amino acid 6 with D-amino acids containing bulky hydrophobic side chains constrains the molecule to the receptor-preferred conformation and results in high binding affinity of both agonists and antagonists with this substitution. A combination of substitutions at Gly^6 and substitution of ethylamide for Gly^{10} further enhances the affinity of GnRH analogs for the GnRH receptor (21, 22).

Target Cell Activation

Activation of target cells through binding of ligand to GnRH receptors is thought to be dependent upon the 3 N-terminal residues of the ligand. Substitutions of the first 3 residues of GnRH analogs with hydrophobic D-amino acids results in GnRH antagonists (23). This type of substitution combined with substitution at position 6 with strong basic amino acids yields potent antagonists of GnRH, but the combination of these two substitutions has been implicated in the release of histamine (24). Further studies of the requirements for target cell activation using reduced-size GnRH analogs (hexapeptides) have suggested that relationships between residue side chains at positions 3 and 6 can change the activity of reduced-size GnRH analogs from agonists to antagonists (25) with the addition of one methylene group at position 3 changing activity from agonistic to antagonistic. Additionally, subtle changes in residue side chains at position 4 can cause steric hindrances involving position 3 to again change activity of GnRH analogs.

Common Analogs of GnRH

The half-life of GnRH in vivo is relatively short (<10 min in humans, 26), as a result of initial degradation of the amino terminal half of the peptide (27). Additionally, GnRH is known to be degraded by a number of enzymes. A pyroglutamate aminopeptidase (cleaves GnRH at $pyroGlu^1$-His^2), a postproline-cleaving enzyme (cleaves GnRH at Pro^9-Gly^{10} amide), and a nonchymotrypsin-like endopeptidase (cleaves GnRH preferentially at Tyr^5-Gly^6, then at His^2-Trp^3; 28–31) have all been isolated from the pituitary gland; however, it is unclear whether these participate in the physiological inactivation of native GnRH (32). Longer half-lives of GnRH analogs have been achieved with hydrophobic D-amino acid substitutions at position 6 (33). Based on substitutions to prolong the half-life and improve the binding activity of GnRH analogs, several highly potent superagonists of GnRH have become commercially available, such as D-Ser(tBu^6) GnRH ethylamide (Buserelin, Hoechst; 34), D-Leu^6-GnRH ethylamide (Leuprolide, TAP; 35), and 3 (2 naphthyl) Ala^6-GnRH (Nafarelin, Syntex; 36). Highly hydrophobic GnRH analogs may have a prolonged biological half-life due to association with binding proteins in serum (37).

Receptors for GnRH

Physical/Chemical Characteristics

The primary site of action of GnRH is the gonadotrope in the anterior pituitary gland; however, binding sites for GnRH have been identified in other tissues. Receptors for GnRH have been observed in the gonads of rats (38, 39) and humans (40), but not in ovine, bovine, or porcine ovaries (41). Additionally, GnRH binding sites have been observed in adrenal (42) and some cancer tissues (43, 44), and in the central nervous system (45–47). Because of the low concentrations of circulating GnRH and its short half-life, it is unlikely that GnRH released from the hypothalamus occupies a sufficient number of receptors in peripheral tissues to have physiological effects, but local synthesis of GnRH and paracrine effects cannot be excluded. It has been suggested that GnRH binding sites in the hypothalamus may participate in behavioral modification (48, 49). Although there is much interest in extrapituitary binding sites for GnRH (50), this review will concentrate on GnRH receptors on pituitary gonadotropes.

The first step in the mechanism of action of GnRH in stimulating gonadotropin release is the binding of GnRH to its receptor on gonadotropes. Receptors for GnRH are found exclusively in the plasma membrane fraction (51). Receptors for GnRH from rat and bovine pituitary plasma membranes are glycoproteins (52, 53), as evidenced by a loss of agonist and antagonist binding after exposure of receptors to neuraminidase and wheat-germ agglutinin. Sialic acid residues on GnRH receptors appear to be required for activation of the receptor as well as for appearance of receptors on the cell surface (53). Binding of GnRH to its receptor appears to be dependent upon the presence of both exterior hydrophilic head groups and fatty acid linked to the β-carbon of phospholipids (54). Additionally, two carboxylic groups and two aromatic amino acids appear to be in the ligand binding portion of the receptor and/or to influence the binding of GnRH (55, 56). It appears that the GnRH receptor is linked to a G-protein (57).

Estimates of the size of the GnRH holoreceptor range from 50,000 to 700,000 kDa, depending upon the conditions used to estimate the size. The zwitterionic detergent CHAPS (3-[-3-cholamidopropyl-dimethylammonio]-1-propanesulfonic acid) has proven useful for solubilization of GnRH receptors that retain their ability to bind ligands (58, 59). Solubilization of GnRH receptors with CHAPS followed by nondenaturing sizing gel exclusion has indicated an apparent molecular weight of the GnRH receptor to be 60,000–150,000 (60, 61). Using covalent labeling of the GnRH receptor with a radiolabeled photoaffinity agonist (^{125}I-Tyr^5-azidobenzoyl-D-Lys^6-GnRH) followed by sodium dodecyl sulfate polyacrylamide gel electrophoresis (SDS-PAGE) and autoradiography, several laboratories working independently have observed specific radioactive labeling at the apparent molecular weight of 60,000 (62, 63). Radiation inactivation (target size analysis) of the functional size of intact GnRH receptors in plasma membranes indicated an apparent molecular weight of 136,000 for the GnRH holoreceptor (64). Although the purification of GnRH receptors and generation of polyclonal antibodies against this receptor have recently been reported, the low abundance of receptor and low titer of the antibodies have hampered further characterization of the GnRH receptor. Therefore, it is unclear whether the 60-kDa component of the GnRH receptor represents the holoreceptor or simply a ligand binding component. It seems likely that the 60-kDa band identified by photoaffinity labeling and Western blotting represents a subunit of the GnRH receptor and that the holoreceptor is made up of this binding subunit and at least 1 other subunit of similar size, which may or may not bind ligand. GnRH receptors have been reported to have been purified to homogeneity by chromatography on wheat germ agglutinin-agarose followed by affinity chromatography using immobilized avidin coupled to biotinylated D-Lys^6-GnRH (65). Analysis of purified radiolabeled GnRH receptors by SDS-PAGE followed by autoradiography indicated two bands of activity at 57 kDa and 59 kDa. Subsequent production of a low-titer polyclonal antibody to GnRH receptors has been reported (59); however, further characterization of GnRH receptors using this antibody has not been published.

Because of the difficulties in purification of GnRH receptors and in generation of useful antibodies against the receptor, the molecular biology of the gene for GnRH receptors remains largely unknown. Recently, however, several laboratories have reported expression of GnRH receptors after injection of pituitary mRNA or mRNA from a pituitary cell line into Xenopus oocytes (66–68). The specific mRNA encoding the GnRH receptor has an apparent size of >28S, which suggests a length of 6–7 kilobases (68). These data were obtained from cells whose origin was a pituitary tumor of a transgenic mouse. Although the cell line expresses GnRH binding sites and produces the α-subunit of the glycoprotein hormones, it is unknown whether this GnRH receptor population has the same characteristics as normally expressed GnRH receptors.

Regulation of the Number of GnRH Receptors

Changes in the number of receptors for GnRH in the pituitary glands of a number of species have been characterized during many physiological conditions. During the estrous cycle of rats, hamsters, ewes, and cows, the maximum number of GnRH receptors was observed during the proestrous period prior to the preovulatory surge of LH (69–74). After the preovulatory surge of LH, the number of GnRH receptors decreases and may require several days to achieve proestrous levels. After removal of the gonads, significant increases in the number of GnRH receptors have been observed (72). In contrast, during pregnancy and lactation, the number of GnRH receptors is less than that observed during the estrous cycle (69, 72). These observations clearly demonstrate regulation of GnRH receptors in vivo.

Numerous treatments in vitro can alter the number of receptors for GnRH in pituitary cell cultures. Treatment of pituitary cell cultures with physiologic concentrations of GnRH results in a biphasic response by the cells with respect to GnRH receptor number (75). Initially, a down-regulation of receptors is observed (<4h posttreatment), followed by an increase in the number of GnRH receptors (9h posttreatment, Fig. 2.1). The initial down-regulation of receptors for GnRH is temporally associated with desensitization of gonadotropes to GnRH, although clearly other mechanisms, including uncoupling of receptors from second messenger systems, contribute to densitization. Homologous down-regulation of GnRH receptors appears to be independent of extracellular calcium, but up-regulation of GnRH receptors is dependent upon extra-cellular calcium and requires protein synthesis (75, 76; Fig. 2.1).

Up-regulation of GnRH receptors by homologous hormone can be mimicked by treatment of pituitary cells with analogs of adenosine 3′,5 monophosphate as well as nonspecific depolarization of pituitary cells with KCl (76) and A23187 (75, 77). Although up-regulation of GnRH receptors indicates the ability of gonadotropes to respond to various external signals with an increased number of plasma membrane recep-tors, this increased receptor number does not increase the sensitivity of gonadotropes to GnRH when LH release is measured as the cellular response (78). Gonadotropes can respond with nearly maximal LH release when only 20% of available GnRH receptors are occupied in vitro (79); and when 50% of receptors are blocked with a GnRH antagonist, ewes can still respond fully to subsequent GnRH administration with

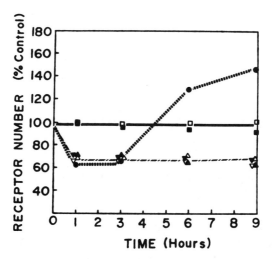

FIGURE 2.1. Effect of incubation with GnRH on receptor number. Two-day pituitary cultures were incubated for the indicated time period with medium alone (open square) or medium containing 3 mM EGTA (solid square), 1 nM GnRH (solid circle), 3 mM EGTA + 1 nM GnRH (open triangle), 0.1 mM D600 + 1 nM GnRH (solid inverted triangle), actinomycin D (1 μg/ml) + 1 nM GnRH (closed triangle), or cycloheximide (1 μg/ml) + 1 nM GnRH (open inverted triangle). After this time period, receptor numbers were determined. Values for standard error of the mean (n = 3–6) were omitted for clarity and were generally 10%. Reprinted by permission from Ref. 75. Copyright by the American Society for Pharmacology and Experimental Therapeutics, 1984.

LH release (80). As indicated above, these data indicate that there are "spare" GnRH receptors when LH release is the sole parameter measured; however, it is unknown if the "spare" receptor conclusion is valid for the other functions of gonadotropes in response to GnRH (i.e., FSH release, receptor synthesis, up-regulation, down-regulation, and gonadotropin biosynthesis).

In addition to regulation of GnRH receptor by homologous hormone, the number of GnRH receptors can be regulated by other hormones, including steroids and protein products from the gonad. As indicated above, removal of the gonads can increase the number of GnRH receptors in vivo when hypothalamic-pituitary connections are intact. In the absence of hypothalamic input, estradiol-17β can increase the number of GnRH receptors (81, 82). Using ovine pituitary gonadotrope cell cultures, Laws et al. (83, 84) have shown that estradiol can increase and progesterone can decrease the number of receptors for GnRH.

Protein products of the gonads have also been shown to influence the number of GnRH receptors. Wang et al. (85) have shown a decreased number of GnRH receptors when rat pituitary cell cultures were treated with inhibin. This group subsequently showed that inhibin was able to block GnRH-stimulated up-regulation of GnRH receptors (86). The effects of inhibin on the basal number of GnRH receptors was shown to be independent of biosynthesis of GnRH receptors (87), but the ability of inhibin to block up-regulation of GnRH receptors was at least partially due to the ability of inhibin to antagonize GnRH-stimulated synthesis of GnRH receptors (87). In direct contrast, Laws et al. (83) observed that treatment of ovine pituitary cell cultures with inhibin significantly increased the number of GnRH receptors. Given these two distinctly separate observations regarding the effects of inhibin on GnRH receptor populations in two different species, clearly, other species will have to be examined before defining a general role of inhibin in regulating the number of pituitary receptors for GnRH.

Fate and Replacement of Occupied GnRH Receptors

The presence of receptors on the cell surface is due to a combination of processes that either contribute to the plasma membrane population (synthesis, recycling, unmasking of receptors) or remove receptors from the cell surface (internalization, degradation, inactivation). After binding of agonist, GnRH receptors form patches in coated pits and are internalized. It appears as if GnRH receptors can undergo microaggregation as part of the target cell activation process. When a GnRH antagonist was allowed to occupy GnRH receptors, no cellular response was observed. However, when antagonist-occupied GnRH receptors are dimerized and bound to an antagonist antibody, the antagonist begins to function as an agonist, indicating that microaggregation of GnRH receptors may be a mechanism involved in target cell activation (88, 89). After aggregation, GnRH receptors are internalized and become associated with lysosomes, suggesting a degradation pathway, and/or become associated with the Golgi complex and LH granules, suggesting a recycling pathway (90–93). Evidence for recycling of GnRH receptors has been presented by Schvartz and Hazum (94) after observing the apparent reappearance of GnRH receptors on the cell surface after internalization. The authors covalently attached a GnRH agonist to GnRH receptors, allowed the complex to be internalized, and subsequently evaluated the susceptibility of this complex to extracellular trypsin treatment. After initial internalization of the agonist-receptor complex, trypsin treatment caused the apparance of a characteristic GnRH receptor fragment indicative of the return of GnRH receptors to the cell surface. Administration of lysosomotropic agents (chloroquine and methylamine) and monensin increased the apparent rate of recycling of GnRH receptors, presumably by reducing the degradation of the agonist-receptor complex in lysosomes. It should be noted that these studies observed the recycling of covalently linked agonist-receptor complexes, which may or may not be routed similarly to normal agonist-receptor complexes. Finally, it appears as if agonist-occupied GnRH receptors are likely routed through the cell differently than antagonist-occupied receptors (95).

Receptors for GnRH, therefore, can be replaced in plasma membranes by recycling and biosynthesis of new GnRH receptors. In using the density-shift technique, the time required for synthesis of one-half of the population of GnRH receptors in rat pituitary cell cultures is 24–28 h (96). Because of the relatively slow basal synthesis rate, GnRH receptors are likely degraded and new receptors synthesized as part of general membrane turnover. Treatment of cells with GnRH stimulates the synthesis of GnRH receptors and reduces the half-time of synthesis to 12 h (97). This stimulation by GnRH of receptor synthesis appears to be independent of extracellular calcium.

Thus, it appears that GnRH receptors follow a common internalization pathway after agonist binding and that the appearance of receptors on the cell surface is at least due to the processes of recycling and hormone-sensitive biosynthesis.

Cellular Mechanisms of GnRH Action

The primary physiological response of GnRH binding by receptors on gonadotropes is the release of gonadotropins. However, there are other cellular responses evoked by GnRH, including down- and up-regulation of GnRH receptors, desensitization of gonadotropes, and gonadotropin- and GnRH receptor-biosynthesis. It appears as if the effects of GnRH are mediated through G-protein-linked mechanisms (98, 99). As several pathways exist for information flow within the gonadotrope, it is likely that one or more second messenger systems may be utilized by the gonadotrope to perform these varied functions in response to GnRH.

LH Release

Studies on the stimulation of LH secretion in response to GnRH first implicated cyclic adenosine 3',5'-monophosphate (cAMP) as the second messenger (100–102). However, the role of cAMP was questioned as several studies could not show significant involvement of cAMP in GnRH-stimulated LH release (103–106). A comprehensive study by Conn et al. (107) demonstrated that LH release in vitro could be uncoupled from cAMP. It is well accepted now that cAMP is not a second messenger in GnRH-stimulated LH release (reviews, 108–110).

Several lines of evidence indicate that calcium functions as a second messenger in acute release of LH in response to GnRH. When extracellular calcium is omitted or chelated, GnRH-stimulated LH release is inhibited (111–117). When calcium is introduced back into media, the release of LH occurs normally (118). As binding of GnRH to its membrane receptors is independent of extracellular calcium (119), an intracellular action of calcium is implicated. Increases in intracellular calcium of gonadotropes by administration of ionphores, liposomes loaded with calcium, or KCl depolarization stimulate the release of LH with similar efficacy to GnRH (115), and this effect is not mimicked by other cations (Mg^{++}, Na^+). Therefore, agents that are thought to provoke an increase in intracellular calcium of gonadotropes also cause LH release.

A second line of evidence for calcium as a second messenger in GnRH-stimulated LH release is the observation that administration of GnRH causes a measurable increase in intracellular calcium. Initially, a transmembrane flux of calcium in response to GnRH was observed (111, 120). Subsequent studies have utilized probes that fluoresce in the presence of calcium, Quin2 and Fura2, to show that GnRH stimulates a transient increase in intracellular calcium levels (121–123) associated with gonadotropin release. This increase in intracellular calcium is not provoked by occupancy of the receptor alone, as the stimulatory actions of GnRH on intracellular calcium levels are not observed after treatment of pituitary cells with a GnRH antagonist.

Further supporting evidence indicating a second messenger role of calcium in GnRH-stimulated LH release is that modulators of calcium channel function can alter gonadotropin release. Treatment of pituitary cells with calcium channel blocking agents such as verapamil and methoxyverapamil can block stimulated LH release (124). These agents also block gonadotropin release in vivo (125, 126). Finally, treatment of pituitary cells with the calcium channel agonist maitotoxin can stimulate the release of LH (127). Calcium ion channels associated with the GnRH receptor appear to be receptor-operated-type channels, as depolarization of the gonadotrope does not occur after stimulation by GnRH (128) although depolarization of gonadotropes with KCl does cause LH release. Based upon studies using calcium channel antagonists, GnRH-sensitive calcium ion channels also possess some of the characteristics of voltage-sensitive calcium channels (124, 129). Taken together these data provide strong evidence that calcium is the second messenger that mediates the acute release of LH in response to GnRH.

Two primary biochemical pathways have been identified in transducing changes in intracellular calcium levels and altered cellular response. The intracellular "calcium receptors," calmodulin and protein kinase C (PKC), have been identified in gonadotropes, and both appear to respond to activation of gonadotropes by GnRH.

Since its identification, PKC has been implicated in numerous sytems for mediation of agonist-induced cellular responses. This enzyme activity is dependent upon calcium and phospholipids (review, 130). Several observations indicate that PKC is involved in GnRH-stimulated functions of the gonadotrope. First, GnRH and GnRH agonists cause the re-distribution of PKC activity from the cytosolic to a particulate fraction of the pituitary both in vivo and in vitro (131–133). Generation of the activators of PKC, calcium and phospholipid, is achieved by phosphoinositide phosphorylation and hydrolysis (reviews, 134, 135). These phosphorylations and subsequent hydrolysis by phospholipase C-type reactions result in the formation of diacylglycerols (DAG) and inositol 1,4,5-trisphosphate (IP_3; 136). Diacylglycerol can function to activate PKC directly. IP_3 causes the release of calcium from intracellular non-mitochondrial stores (137) and may regulate plasma membrane calcium channels as well (138). GnRH stimulates the turnover of the poly-phosphoinositide cycle (139, 140), suggesting stimulation of the phospholipase C-type reaction and generation of the activators of PKC. Additionally, as described above, if intracellular calcium levels are increased in gonadotropes, LH release is stimulated. Gonadotropes can respond to administration of synthetic diacylglycerols with enhanced LH release (141, 142). The stimulation of LH release by administration of protein kinase activators appears independent of extracellular calcium, as evidenced by chelation of extracellular calcium, antagonism of calcium channels or coculture with calmodulin inhibitors (141, 143)—and, in fact, is synergistically enhanced in the presence of calcium ionophores (142). Finally, administration of phorbol esters (i.e., phorbol myristate acetate; PMA) that can directly activate PKC also causes LH release. These data strongly implicated a role for PKC in GnRH-stimulated LH release.

There are, however, a number of observations that question the involvement of PKC. First, PKC activators do not stimulate LH release to the same extent as GnRH (141, 142, 144). Additionally, administration of PKC activators (PMA) and GnRH results in an additive stimulation of LH release, suggesting independent mechanisms of action (140). The most definitive studies to indicate a dissociation between PKC activity and GnRH-stimulated LH release have been obtained through the use of cells that have been depleted of PKC activity. Because of the lack of useful specific inhibitors of PKC, protocols were developed to "down-regulate" PKC activity in order to study cellular responses in the absence of PKC activity. After exposure of pituitary cells to high doses of PMA (relative to those sufficient to stimulate LH release) for several hours, PKC was depleted from these cells as evidenced by (1) no measurable PKC phosphorylating activity, (2) no PKC activity as measured by the ability of PMA to stimulate LH release, (3) no demonstrable binding sites for phorbol esters (PKC is an intracellular "receptor" for phorbol esters), and (4) absence of any immunologically detectable PKC (145). Using pituitary cells depleted of PKC activity, McArdle et al. (146) showed that LH release in response to GnRH or calcium ionophore was intact. The absolute levels of LH release in PKC-depleted cells were less than in PKC-intact cells, because of PMA treatment for depletion of PKC caus-

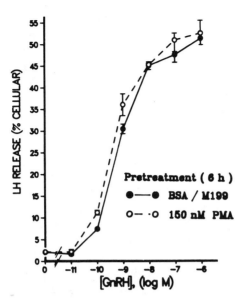

FIGURE 2.2. Effect of protein kinase C depletion on the LH releasing effect of GnRH. Cells were pretreated with medium 199/0.3% BSA (BSA/M199) or phorbol myristate acetate (PMA), washed, and incubated for 12 h in plating medium. The cells were then challenged for 3 h with the indicated concentrations of GnRH. Depletion of protein kinase C reduced cellular LH from 139.4 ± 5.0 ng/75 μl to 91.7 ± 4.2 ng/75 μl (n = 9). Values shown are the mean ± SE of 3 duplicate determinations (n = 3) and are representative of those obtained in 4 similar experiments. Adapted by permission from Ref. 146. Copyright by the American Society for Biochemistry and Molecular Biology, 1987.

ing LH release during pretreatment. Consequently, PKC-depleted cells contained less LH than control cells. When results are corrected for cellular content of LH, it is clear that absence of PKC activity does not affect GnRH-stimulated LH release (Fig. 2.2). These and other observations (144, 147, 148) provide strong evidence that PKC does not mediate the effects of GnRH to stimulate acute LH release.

An alternative calcium-sensitive system is the calmodulin pathway. Calmodulin is a ubiquitous calcium-binding protein that, upon activation by calcium, can regulate the activity of many regulatory enzymes such as adenylate cyclase, phosphorylase kinase, myosine light chain kinase, calcineurin, and phosphodiesterase (149). Additionally, several cytoskeletal proteins, likely involved in the cellular secretion mechanism, can be regulated by calmodulin (150). Administration of GnRH to ovariectomized rats causes redistribution of calmodulin, as measured by radioimmunoassay, from the cytosolic to the plasma membrane fraction of pituitary tissue (151). Moreover, calmodulin associates with patches of agonist-occupied GnRH receptors on gonadotropes (152). In addition to these observations of physical associations of calmodulin and GnRH receptors, biochemical evidence also supports a role for calmodulin in the action of GnRH. Administration of agents that inhibit the activity of calmodulin (pimozide, penfluoridol, chlorpromazine, chlordiazpoxide, and naphthalene sulfonimides) can inhibit GnRH-stimulated LH release (153, 154). Notably, these calmodulin inhibitors show similar actions in gonadotropes, even though they are from different classes of calmodulin inhibitors. These calmodulin inhibitors can block LH release stimulated by calcium ionophores (142), suggesting that calmodulin is required for GnRH- and ionophore-stimulated LH release. Five major calmodulin-binding components in gonadotropes have been suggested through utilization of a calmodulin gel overlayer assay that evaluates calcium-dependent calmodulin binding to cellular products after SDS-PAGE (155). Subsequent work toward identifying these calmodulin components has suggested the presence of spectrin, caldesmon, and calcineurin as three of the calmodulin-binding proteins present in the pituitary gonadotrope (156). These data provide strong evidence for a role of calmodulin in GnRH-stimulated LH release. Unequivocal evidence and specific calmodulin-activated protein function and actions await further study.

Biosynthesis of LH

In addition to stimulating the release of LH, GnRH is also required for biosynthesis of LH. LH is composed of 2 subunits, α and β. The α-subunit is common for LH, FSH, thyroid stimulating hormone, and human chorionic gonadotropin. The β-subunit differs between these glycoprotein hormones and confers biological specificity (157). With the complex nature of LH, there are several specific processes related to biosynthesis that are regulated, including mRNA production for both subunits, translation, subunit assembly, and glycosylation. GnRH stimulates and is required for normal production of mRNA for the β-subunit of LH (158–160). In pituitary cell cultures, PKC appears to be required for GnRH-stimulated β-subunit mRNA production (158). There are conflicting reports whether GnRH stimulates translation of the α- and β-subunits. Starzec et al. (161, 162) have shown that GnRH stimulates translation of both the α- and β-subunits of LH; however, this was not observed by others (163, 164). Moreover, Starzec et al. (162) have suggested that GnRH-stimulated translation of LH can be mimicked by cAMP analogs and phorbol esters in a nonadditive manner indicative of a similar mechanism of action. Lastly, glycosylation of LH is regulated by GnRH (163, 164). Glycosylation of LH can be stimulated by phorbol esters and diacylglycerol (165). Additionally, D600 (a calcium entry blocker) and pimozide (calmodulin inactivator) can prevent GnRH-stimulated glycosylation of LH (163). These data indicate the calcium

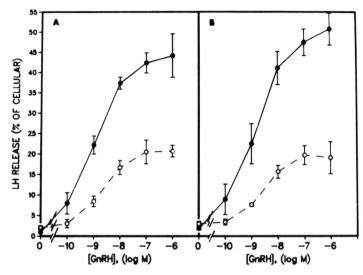

FIGURE 2.3. Homologous desensitization to GnRH is not inhibited by protein kinase C depletion. Pituitary cells were depleted of protein kinase C activity on the second day of culture with 500 nM phorbol myristate acetate in medium containing 0.5% DMSO (B) or with vehicle alone (A). They were then washed and maintained in plating medium for 12 h before being washed and challenged for 6 h with 10^{-7} M GnRH (○) or with medium alone (●). The cells were then washed again, and challenged for 3 h with the indicated concentrations of GnRH. The values shown are the mean ± SE of those obtained in 4 separate experiments. Reprinted by permission from Ref. 176, © by The Endocrine Society, 1987.

requirement for LH glycosylation and suggest mediation by calmodulin and/or PKC.

The difficulty in describing a single mechanism for GnRH-stimulated biosynthesis of LH is clear. However, it appears as if LH biosynthesis, in part, is regulated in a similar manner to that of GnRH-stimulated release of LH, as calcium and calmodulin are required for glycosylation; yet the stimulatory action of GnRH on the production and translation of individual subunits and their mRNAs is different from LH release, as PKC may mediate mRNA production and translation.

Desensitization

Gonadotropes, like many hormone-responsive cell types, can become refractory to specific hormones. Desensitization is the condition in which cellular responsiveness to a subsequent stimulation by the same hormone is decreased (Fig. 2.3, 166–169). Desensitization of the pituitary gland to GnRH and its analogs has been exploited for its clinical value. Long-term exposure to GnRH analogs can result in virtually the complete cessation of LH and FSH release as well as subsequent gonadal steroid secretion. This "chemical castration" has proven useful for treatment of individuals with steroid-dependent neoplasia as well as for controlling ovarian follicular development in patients for in vitro fertilization. The loss of responsiveness of gonadotropes to GnRH after prior exposure can be dissociated from the mechanism of LH release. As indicated above, GnRH-stimulated LH release is dependent upon extracellular calcium. When extracellular calcium is chelated during exposure to GnRH, gonadotropes still become desensitized (170, 171). Additionally, desensitization to GnRH can neither be provoked by calcium ionophores nor blocked by addition of calcium channel antagonists (170). Desensitization of gonadotropes to GnRH can be achieved after a brief exposure to GnRH (20 min) and last for at least 12 h after a single exposure (171). Occupancy of the GnRH receptor alone is insufficient to cause desensitization, as administration of antagonists of GnRH does not induce desensitization. Microaggregation of GnRH receptors, dimerization by antibody-antagonist-receptor complexes, does appear to be sufficient stimulus for desensitization (172); however, internalization of occupied GnRH receptors is not required (173). Desensitization of gonadotropes to GnRH is also associated with a loss of responsiveness to maitotoxin, which activates calcium ion channels, indicating that loss of activation of calcium ion channels by GnRH may contribute to desensitization (127, 174). Desensitization of gonadotropes has also been shown to be affected by changes in membrane fluidity (174, 175). Finally, desensitization occurs normally in gonadotropes depleted of PKC and is not induced by activators of PKC, suggesting a lack of involvement of PKC in mediating desensitization (Fig. 2.3, 176). Therefore, it appears that after binding of GnRH to its receptors, receptors undergo microaggregation which stimulates LH release and desensitization. Subsequent known effects of GnRH (i.e., calcium entry) are required for LH release but are not required for desensitization. Down-regulation of GnRH receptors has been suggested to participate in cellular desensitization. Clearly, down-regulation of receptors could reduce the sensitivity of gonadotropes to GnRH in the short term; however, there also appears to be uncoupling of the receptor-effector system which contributes to desensitization.

Regulation of GnRH Receptor Populations

As indicated above, GnRH can stimulate many alterations in the numbers of its own receptors, including down- and up-regulation, unmasking of receptors, and biosynthesis of receptors. Although these varied effects are all the result of GnRH stimulation, it appears as though these alterations are independently regulated.

Down-regulation of GnRH receptors occurs within the first 3–4 h of GnRH treatment. GnRH antagonists do not induce down-regulation, indicating that this effect is not due simply to occupancy of the GnRH receptor. Down-regulation appears to be independent of calcium flux caused by GnRH, as chelation of extracellular calcium does not interfere with down-regulation of GnRH receptors (75). Moreover, down-regulation is not evoked by agents that raise intracellular calcium (75). In gonadotropes exposed to high concentrations of phorbol esters to activate PKC, there is decreased binding of GnRH agonist, which suggests a role in down-regulation (176); however, treatment of gonadotropes that are depleted of PKC activity with GnRH is followed by normal down-regulation of GnRH receptors (176). These data suggest that down-regulation of GnRH receptors utilizes a different intracellular second messenger system than does GnRH-stimulated release of LH.

Up-regulation of GnRH receptors in response to homologous hormone occurs several hours after down-regulation. Again, occupancy of the receptor alone is not responsible for up-regulation, as GnRH antagonists cannot substitute for GnRH agonists in causing this effect. In direct contrast to down-regulation, up-regulation of GnRH receptors is dependent upon extracellular calcium and can be stimulated by agents that elevate intracellular calcium levels (75–77). Additionally, up-regulation of GnRH receptors requires protein synthesis as well as microtubule function (77). Depolarization of gonadotropes by KCl administration can stimulate up-regulation (76), and these effects can be observed after treatment of gonadotropes with analogs of cAMP (76). Recent evidence suggests there are at least two mechanisms that contribute to up-regulation of GnRH receptors. Treatment of gonadotropes with GnRH significantly stimulates the synthesis rate of GnRH receptors (97). This stimulatory effect of GnRH is found to occur normally even when extracellular calcium is chelated and can not be caused by the administration of calcium ionophore. Therefore GnRH-stimulated synthesis of its own receptors is independent of extracellular calcium, but up-regulation of GnRH receptors is dependent on extracellular calcium. Presumably, stimulation of the synthesis of GnRH receptors contributes to up-regulation, but is independent of calcium, suggesting more than one mechanism of up-regulation. Treatment of cells with phorbol esters can lead to increases in receptor numbers; however, this appears to be unmasking of GnRH receptors that are already present on gonadotropes and requires the simultaneous administration of the phorbol ester and GnRH agonist (177). As the effect of phorbol ester to unmask GnRH receptors occurs within 20 min of treatment, the observed effects of phorbol esters are likely not similar to the up-regulation induced by GnRH. Moreover, these "phorbol ester-unmasked" GnRH receptors appear to be selectively uncoupled to phosphoinositide metabolism (63) and to have a rate of synthesis similar to that of GnRH receptors

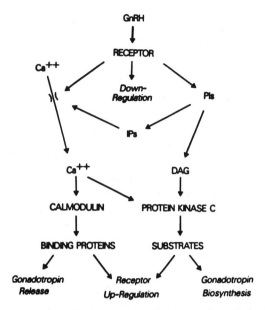

FIGURE 2.4. Pathways of GnRH action. (PIs = phosphoinositides; IPS = inositol phosphates; DAG = diacylglycerol.) From Ref. 178; Copyright © 1988; reprinted by permission of Wiley-Liss, a division of John Wiley and Sons, Inc.

normally present on gonadotropes (96). These observations indicate that unmasking of GnRH receptors by phorbol esters and GnRH-stimulated up-regulation are probably two separate events. It is clear from the many varied observations involving the up-regulation of GnRH receptors that up-regulation is a complex process and is likely mediated, in part, by several intracellular mechanisms that we are just beginning to identify.

Summary and Conclusions

Hypothalamic GnRH controls the release of gonadotropins from the pituitary gland. The effect of GnRH to stimulate gonadotropin release is used to improve reproductive function and efficiency. Long-term administration of GnRH or its analogs can result in reduction of LH and FSH release with a concomitant decrease in sex steroid production. This characteristic forms the basis for one of the primary clinical uses of GnRH analogs, treatment of steroid-dependent neoplasia. In addition to effects on gonadotropin release, GnRH also regulates gonadotropin biosynthesis, up- and down-regulation of GnRH receptors, desensitization, GnRH receptor biosynthesis, and gonadotropin subunit mRNA production. These varied effects of GnRH appear to be mediated by interaction of different intracellular second messenger systems (Fig. 2.4). Thus,

GnRH actions illustrate the ability of a single hormone utilizing a single receptor type to activate several different intracellular mechanisms within a single cell type.

References

1. Yang-Feng TL, Seeburg PH, Francke U. Human luteinizing hormone-releasing hormone gene (LHRH) is located on short arm of chromosome 8 (region 8p11.2-p21). Somatic Cell Mol Genet 1986;12:95–100.
2. Seeburg PH, Adelson JP. Characterization of cDNA for precursor of human luteinizing hormone releasing hormone. Nature 1984;311:666–8.
3. Adelman JP, Mason AJ, Hayflick JS, Seeburg PH. Isolation of the gene and hypothalamic cDNA for the common precursor of gonadotropin-releasing hormone and prolactin-inhibiting factor in human and rat. Proc Natl Acad Sci USA 1986;83:177–83.
4. Seeburg PH, Mason AJ, Stewart TA, Nikolics K. The mammalian GnRH gene and its pivotal role in reproduction. Recent Prog Horm Res 1987;43:69–91.
5. Mason AJ, Hayflick JS, Zoeller T, et al. Truncating the gonadotropin releasing hormone gene is responsible for hypogonadism in the hpg mouse. Science 1986;234:1366–71.
6. Schally AV, Arimura A, Baba Y, et al. Isolation and properties of the FSH and LH-releasing hormone. Biochem Biophys Res Commun 1971;43:393–9.
7. Matsuo J, Baba Y, Nair RMG, Arimura A, Schally AV. Structure of the porcine LH- and FSH-releasing hormone: I. The proposed amino acid sequence. Biochem Biophys Res Commun 1971;43:1334–9.
8. Burgus R, Butcher M, Amoss M, et al. Primary structure of the ovine hypothalamic luteinizing hormone-releasing factor (LRF). Proc Natl Acad Sci USA 1972;69:278–82.
9. King JA, Millar RP. Structure of chicken hypothalamic luteinizing hormone-releasing hormone: I. Structural determination on partially purified material. J Biol Chem 1982;257:10722–8.
10. King JA, Millar R. Structure of chicken hypothalamic luteinizing hormone-releasing hormone: II. Isolation and characterization. J Biol Chem 1982;257:10729–32.
11. Miyamoto K, Hasegawa Y, Nomura M, Igarashi M, Kangawa K, Matsuo H. Identification of the second gonadotropin-releasing hormone in chicken hypothalamus: evidence that gonadotropin secretion is probably controlled by two distinct gonadotropin-releasing hormones in avian species. Proc Natl Acad Sci USA 1984;81:3874–8.
12. Sherwood NM, Eiden L, Brownstein M, Spiess J, Rivier J, Vale WW. Characterization of a teleost gonadotropin-releasing hormone. Proc Natl Acad Sci USA 1983;80:2794–8.
13. Sherwood NM, Sower SA, Marshak DR, Fraser BA, Brownstein MJ. Primary structure of gonadotropin-releasing hormone from lamprey brain. J Biol Chem 1986;261:4812–41.
14. Sherwood NM. Evolution of a neuropeptide family: gonadotropin-releasing hormone. Am Zool 1986;26:1041–54.

15. Millar RP, King JA. Evolution of gonadotropin-releasing hormone: multiple usage of a peptide. NIPS 1988;3:49–53.
16. Karten MJ, Rivier JE. Gonadotropin-releasing hormone analog design: structure-function studies toward the development of agonists and antagonists: rationale and perspective. Endocr Rev 1986;7:44–66.
17. Monahan MW, Amoss MS, Anderson HA, Vale W. Synthetic analogs of the hypothalamic luteinizing hormone factor with measured agonist or antagonist properties. Biochemistry 1973;12:4616–20.
18. Coy DH, Seprodi J, Vilchez-Martinez JA, Pedroza E, Gardner J, Schally AV. Structure function studies and prediction of conformational requirements for LH-RH. In: Collin R, Barbeau A, Ducharme JR, Rockefort JG, eds. Central nervous system effects of hypothalamic hormones and other peptides. New York: Raven Press, 1979:317–23.
19. Nikolics K, Coy DH, Vilchez-Martinez JA, Coy EJ, Schally AV. Synthesis and biological activity of position 1 analogs of LH-RH. Int J Pept Protein Res 1977;9:57–62.
20. Momany FA. Conformational energy analysis of the molecule, luteinizing hormone-releasing hormone: I. Native decapeptide. J Am Chem Soc 1975;98:2990–6.
21. Fujino M, Kobayashi S, Obayashi M, et al. Structure-activity relationships in the C-terminal part of luteinizing hormone releasing hormone (LH-RH). Biochem Biophys Res Commun 1972;49:863–9.
22. Fujino M, Fukuda T, Shinagawa S, Kobayashi S, Yamazaki I, Nakayama R. Synthetic analogs of luteinizing hormone releasing hormone (LH-RH) substituted in position 6 and 10. Biochem Biophys Res Commun 1974;60:406–13.
23. Conn PM, Rogers DC, Seay S, et al. Receptor-effector coupling in the pituitary gonadotrope. In: McKerns KW, Naor Z, eds. Biochemical endocrinology. New York: Plenum Press, 1984:153–73.
24. Hook WA, Karten M, Siraganian RP. Histamine release by structural analogs of LHRH [Abstract]. Fed Proc 1985;44:1323 (abstract #5336).
25. Haviv F, Palabrica CA, Bush EN, et al. Active reduced size hexapeptide analogues of luteinizing hormone-releasing hormone. J Med Chem 1989;32:2340–4.
26. Bennett HPJ, McMartin C. Peptide hormones and their analogues: distribution, clearance from the circulation, and inactivation in vivo. Pharmacol Rev 1979;30:247–92.
27. Griffiths EC, Kelly AJ. Mechanism of inactivation of hypothalamic regulatory hormones. Mol Cell Endocrinol 1979;14:3–17.
28. Horsthemke B, Bauer K. Substrate specificity of an adenohypophyseal endopeptidase capable of hydrolyzing luteinizing hormone-releasing hormone: preferential cleavage of peptide bonds involving the carboxyl terminus of hydrophobic and basic amino acids. Biochemistry 1982;21:1033–6.
29. Tate SS. Purification and properties of a bovine brain thyrotropin-releasing-factor deamidase, a post proline cleaving enzyme of limited specificity. Eur J Biochem 1981;118:17–23.
30. Knisatschek H, Bauer K. Characterization of "thyroliberin deaminating enzyme" as a post-proline-cleaving enzyme. J Biol Chem 1979;254:10936–43.

31. Horsthemke B, Bauer K. Characterization of a nonchymotrypsin-like endopeptidase from anterior pituitary that hydrolyzes luteinizing hormone-releasing hormone at the tyrosyl-glycine and histidyl-tryptophan bonds. Biochemistry 1981;19:2867–73.
32. Handelsman DJ, Swerdloff RS. Pharmacokinetics of gonadotropin-releasing hormone and its analogs. Endocr Rev 1986;7:95–105.
33. Coy DH, Vilchez-Martinez JA, Coy EJ, Schally AV. Analogs of luteinizing hormone-releasing hormone with increased biological activity produced by D-amino acid substitutions in position 6. J Med Chem 1976;19:423–5.
34. Coy DH, Coy EJ, Schally AV, Vilchez-Martinez JA, Hirotsu Y, Arimura A. Synthetic and biological properties of [D-Ala-6-DES-Gly-NH$_2$-10]-LH-RH ethylamide, a peptide with greatly enhanced LH- and FSH-releasing activity. Biochem Biophy Res Commun 1974;57:335–40.
35. Vilchez-Martinez JA, Coy DH, Arimura A, Coy EJ, Hirotsu Y, Schally AV. Synthesis and biological properties of [Leu-6]-LH-RH and [D-Leu-6, DES Gly NH$_2$-10]-LH-RH ethylamide. Biochem Biophys Res Commun 1974;59:1226–32.
36. Nestor JJ, Ho TL, Tahilramani R, McRae GI, Vickery BH. Long acting LHRH agonists and antagonists. In: Labri F, Belanger A, Dupont A, eds. LHRH and its analogues: basic and clinical aspects. Amsterdam: Excerpta Medica, 1984:24–35.
37. Danforth DR, Gordon K, Leal JA, Williams RF, Hodgen GD. Extended presence of antide (Nal-Lys GnRH antagonist) in circulation: prolonged duration of gonadotropin inhibition may derive from antide binding to serum proteins. J Clin Endocrinol Metab 1990;70:554–6.
38. Clayton RN, Harwood JP, Catt KJ. Gonadotropin-releasing hormone analogue binds to luteal cells and inhibits progesterone production. Nature 1979;282:90–2.
39. Jones PBC, Conn PM, Marian J, Hsueh AJW. Binding of gonadotropin-releasing hormone agonist to rat ovarian granulosa cells. Life Sci 1980;27:2125–32.
40. Latouche J, Crumeyrolle-Arias M, Jordon D, et al. GnRH receptors in human granulosa cells: anatomical localization and characterization by autoradiographic study. Endocrinology 1989;125:1739–41.
41. Brown JL, Reeves JJ. Absence of specific luteinizing hormone releasing hormone receptors in ovine, bovine or porcine ovaries. Biol Reprod 1983;29:1179–82.
42. Eidne KA, Hendricks DT, Millar RP. Demonstration of a 60K molecular weight luteinizing hormone-releasing hormone receptor in solubilized adrenal membrane by a ligand-immunoblotting technique. Endocrinology 1985;116:1792–5.
43. Eidne KA, Flanagan CA, Millar RP. Gonadotropin releasing hormone binding sites in human breast carcinoma. Science 1985;229:989–91.
44. Fekete M, Zalanti A, Schally AV. Presence of membrane binding sites for [D-Trp^6]-luteinizing hormone-releasing hormone in experimental pancreatic cancer. Cancer Lett 1989;45:87–91.
45. Reubi JC, Palcios JM, Maurer R. Specific luteinizing-hormone-releasing hormone receptor binding sites in hippocampus and pituitary: an autoradiographical study. Neuroscience 1987;21:847–56.

46. Jennes L, Dalati B, Conn PM. Distribution of gonadotropin releasing hormone agonist binding sites in the rat central nervous system. Brain Res 1988;452:156–64.
47. Jennes L, Janovick J, Braden T, Conn PM. Gonadotropin releasing hormone binding sites in rat hippocampus: different structure/binding relationships compared to the anterior pituitary. Mol Cell Neurosci 1990;1:121–7.
48. Moss RL, McCann S. Induction of mating behavior in rats by luteinizing hormone-releasing hormone. Science 1973;181:177–9.
49. Pfaff DW. Luteinizing hormone-releasing factor potentiates lordosis behavior in hypophysectomized ovariectomized female rats. Science 1973;182:1148–9.
50. Hsueh AJW, Jones PB. Extrapituitary actions of gonadotropin-releasing hormone. Endocr Rev 1981;2:437–61.
51. Marian J, Conn PM. Subcellular localization of the receptor for gonadotropin-releasing hormone in pituitary and ovarian tissue. Endocrinology 1983;112:104–12.
52. Hazum E. GnRH-receptor of rat pituitary is a glycoprotein: differential effect of neuroaminidase and lectins on agonists and antagonists binding. Mol Cell Endocrinol 1982;26:217–22.
53. Schvartz I, Hazum E. Tunicamycin and neuraminidase effects on luteinizing hormone (LH)-releasing hormone binding and LH release from rat pituitary cells in culture. Endocrinology 1985;116:2341–6.
54. Hazum E, Garritsen A, Keinan D. Role of lipids on gonadotropin releasing hormone agonist and antagonist binding to rat pituitary. Biochem Biophys Res Commun 1982;105:8–13.
55. Keinan D, Hazum E. Mapping of gonadotropin releasing hormone receptor binding site. Biochemistry 1985;24:7728–32.
56. Hazum E. Binding properties of solubilized gonadotropin releasing hormone receptor: role of carboxylic groups. Biochemistry 1987;26:7011–4.
57. Perrin MH, Haas Y, Porter J, Rivier J, Vale W. The gonadotropin-releasing hormone pituitary receptor interacts with a guanosine triphosphate binding protein: differential effects of guanyl nucleotides on agonist and antagonist binding. Endocrinology 1989;124:798–804.
58. Perrin MM, Haas Y, Rivier JE, Vale WW. Solubilization of the gonadotropin-releasing hormone receptor from bovine pituitary plasma membranes. Endocrinology 1983;112:1538–40.
59. Hazum E, Schvartz I, Popliker M. Production and characterization of antibodies to gonadotropin-releasing hormone receptors. J Biol Chem 1987; 262:531–4.
60. Iwashita M, Hirota J, Izumi S-I, Chen H-C, Catt KJ. Solubilization and characterization of the rat pituitary gonadotrophin-releasing hormone receptor. J Mol Endocrinol 1988;1:187–96.
61. Ogier SA, Mitchell R, Fink G. Solubilization of a large molecular weight form of the rat LHRH receptor. J Endocrinol 1987;115:151–9.
62. Hazum E. Photoaffinity labeling of luteinizing hormone receptor of rat pituitary membrane preparations. Endocrinology 1981;109:1281–3.
63. Huckle WR, Hawes BE, Conn PM. Protein kinase C-mediated gonadotropin releasing hormone sequestration is associated with uncoupling of phosphoinositide turnover hydrolysis. J Biol Chem 1989;264:8619–26.

64. Conn PM, Venter JC. Radiation inactivation (target size analysis) of the gonadotropin-releasing hormone receptor: evidence for a high molecular weight complex. Endocrinology 1985;116:1324–6.

65. Hazum E, Schvartz I, Waksman Y, Keinan D. Solubilization and purification of rat pituitary gonadotropin-releasing hormone receptor. J Biol Chem 1986;261:13043–8.

66. Eidne KA, McNiven AI, Taylor PL, et al. Functional expression of rat pituitary gonadotropin-releasing hormone receptors in Xenopus oocytes. J Mol Endocrinol 1988;1:R9–R12.

67. Yoshida S, Plant S, Taylor PL, Eidne KA. Chloride channels mediate the response to gonadotropin-releasing hormone (GnRH) in Xenopus oocytes injected with rat anterior pituitary mRNA. Mol Endocrinol 1989;3:1953–60.

68. Sealfon SC, Gillo B, Mundomattom S, et al. Gonadotropin releasing hormone receptor expression in Xenopus oocytes. Mol Endocrinol 1990;4:119–24.

69. Clayton RN, Solano AR, Garcia-Vila A, Dufau ML, Catt KJ. Regulation of pituitary receptors for gonadotropin releasing hormone during the rat estrous cycle. Endocrinology 1980;107:699–706.

70. Savoy-Moore RT, Schwartz NB, Duncan JA, Marshall JC. Pituitary gonadotropin-releasing hormone receptors during the rat estrous cycle. Science 1980;209:942–4.

71. Adams TE, Spies HG. Binding characteristics of gonadotropin-releasing hormone receptors throughout the estrous cycle of the hamster. Endocrinology 1981;108:2245–53.

72. Marian J, Cooper RL, Conn PM. Regulation of the rat pituitary gonadotropin-releasing hormone receptor. Mol Pharmacol 1981;19:339–405.

73. Crowder ME, Nett TM. Pituitary content of gonadotropins and receptors for gonadotropin-releasing hormone (GnRH) and hypothalamic content of GnRH during the periovulatory period of the ewe. Endocrinology 1984;114:234–9.

74. Nett TM, Cermak D, Braden T, Manns J, Niswender GD. Pituitary receptors for GnRH and estradiol, and pituitary content of gonadotropins in beef cows: I. Changes during the estrous cycle. Dom Anim Endocrinol 1987;4:123–32.

75. Conn PM, Rogers DC, Seay SG. Biphasic regulation of the gonadotropin-releasing hormone receptor by receptor microaggregation and intracellular Ca^{2+} levels. Mol Pharmacol 1984;25:51–5.

76. Young LS, Naik SI, Clayton RN. Adenosine $3',5'$-monophosphate derivatives increase gonadotropin-releasing hormone receptors in cultured pituitary cells. Endocrinology 1984;114:2114–22.

77. Young LS, Naik SI, Clayton RN. Pituitary gonadotrophin-releasing hormone receptor up-regulation in vitro: dependence on calcium and microtubule function. J Endocrinol 1985;107:49–56.

78. Young LS, Naik SI, Clayton RN. Increased gonadotrophin releasing hormone receptors on pituitary gonadotrophs: effect on subsequent LH secretion. Mol Cell Endocrinol 1985;41:69–78.

79. Naor Z, Clayton RN, Catt KJ. Characterization of gonadotropin-releasing hormone receptors in cultured rat pituitary cells. Endocrinology 1980;107:1144–52.

80. Wise ME, Nieman D, Stewart J, Nett TM. Effect of number of receptors for gonadotropin-releasing hormone on the release of luteinizing hormone. Biol Reprod 1984;31:1007–13.

81. Clarke IJ, Cummins JT, Crowder ME, Nett TM. Pituitary receptors for gonadotropin-releasing hormone in relation to changes in pituitary and plasma gonadotropins in ovariectomized hypothalamo/pituitary-disconnected ewes: II. A marked rise in receptor number during the acute feedback effects of estradiol. Biol Reprod 1988;39:349–54.

82. Gregg DW, Nett TM. Direct effects of estradiol-17β on the number of gonadotropin-releasing hormone receptors in the ovine pituitary. Biol Reprod 1989;40:288–93.

83. Laws SC, Beggs MJ, Webster JC, Miller WL. Inhibin increases and progesterone decreases receptors for gonadotropin-releasing hormone in ovine pituitary culture. Endocrinology 1990;127:373–80.

84. Laws SC, Webster JC, Miller WL. Estradiol alters the effectiveness of gonadotropin-releasing hormone (GnRH) in ovine pituitary cultures: GnRH receptors versus responsiveness to GnRH. Endocrinology 1990;127:381–6.

85. Wang QF, Farnworth PG, Findlay JK, Burger HG. Effect of 31K bovine inhibin on the specific binding of gonadotropin-releasing hormone to rat anterior pituitary cells in culture. Endocrinology 1988;123:2161–6.

86. Wang QF, Farnworth PG, Findlay JK, Burger HG. Inhibitory effect of pure 31-kilodalton bovine inhibin on gonadotropin-releasing hormone (GnRH)-induced up-regulation of GnRH binding sites in cultured rat anterior pituitary cells. Endocrinology 1989;124:363–8.

87. Braden TD, Farnworth PG, Burger HG, Conn PM. Regulation of the synthetic rate of gonadotropin-releasing hormone receptors in rat pituitary cell cultures by inhibin. Endocrinology 1990;127:2387–92.

88. Conn PM, Rogers DC, Stewart JM, Niedal J, Sheffield T. Conversion of a gonadotropin-releasing hormone antagonist to an agonist. Nature 1982; 296:653–5.

89. Conn PM. Ligand dimerization: a technique for assessing receptor-receptor interactions. Methods Enzymol 1983;103:49–58.

90. Pelletier G, Dube D, Guy J, Sequin C, Lefebvre FA. Binding and internalization of a luteinizing hormone-releasing hormone agonist by rat gonadotrophic cells: a radiographic study. Endocrinology 1982;111:1068–76.

91. Duello TM, Nett TM, Farquhar MG. Fate of a gonadotropin-releasing hormone agonist internalized by rat pituitary gonadotrophs. Endocrinology 1983;112:1–10.

92. Jennes L, Stumpf WE, Conn PM. Internalization pathways of electron opaque gonadotropin-releasing hormone derivatives bound by cultured gonadotropes. Endocrinology 1983;113:1683–9.

93. Hazum E, Conn PM. Molecular mechanism of gonadotropin-releasing hormone (GnRH) action: I. The GnRH receptor. Endocr Rev 1988;9: 379–85.

94. Schvartz I, Hazum E. Internalization and recycling of receptor-bound gonadotropin-releasing hormone agonist in pituitary gonadotropes. J Biol Chem 1987;262:17046–50.

95. Jennes L, Coy D, Conn PM. Receptor-mediated uptake of GnRH agonist and antagonists by cultured gonadotropes: evidence for differential intracellular routing. Peptides 1986;7:459–63.

96. Braden TD, Hawes BE, Conn PM. Synthesis of gonadotropin-releasing hormone receptors by gonadotrope cell cultures: both preexisting receptors and those unmasked by protein kinase-C activators show a similar synthetic rate. Endocrinology 1989;125:1623–9.

97. Braden TD, Conn PM. Altered rate of synthesis of gonadotropin-releasing hormone receptors: effects of homologous hormone appear independent of extracellular calcium. Endocrinology 1990;126:2577–82.

98. Andrews WV, Staley DD, Huckle WR, Conn PM. Stimulation of luteinizing hormone (LH) release and phospholipid breakdown by guanosine triphosphate in permeabilized pituitary gonadotropes: antagonist action suggests association of a G-protein and gonadotropin-releasing hormone receptor. Endocrinology 1986;119:2537–46.

99. Waters SB, Hawes BE, Conn PM. Stimulation of luteinizing hormone release by sodium fluoride is independent of protein kinase-C activity and unaffected by desensitization to gonadotropin-releasing hormone. Endocrinology 1990;126:2583–91.

100. Borgeat P, Chavaney G, Dupont A, Labrie F, Arimura A, Schally AV. Stimulation of adenosine 3′,5′-cyclic monophosphate accumulation in anterior pituitary gland in vitro by synthetic luteinizing hormone-releasing hormone. Proc Natl Acad Sci USA 1972;69:2677–81.

101. Menon KMJ, Cuanaga KP, Azhar S. GnRH action in rat anterior pituitary gland: regulation of protein, glycoprotein and LH synthesis. Acta Endocrinol 1977;86:473–88.

102. Adams TE, Wagner TOF, Sawyer HR, Nett TM. GnRH interactions with anterior pituitary: II. Cyclic AMP as an intracellular mediator in the GnRH activated gonadotroph. Biol Reprod 1979;21:735–47.

103. Naor Z, Koch Y, Chobsieng P, Zor U. Pituitary cyclic AMP production and mechanisms of luteinizing hormone release. FEBS Lett 1975;58:318–21.

104. Naor Z, Zor U, Meidan R, Koch Y. Sex differences in pituitary cyclic AMP response to gonadotropin-releasing hormone. Am J Physiol 1978;235:E37–E41.

105. Ratner A, Wilson MC, Srivastave L, Peake GT. Dissociation between LH release and pituitary cyclic nucleotide accumulation in response to synthetic LH releasing hormone in vivo. Neuroendocrinology 1976;20:35–42.

106. Rigler GL, Peake GT, Ratner A. Effect of luteinizing hormone releasing hormone on accumulation of pituitary cyclic AMP and GMP in vitro. J Endocrinol 1978;76:367–8.

107. Conn PM, Morrell DV, Dufau ML, Catt KJ. Gonadotropin-releasing hormone action in cultured pituicytes: independence of luteinizing hormone release and adenosine 3′,5′-monophosphate production. Endocrinology 1979;104:448–53.

108. Conn PM, Huckle WR, Andrews WV, McArdle CA. The molecular mechanism of action of gonadotropin releasing hormone (GnRH) in the pituitary. Recent Prog Horm Res 1987;43:29–68.

109. Conn PM, McArdle CA, Andrews WV, Huckle WR. The molecular basis of gonadotropin releasing hormone (GnRH) action in the pituitary gonadotrope. Biol Reprod 1987;36:17–35.

110. Huckle WR, Conn PM. Molecular mechanism of gonadotropin releasing hormone action: II. The effector system. Endocr Rev 1988;9:387–95.

111. Hopkins CR, Walker AM. Calcium as a second messenger in the stimulation of luteinizing hormone secretion. Mol Cell Endocrinol 1978;12:189–208.

112. Wakabayashi K, Kamberi IA, McCann SM. In vitro response of the rat pituitary to gonadotropin releasing factors and to ions. Endocrinology 1969; 85:1046–56.

113. Samli MH, Geshwind II. Some effects of energy-transfer inhibitors and of Ca^{2+}-free and K^+-enhanced media on the release of LH from the rat pituitary gland in vitro. Endocrinology 1968;82:225–31.

114. Adams TE, Nett TM. Interactions of GnRH with the pituitary: III. Role of divalent cations, microtubules and microfilaments in the GnRH activated gonadotroph. Biol Reprod 1979;21:1073–86.

115. Marian J, Conn PM. Gonadotropin releasing hormone stimulation of cultured pituitary cells requires calcium. Mol Pharmacol 16:196–201.

116. Stern JE, Conn PM. Perifusion of rat pituitaries: requirements of optimal GnRH-stimulated LH release. Am J Physiol 1981;240:E504–9.

117. Conn PM, Rogers DC, Sandhu FS. Alteration of the intracellular calcium level stimulated gonadotropin release from cultured rat anterior pituitary cells. Endocrinology 1979;105:1122–7.

118. Bates MD, Conn PM. Calcium mobilization in the pituitary gonadotrope: relative roles of intra- and extracellular sources. Endocrinology 1984;115: 1380–5.

119. Marian J, Conn PM. The calcium requirement of GnRH-stimulated LH release is not mediated through specific action on the receptor. Life Sci 1980;27:87–92.

120. Conn PM, Kilpatrick D, Kirshner N. Ionophoretic Ca^{2+} mobilization in rat gonadotropes and bovine adrenomedullary cells. Cell Calcium 1980;1: 129–33.

121. Clapper D, Conn PM. Gonadotropin-releasing hormone stimulation of pituitary gonadotrope cells produces an increase in intracellular calcium. Biol Reprod 1985;32:269–78.

122. Chang JP, McCoy EE, Graeter J, Tasaka K, Catt KJ. Participation of voltage-dependent calcium channels in the action of gonadotropin-releasing hormone. J Biol Chem 1986;261:9105–8.

123. Leong DA. Spatial mapping of cytosolic calcium oscillations in single gonadotropes [Abstract]. Seventy-first annual meeting of the Endocrine Society, Seattle, WA, 1989:24 (abstract #7).

124. Conn PM, Rogers DC, Seay SG. Structure-function relationships of calcium ion channel antagonists at the pituitary gonadotrope. Endocrinology 1983; 113:1592–5.

125. Barbino A, DeMarinis L. Calcium antagonists and hormone release: II. Effects of verapamil on basal, gonadotropin-releasing hormone, and thryotropin-releasing hormone induced pituitary hormone release in normal subjects. J Clin Endocrinol Metab 1980;51:749–53.

126. Veldhuis JD, Borges JLC, Drake CR, Rogal AD, Kaiser DL, Thorner MO. Divergent influences of the structurally dissimilar calcium entry blockers diltiazem and verapamil on thyrotropin- and gonadotropin-releasing hormone-stimulated anterior pituitary hormone secretion in man. J Clin Endocrinol Metab 1985;60:144–9.

127. Conn PM, Staley DD, Yasumoto T, Huckle WR, Janovick J. Homologous desensitization with gonadotropin-releasing hormone (GnRH) also dim-

inishes gonadotrope responsiveness to maitotoxin: a role for the GnRH receptor regulated calcium ion channel in mediation of cellular desensitization. Mol Endocrinol 1987;1:154–9.

128. Mason WT, Waring DW. Electrophysiological recording from gonadotrophs: evidence for Ca^{2+} channels mediated by gonadotropin-releasing hormone. Neuroendocrinology 1985;41:258–68.

129. Stojilkovic SS, Izumi S, Catt KJ. Participation of voltage-sensitive calcium channels in pituitary hormone release. J Biol Chem 1988;263:13054–61.

130. Nishizuka Y. Studies and perspectives of protein kinase C. Science 1986; 233:305–12.

131. Naor Z, Zer J, Zakut H, Hermon J. Characterization of pituitary calcium-activated, phospholipid-dependent protein kinase: redistribution by gonadotropin releasing hormone. Proc Natl Acad Sci USA 1985;82:8203–7.

132. Hirota K, Hirota T, Aguilera G, Catt KJ. Hormone induced redistribution of calcium-activated phospholipid dependent protein kinase in pituitary gonadotrophs. J Biol Chem 1985;260:3243–6.

133. McArdle CA, Conn PM. Hormone-stimulated redistribution of gonadotrope protein kinase C in vivo: dependence on Ca^{2+} influx. Mol Pharmacol 1986; 29:570–6.

134. Nishizuka Y. Turnover of inositol phospholipids and signal transduction. Science 1984;225:1365–70.

135. Rana RS, Hokin LE. Role of phosphoinositides in transmembrane signaling. Physiol Rev 1990;70:115–64.

136. Berridge MJ. Inositol phosphate and diacylglycerol as second messengers. Biochem J 1984;220:345–60.

137. Streb H, Irvine RJ, Berridge MJ, Schulz I. Release of calcium from a nonmitochondrial intracellular store in pancreatic acinar cells by inositol 1,4,5-trisphosphate. Nature 1983;306:67–9.

138. Kuno M, Gardner P. Ion channels activated by inositol 1,4,5-trisphosphate in plasma membranes of T-lymphocytes. Nature 1987;326:301–4.

139. Andrews WV, Conn PM. Gonadotropin-releasing hormone stimulates mass changes in phosphoinositides and diacylglycerol accumulation in purified gonadotrope cell cultures. Endocrinology 1986;118:1148–58.

140. Huckle WR, Conn PM. The relationship between gonadotropin-releasing hormone-stimulated luteinizing hormone release and inositol phosphate production: studies with calcium antagonists and protein kinase C activators. Endocrinology 1987;120:160–9.

141. Conn PM, Ganong BR, Ebeling J, Staley D, Neidel JE, Bell BM. Diacylglycerols release LH: structure-activity relations reveal a role for protein kinase C. Biochem Biophys Res Commun 1985;126:532–9.

142. Harris CE, Staley D, Conn PM. Diacylglycerols and protein kinase C: potential amplifying mechanism for Ca^{2+} mediated gonadotropin-releasing hormone-stimulated luteinizing hormone release. Mol Pharmacol 1985; 27:532–6.

143. Naor Z, Eli Y. Synergistic stimulation of luteinizing hormone (LH) release by protein kinase C activators and Ca^{2+}-ionophore. Biochem Biophys Res Commun 1985;130:848–53.

144. Lewis CE, Richards PSM, Moris JF. Heterogeneity of responses to LH-releasing hormone and phorbol ester among rat gonadotrophs: a study using a reverse haemolytic plaque assay for LH. J Mol Endocrinol 1989;2:55–63.

145. McArdle CA, Conn PM. The use of protein kinase C-depleted cells for investigation of the role of protein kinase C in stimulus-response coupling in the pituitary. Methods Enzymol 1989;168:287–301.
146. McArdle CA, Huckle WR, Conn PM. Phorbol esters reduce gonadotrope responsiveness to protein kinase C activators but not to Ca^{2+}-mobilizing secretagogues: does protein kinase C mediate gonadotropin-releasing hormone action? J Biol Chem 1987;262:5028–35.
147. Beggs MJ, Miller WL. GnRH-stimulated LH release from ovine gonadotrophs in culture is separate from phorbol ester stimulated LH release. Endocrinology 1989;124:667–74.
148. van der Merwe PA, Millar RP, Davidson JS. Calcium stimulated luteinizing-hormone (lutropin) exocytosis by a mechanism independent of protein kinase C. Biochem J 1990;268:493–8.
149. Means AR, Dedman JR. Calmodulin, an intracellular calcium receptor. Nature 1980;285:73–7.
150. Chafouleas JG, Guerriero V, Means AR. Possible regulatory roles of calmodulin and myosin light chain kinase in secretion. In: Conn PM, ed. Cellular regulation of secretion and release. New York: Academic Press, 1985;445–58.
151. Conn PM, Chafouleas JG, Rogers D, Means AR. Gonadotropin-releasing hormone stimulates calmodulin redistribution in rat pituitary. Nature 1981; 292:264–5.
152. Jennes L, Bronson D, Stumpf WE, Conn PM. Evidence for an association between calmodulin and membrane patches containing gonadotropin-releasing hormone-receptor complexes in cultured gonadotropes. Cell Tissue Res 1985;239:311–5.
153. Conn PM, Rogers DC, Sheffield T. Inhibition of gonadotropin-releasing hormone-stimulated luteinizing hormone release by pimozide: evidence for a site of action after calcium mobilization. Endocrinology 1981;109:1122–6.
154. Conn PM, Bates MD, Rogers DC, Seay SG, Smith WA. GnRH-receptor-effector-response coupling in the pituitary gonadotrope: a Ca^{2+}-mediated system. In: Fotherby K, Pal SB, eds. The role of drugs and electrolytes in hormogenesis. Berlin: Walter de Gruyer, 1984;85–103.
155. Wooge CH, Conn PM. Characterization of calmodulin-binding components in the pituitary gonadotrope. Mol Cell Endocrinol 1988;56:41–51.
156. Natarajan K, Ness J, Wooge CH, Janovick J, Conn PM. Specific identification and subcellular localization of three calmodulin-binding proteins in the rat gonadotrope: spectrin, caldesmon, and calcineurin. Biol Reprod 1991; 44:43–52.
157. Pierce JC, Parsons TF. Glycoprotein hormones: structure and function. Annu Rev Biochem 1981;50:465–95.
158. Andrews WV, Maurer RA, Conn PM. Stimulation of rat luteinizing hormone-β messenger RNA levels by gonadotropin releasing hormone: apparent role for protein kinase C. J Biol Chem 1988;263:13755–61.
159. Hamernik DL, Nett TM. Gonadotropin-releasing hormone increases the amount of messenger ribonucleic acid for gonadotropins in ovariectomized ewes after hypothalamic-pituitary disconnection. Endocrinology 1988; 122:959–66.

160. Lalloz MRA, Detta A, Clayton RN. Gonadotropin-releasing hormone is required for enhanced luteinizing hormone subunit gene expression in vivo. Endocrinology 1988;122:1681–8.
161. Starzec A, Counis R, Jutisz M. Gonadotropin-releasing hormone stimulates the synthesis of the polypeptide chains of luteinizing hormone. Endocrinology 1986;119:561–5.
162. Starzec A, Jutisz M, Counis R. Cyclic adenosine monophosphate and phorbol ester, like gonadotropin-releasing hormone, stimulate the biosynthesis of luteinizing hormone polypeptide chains in a nonadditive manner. Mol Endocrinol 1989;3:618–24.
163. Liu T-C, Jackson GL. Synthesis and release of luteinizing hormone in vitro by rat anterior pituitary cells: effects of gallopamil hydrochloride (D600) and pimozide. Endocrinology 1985;117:1608–14.
164. Vogel DL, Magner JA, Sherins RJ, Weintraub BD. Biosynthesis, glycosylation, and secretion of rat luteinizing hormone α- and β-subunits: differential effects of orchidectomy and gonadotropin-releasing hormone. Endocrinology 1986;119:202–13.
165. Liu T-C, Jackson GL. Stimulation by phorbol ester and diacylglycerol of luteinizing hormone glycosylation and release by rat anterior pituitary cells. Endocrinology 1987;121:1589–95.
166. deKoning JA, van Dietan MJ, van Rees GP. Refractoriness of the pituitary gland after continuous exposure to luteinizing hormone releasing hormone. J Endocrinol 1978;79:311–8.
167. Smith MA, Vale W. Desensitization to gonadotropin-releasing hormone observed in superfused pituitary cells on cytodex beads. Endocrinology 1981;108:752–9.
168. Badger TM, Loughlin JS, Nadaff PG. The luteinizing hormone-releasing hormone (LHRH)-desensitized rat pituitary: luteinizing hormone-responsiveness to LHRH in vitro. Endocrinology 1983;112:793–9.
169. Keri G, Nikolics K, Teplan I, Molnar J. Desensitization of luteinizing hormone release in cultured pituitary cells by gonadotropin-releasing hormone. Mol Cell Endocrinol 1983;30:109–20.
170. Smith WA, Conn PM. GnRH-mediated desensitization of the pituitary gonadotrope is not calcium dependent. Endocrinology 1983;112:408–10.
171. Jinnah HA, Conn PM. Gonadotropin-releasing hormone-mediated desensitization of cultured rat anterior pituitary cells can be uncoupled from luteinizing hormone release. Endocrinology 1986;118:2599–604.
172. Smith WA, Conn PM. Microaggregation of the gonadotropin-releasing hormone-receptor: relation to gonadotrope desensitization. Endocrinology 1984;114:553–9.
173. Gorospe WC, Conn PM. Agents that decrease gonadotropin-releasing hormone (GnRH) receptor internalization do not inhibit GnRH-mediated gonadotrope desensitization. Endocrinology 1987;120:222–9.
174. Gorospe WC, Conn PM. Restoration of the LH secretory response in desensitized gonadotropes. Mol Cell Endocrinol 1988;59:101–10.
175. Gorospe WC, Conn PM. Membrane fluidity regulated development of gonadotrope desensitization to GnRH. Mol Cell Endocrinol 1987;53:131–40.

176. McArdle CA, Gorospe WC, Huckle WR, Conn PM. Homologous down-regulation of gonadotropin-releasing hormone receptors and desensitization of gonadotropes: lack of dependence on protein kinase C. Mol Endocrinol 1987;1:420–9.
177. Huckle WR, McArdle CA, Conn PM. Differential sensitivity of gonadotropin-releasing hormone receptors to activators of protein kinase C: a marker for receptor activators. J Biol Chem 1988;263:3296–302.
178. Huckle WR, Conn PM. The role of protein kinase C in pituitary gonadotropin releasing hormone action. In: Lakowski JM, Perez-Polo JR, Rassin DK, eds. Neural control of reproductive function. New York: Alan Liss, 1988:441–6.

3

Regulation of Gonadotropin Gene Expression by Gonadotropin Releasing Hormone

JOHN C. MARSHALL, ALAN C. DALKIN, AND
DANIEL J. HAISENLEDER

Pituitary luteinizing hormone and follicle stimulating hormone are composed of a common alpha and different beta subunits (1), which are coded for by 3 separate genes (2). Both hormones are secreted by the pituitary gonadotrope cells, and gonadotropin releasing hormone appears to be the major regulator of LH and FSH synthesis and secretion. GnRH is secreted by the hypothalamus in a pulsatile manner (3, 4), and this pattern of stimulus appears to be essential for maintaining gonadotropin production and secretion (5–7). GnRH secretion changes in different physiologic circumstances, and alterations in both the amplitude and frequency of GnRH pulses occur in normal physiology (8–15). These changes in GnRH stimulation are accompanied by differential release of LH and FSH, and it appears that a single gonadotropin releasing hormone is responsible for differential secretion of LH and FSH by the gonadotrope. The pattern of GnRH secretion and gonadotrope responses to GnRH can be modified by gonadal steroids and by peptides such as inhibin and activin. Thus, it appears that regulation of LH and FSH synthesis and secretion results from changes in the pattern of the GnRH pulse stimulus together with direct actions of gonadal steroids and of peptides on the gonadotrope cell.

In this chapter we examine the role of GnRH in regulating gonadotropin subunit gene expression and gonadotropin secretion. We shall examine physiologic data obtained by quantitation of steady-state mRNAs in studies in rats and shall also examine the direct role of GnRH pulse patterns in regulating gene transcription and mRNA expression. Steady-state mRNA concentrations were measured in dot/blot hybridizations using cDNA clones originally provided by Dr. W.W. Chin (rat alpha and LH beta; 16, 17) and Dr. R.A. Maurer (FSH beta; 18). Studies of changes in alpha, LH beta, and FSH beta gene transcription rates were made in collaborative experiments with Dr. M.A. Shupnik (19).

Regulation of Gonadotropin Subunit mRNAs In Vivo

Gonadal Regulation of Subunit mRNA Expression

Both serum LH and FSH and subunit mRNAs increase in male and female rats after gonadectomy. Recent studies of mRNA concentrations have shown that the timing and magnitude of the increases differ (20–23), and this suggests that mechanisms are present that can differentially regulate subunit gene expression. After ovariectomy, serum LH and alpha and LH beta mRNAs do not increase until 4–7 days later. Alpha mRNA plateaus after 14 days (5-fold increase), while LH beta mRNA increases through 30 days (15-fold rise). In contrast to these slower progressive increases, FSH beta mRNA rises rapidly to a plateau (4-fold increase) after 4 days. In males, orchidectomy results in increased alpha and LH beta mRNA within 24 h. Again, alpha mRNA plateaus after 2 weeks and LH beta mRNA continues to rise through 30 days. FSH beta mRNA also increases more rapidly after orchidectomy, but after peak levels are achieved (2-fold increase) at 7 days, FSH beta mRNA plateaus or even declines (24).

In male rats, replacement of testosterone (T) at the time of castration prevents the increase in alpha, LH beta, and FSH beta mRNAs (25). In previously castrated males, replacement of physiologic concentrations of testosterone (approximately 3 ng/ml) by subcutaneous implants suppresses subunit mRNAs to values similar to those in intact males (26). In other studies, in which T was given in higher doses by injection, FSH beta mRNA was not fully suppressed in castrated animals, which may reflect the different manner of T replacement or the higher concentration of T achieved (27). Testosterone may exert direct actions on FSH beta mRNA stability. When a GnRH antagonist is given to castrated male rats to block endogenous GnRH action, FSH beta mRNA concentrations fall with a half disappearance time of approximately 20 h. When the same experiment is repeated in the presence of T, steady-state FSH beta mRNA declines more slowly (approximately 50 h), suggesting that T may prolong transcription or stabilize FSH beta mRNA. The latter suggestion appears more likely, as the transcription rate of FSH beta mRNA was not increased by testosterone in GnRH antagonist-treated animals (28).

In ovariectomized female rats, estradiol (E_2) also suppresses subunit mRNAs, but differential effects have also been observed. All three subunit mRNAs were suppressed by pharmacologic E_2 replacement (22, 24). However, when E_2 was replaced at physiologic concentrations (40–50 pg/ml) by implants placed 7 days after ovariectomy, both beta subunit mRNAs were only partially suppressed and alpha mRNA was unchanged. In short-term (2 days) ovariectomized females, E_2 prevented the increase in LH beta, alpha mRNA still increased, and FSH beta mRNA was only partially suppressed. Similarly, when both E_2 and progesterone were given at ovariectomy, the increase in FSH beta mRNA was only partly prevented, and levels remained significantly above those in intact animals even when a GnRH antagonist was administered in addition. Thus, FSH beta mRNA concentrations increase after ovariectomy even when the effects of enhanced endogenous GnRH secretion are blocked. This suggests that other ovarian compounds, possibly members of the inhibin family, are involved in suppressing FSH beta mRNA expression in intact female rats (26).

In general, replacement of physiologic concentrations of gonadal steroids results in suppression of subunit mRNA concentrations, but the degree and time course of this action appear to depend on the amount and manner of steroid replacement. Similarly, the mechanisms of steroid hormone action may involve changes in both GnRH secretion and modification of the effects of GnRH on the gonadotrope. T and E_2 act to suppress pulsatile GnRH secretion (29, 30) and also modify responses to GnRH (31). P reduces in vivo GnRH secretion (32), and in vitro directly reduces FSH beta gene transcription in ovine cells (33). Thus, evidence suggests that steroids and also peptides such as inhibin, activin, and follistatin can act directly on the gonadotrope (34–37) and that in vivo steroids can also modify the pattern of GnRH secretion. Although the interrelationships of these actions in normal physiology remain unknown, it is probable that gonadal steroids regulate subunit gene expression both by modifying GnRH secretion and by direct actions on the gonadotrope cells.

Subunit mRNA Regulation During the Rat Estrous Cycle

In 4-day cycling female rats, serum LH and FSH secretion remains low except during the preovulatory surge on proestrus afternoon and evening (38). Studies have correlated serum gonadotropins with steady-state concentrations of alpha, LH beta, and FSH beta mRNAs (39, 40). On metestrus morning, FSH beta mRNA levels were increased (2-fold), and gradually fell to basal by evening. Alpha and LH beta mRNAs were stable on metestrus, but on diestrus, both transiently increased (2-fold) while FSH beta mRNA was unchanged. On both metestrus and diestrus, these changes in mRNA concentrations occurred when serum gonadotropin concentrations remained low. On the afternoon of proestrus, LH beta mRNA increased prior to the preovulatory rise in serum LH. FSH beta mRNA also increased, but reached maximum concentrations (4-fold increase) after the beginning of the serum FSH surge. Alpha mRNA was unchanged during the gonadotropin surges. Thus, in cycling females both coordinate and differential regulation of subunit gene expression occurs. Alpha and LH beta mRNA increase coordinately on diestrus, and both beta subunit mRNAs increase during the proestrus gonadotropin surges. In contrast, the increase in FSH beta mRNA on metestrus occurred when both alpha and LH beta mRNAs were stable.

The mechanisms regulating subunit mRNA expression during the estrous cycle remain unknown. During the cycle the pattern of pulsatile GnRH secretion changes, and both the amplitude and the frequency of GnRH pulses increase during the proestrus LH surge (41, 42). Secretion of LH and FSH can also be modified by changes in circulating E_2 and P during the cycle (32, 38, 43). At present few data are available in female rats, but it is likely that changes in the GnRH pulse pattern, probably modified by direct actions of ovarian steroids and peptides, act to differentially regulate subunit gene expression. In this regard, inhibins from the ovary may be particularly important. Inhibin can selectively inhibit FSH release and also reduce FSH beta mRNA in vitro (44–46). In addition, plasma inhibin levels during the estrous cycle showed a generally inverse relationship to plasma FSH and to FSH beta subunit mRNA concentrations. The decline in FSH beta mRNA during metestrus was associated with a rise in plasma inhibin, and plasma inhibin fell on the evening of proestrus when FSH beta mRNA increased rapidly (47).

Further data to support a role of the ovary are found from studies performed during the daily LH surge in ovariectomized-estradiol replaced rats. During the evening LH surge alpha mRNA increased 2-fold, but LH beta mRNA was unchanged (48). Thus, when plasma E_2 is stable, and progesterone and ovarian peptides are absent, a different pattern of alpha and LH beta mRNA changes is found compared to the afternoon LH surge on proestrus. It remains unclear whether these differences reflect altered GnRH secretion or altered responses to GnRH.

Regulation of Subunit Gene Expression by GnRH Pulses

Evidence has accumulated that emphasizes the critical role of a pulsatile GnRH stimulus in maintaining gonadotropin secretion. LH and FSH secretion is maintained by GnRH pulses, whereas continuous GnRH desensitizes the gonadotrope (5, 49). Interestingly, alpha mRNA is increased in desensitized gonadotropes, while LH beta mRNA is unchanged or decreased (50, 51). These data suggest an important role for GnRH pulses in regulating subunit mRNAs. Recent studies have demonstrated that a pulsatile stimulus is required for stimulation of LH beta transcription, whereas alpha transcription is increased by a continuous GnRH stimulus (52). GnRH appears to be critical for maintaining subunit gene expression, and studies using GnRH antagonists in castrated rats have shown that all three subunit mRNAs are suppressed by varying degrees (34, 53). These data have emphasized the importance of a pulsatile GnRH signal and suggest that the pattern of GnRH stimulation may be a factor that determines regulation of the gonadotropin subunit genes.

We have used a GnRH-deficient rat model and delivered exogenous GnRH pulses at various amplitudes and frequencies to examine the role of GnRH pulse patterns. Castrated male rats were replaced with sub-cutaneous implants containing T, to produce serum T concentrations of 2.5–3 ng/ml. Continuous delivery of testosterone in this manner prevents the postcastration rise in gonadotropins and GnRH receptors, which in turn suggests that the postcastration increase in GnRH secretion is reduced or abolished (54). In addition, 75% of castrated-testosterone replaced rats have less than 4 LH (GnRH) pulses in 24 h (55). Thus, the castrated-T replaced rat is relatively GnRH-deficient and is a convenient model in which to study the effects of GnRH pulse patterns when plasma T is stable.

The Role of GnRH Pulse Amplitude

In castrated rats, LH (GnRH) pulses occur every 30 min, and thus for studies that examined pulse amplitude we administered exogenous GnRH pulses every 30 min to castrated-T replaced rats. GnRH pulses were continued for 24–48 h, and the LH response to GnRH, pituitary GnRH receptor number, and subunit mRNA concentrations was measured. GnRH receptors, LH beta mRNA, and the LH response to the last GnRH pulse were all maximal after 25-ng GnRH pulses, and lower or higher amplitude pulses were less effective. In contrast, doses of GnRH across a wide range (10–250 ng/pulse) increased both alpha and FSH beta mRNAs (56–58). Similar differential effects of amplitude appear to occur in female rats. Ovariectomized-E_2 replaced females were given GnRH pulses every 30 min and increases in mRNAs were noted. Of interest, both LH and FSH beta mRNAs were increased by lower GnRH doses (0.5–25 ng/pulse) than were required in males. As in males, higher doses per pulse did not increase beta mRNAs, but alpha mRNA continued to increase (59). Thus in both sexes, the amplitude of the GnRH pulse stimulus appears to exert differential effects on steady-state subunit mRNA concentrations. Alpha and FSH beta mRNAs appear to be rela-tively independent of GnRH pulse amplitude. LH beta mRNA ex-pression, however, is highly sensitive to changes in GnRH amplitude, and maximum responses only occur over a narrow range of GnRH dose/pulse.

As noted above, gonadal steroids may exert direct effects on gon-adotrope responses to GnRH, and recent studies have suggested that testosterone can modify mRNA responses to GnRH pulse stimuli. Testosterone replacement, in concentrations to cover the physiologic range, was used in association with an optimal GnRH pulse stimulus (25 ng/pulse every 30 min). Alpha mRNA responses tended to be lower in the presence of higher concentrations of T, and LH beta mRNA responses to the higher GnRH pulse doses (75–250 ng/pulse) were also reduced. FSH beta mRNA concentration was increased by physiologic T in the absence of GnRH stimuli, perhaps reflecting an effect of T in stabilizing FSH beta mRNA. In response to GnRH pulses, FSH beta mRNA increased similarly in the presence of low or high T concentrations at all GnRH amplitudes (58).

Alpha mRNA is present in both thyrotrope and gonadotrope cells, and mRNA responses were examined in castrated-T replaced rats given triiodothyronine (T_3) to suppress thyrotrope alpha (60). T_3 reduced alpha mRNA by 50%, suggesting that half of the pituitary alpha mRNA is present in thyrotropes. GnRH pulses (25 ng every 30 min) increased alpha mRNA in T_3-treated rats. The alpha mRNA response was of similar magnitude in control and T_3-treated rats, indicating that GnRH was stimulating alpha mRNA of gonadotrope origin (61). These studies also indicated different time courses of GnRH action of subunit mRNAs. FSH beta mRNA increased more rapidly (8–12 h) than alpha (12–16 h), whereas LH beta mRNA did not show a measurable increase (2-fold) until after 18–24 h of GnRH pulses.

The Role of GnRH Pulse Frequency

The castrated-T replaced male rat model was also used to study subunit mRNA responses to GnRH pulses given at constant amplitude but different frequencies. GnRH (25 ng/pulse) was given at intervals between 8 and 480 min for 24–48 h. GnRH pulses given at intervals of less than 120 min increased the number of GnRH membrane receptors, and acute LH release was maximal after pulses given every 15–60 min. A frequency of 1 pulse every 30 min produced maximum responses of GnRH receptors and alpha and LH beta mRNAs, and these increased to levels similar to those found in castrated males (62, 63). In later studies, we examined alpha, LH beta, and FSH beta mRNA expression in the same rat pituitaries. Fast-frequency GnRH stimuli (every 8 min) maximally increased alpha mRNA, and LH beta mRNA was also increased. Pulses every 30 min (the spontaneous frequency present in castrated rats) increased all three subunit mRNAs. Of interest, slow-pulse stimuli (every 120 min or slower) maintained the elevated level of FSH beta mRNA but did not increase alpha or LH beta mRNAs (64).

Similar effects of GnRH pulse frequency have been reported in sheep (65), where 30-min pulses increased alpha and 60-min pulses increased all three subunit mRNAs. The preferential effect of slower-frequency GnRH on FSH beta mRNA was not observed in this model. This may reflect a different steroid action, as progesterone was used to inhibit endogenous GnRH and progesterone inhibits FSH beta transcription in vitro (33). GnRH pulse frequency appears to regulate the concentration of steady-state mRNAs by an effect at the level of gene transcription (52, 66). As noted earlier, in vitro studies have emphasized the requirement for a pulsatile stimulus to initiate LH beta transcription. The role of GnRH frequency was studied in vivo using the castrated-T replaced rat model. Pulses were given for 4 h prior to removing the pituitaries and measuring transcription rates. Alpha gene transcription was increased by fast-frequency GnRH pulses (every 8 or 30 min), but not by pulses given every 120 min. LH beta transcription was only increased after 30-min GnRH pulses, and FSH beta transcription was only elevated by the slower (every 120 min) pulses. Thus these in vivo studies of gene transcription rates are in general accord with earlier data measuring cytosolic steady-state mRNA concentrations, suggesting that the predominant effects of GnRH amplitude and frequency are exerted at the transcriptional level. A pulsatile GnRH stimulus appears to be essential to increase subunit transcription rates, as a continuous GnRH infusion did not increase LH beta or FSH beta transcription rates above control values (66).

These data in rats indicate that changes in both the amplitude and the frequency of GnRH pulsatile stimulation can effect differential expression of the gonadotropin subunit genes. The above data were obtained in the presence of testosterone alone, and the patterns of differential regulation may well be different in a different steroid/gonadal peptide milieu. These data also suggest that the ability to change GnRH pulse stimuli may be important in normal physiology. In prepubertal children, GnRH is secreted at a slow frequency (approximately 1 pulse every 3 h) and exogenous GnRH effects predominant FSH secretion. During puberty the amplitude and frequency of GnRH secretion increase to approximately 1 pulse/h, and this is associated with predominant LH secretion in response to exogenous GnRH (10). Thus, in humans and in primates slow-frequency GnRH stimuli are associated with enhanced FSH secretion and faster-frequency stimuli with LH release. The above data in rodents suggest that these effects of GnRH frequency are exerted in large part on the transcription of the gonadotropin subunit genes.

Summary

Studies in rodents have shown that subunit mRNA expression can occur in both coordinate and differential manners in normal physiology. Gonadal steroids and peptides may regulate GnRH secretion, but also exert direct actions on the gonadotrope to modify mRNA concentrations. Of interest, simultaneous increases of all 3 subunit mRNAs do not occur in intact animals, but both coordinate and differential changes in beta subunit mRNAs occur during the estrous cycle. Steady-state mRNA concentrations may be increased at times when gonadotropin secretion is low, suggesting different regulation of secretion and subunit gene expression.

The pattern of the GnRH stimulus can differentially modulate expression of subunit mRNAs, and this effect appears to be exerted predominantly at the transcriptional level. As the pattern of GnRH secretion changes in vivo, this suggests an important role for changes in GnRH pulse secretion as a means of regulating gonadotropin synthesis and release. Changes in the pattern of pulsatile GnRH stimulation may be one mechanism by which a single gonadotropin-releasing hormone can effect differential regulation of the three gonadotropin subunit genes.

References

1. Pierce JG, Parsons TF. Glycoprotein hormones: structure and function. Annu Rev Biochem 1981;50:465.
2. Chin WW. Glycoprotein hormone genes. In: Habener JF, ed. Genes encoding hormones and regulatory peptides. Clifton, NJ: Human Press, 1987;137.
3. Clarke IJ, Cummins JT. Temporal relationship between gonadotropin-releasing hormone (GnRH) and luteinizing hormone (LH) secretion in ovariectomized ewes. Endocrinology 1982;111:1737.
4. Urbanski HF, Pickle RL, Ramirez UD. Simultaneous measurement of GnRH, LH and FSH in the ovariectomized rat. Endocrinology 1988;123:413.
5. Belchetz PE, Plant TM, Nakai Y, Keogh EG, Knobil E. Hypophyseal responses to continuous and intermittent delivery of hypothalamic gonadotropin-releasing hormone. Science 1978;202:631.
6. Bergquist C, Nillius SJ, Wide L. Inhibition of ovulation in women by intranasal treatment with a LHRH agonist. Contraception 1979;19:497.
7. Marshall JC, Kelch RP. Gonadotropin-releasing hormone: role of pulsatile secretion in the regulation of reproduction. N Engl J Med 1986;315:1459.
8. Santen RJ, Bardin CW. Episodic luteinizing hormone secretion in man. J Clin Invest 1973;52:2617.
9. Yen SSC, Tsai CC, Naftolin F, Vandenberg G, Ajabor L. Pulsatile patterns of gonadotropin release in subjects with and without ovarian function. J Clin Endocrinol Metab 1972;34:671.
10. Hale PM, Khoury S, Foster CM, et al. Increased LH pulse frequency during sleep in early to mid-pubertal boys: effects of testosterone infusion. J Clin Endocrinol Metab 1988;66:785.
11. Wu FCW, Butler GE, Kelnar CJH, Sellar RE. Patterns of pulsatile LH secretion before and during the onset of puberty in boys: a study using an immunoradiometric assay. J Clin Endocrinol Metab 1990;70:629.
12. Backstrom CT, McNeilly AS, Leask RM, Baird DT. Pulsatile secretion of LH, FSH, prolactin, estradiol and progesterone during the human menstrual cycle. Clin Endocrinol (Oxf) 1982;17:29.
13. Reame N, Sauder SE, Kelch RP, Marshall JC. Pulsatile gonadotropin secretion during the human menstrual cycle—evidence for altered frequency of gonadotropin-releasing hormone secretion. J Clin Endocrinol Metab 1984; 59:328.

14. Crowley WF, Filicori M, Spratt DI, Santoro NF. The physiology of GnRH secretion in men and women. Recent Prog Horm Res 1985;41:473.

15. Yen SSC, Tsai CC, Naftolin S, Vandenberg G, Ajabor L. Pulsatile patterns of gonadotropin-release in subjects with and without ovarian function. J Clin Endocrinol Metab 1972;34:671.

16. Godine JE, Chin WW, Habener JF. Alpha subunit of rat pituitary glycoprotein hormone: primary structure of the precursor determined from the nucleotide sequence of cloned cDNAs. J Biol Chem 1982;257:8368.

17. Jameson JL, Chin WW, Hollenberg AM, Chang AS, Habener JF. The gene encoding the beta subunit of rat LH. J Biol Chem 1983;259:15474.

18. Maurer RA. Molecular cloning and nucleotide sequence analysis of the cDNA for the beta subunit of rat follicle-stimulating hormone. Mol Endocrinol 1987;1:717.

19. Shupnik MA, Gharib SD, Chin WW. Divergent effects of estradiol on gonadotropin gene transcription in pituitary fragments. Mol Endocrinol 1989; 3:474.

20. Corbani M, Counis R, Stazzei A, Jutisz M. Effect of gonadectomy on pituitary levels of mRNA encoding gonadotropin subunits and secretion of LH. Mol Cell Endocrinol 1984;35:83.

21. Abbot SD, Docherty K, Roberts JL, Tepper MA, Chin WW, Clayton RN. Castration increases LH subunit mRNA levels in male rat pituitaries. J Endocrinol 1985;107:R1–R4.

22. Gharib SD, Bower SM, Need LR, Chin WW. Regulation of rat LH subunit mRNAs by gonadal steroid hormones. J Clin Invest 1986;77:582–9.

23. Papavasiliou SS, Zmeili S, Herbon L, Duncan-Weldon J, Marshall JC, Landefeld TD. Alpha and LH beta mRNA of male and female rats after castration: quantitation using an optimized RNA dot blot hybridization assay. Endocrinology 1986;119:691.

24. Gharib SD, Wierman ME, Badger TM, Chin WW. Sex steroid hormone regulation of FSH subunit mRNA levels in the rat. J Clin Invest 1987;80:249.

25. Papavasiliou SS, Zmeili SM, Khoury S, Landefeld TD, Chin WW, Marshall JC. GnRH differentially regulates expression of the genes for LH alpha and beta subunits in male rats. Proc Natl Acad Sci USA 1986;83:4026.

26. Dalkin AC, Haisenleder DJ, Ortolano GA, Suhr A, Marshall JC. Gonadal regulation of gonadotropin subunit gene expression: evidence for regulation of FSH beta mRNA by nonsteroidal hormones in female rats. Endocrinology 1990;127:798.

27. Wierman ME, Gharib SD, LaRovere JM, Badger TM, Chin WW. Selective failure of androgens to regulate follicle-stimulating hormone beta mRNA levels in the male rat. Mol Endocrinol 1988;2:492.

28. Paul SJ, Ortolano GA, Haisenleder DJ, Stewart JM, Shupnik MA, Marshall JC. Gonadotropin subunit mRNA concentrations after blockade of GnRH action: testosterone selectively increases FSH beta mRNA by post transcriptional mechanisms. Mol Endocrinol 1991.

29. Steiner RA, Bremner WJ, Clifton DK. Regulation of LH pulse frequency and amplitude by testosterone in the adult male rat. Endocrinology 1982; 111:2055.

30. Sarkar DK, Fink G. LHRH in pituitary stalk plasma from long term ovariectomized rats: effects of steroids. J Endocrinol 1980;86:511.

31. Shupnik MA, Gharib SD, Chin WW. Estrogen suppresses rat gonadotropin gene transcription in vivo. Endocrinology 1988;122:1842.
32. Leipheimer RE, Bona-Gallo A, Gallo RV. Ovarian steroid regulation of basal pulsatile LH release between the morning of proestrus and estrus in the rat. Endocrinology 1986;118:2083.
33. Phillips CL, Lin LN, Wu JC, Guzman K, Milsted A, Miller WL. 17 β-estradiol and progesterone inhibit transcription of the genes encoding the subunits of ovine FSH. Mol Endocrinol 1988;2:641.
34. Perheentupa A, Huhtaniemi I. Gonadotropin gene expression and secretion in GnRH antagonist treated male rats—effects of sex steroid replacement. Endocrinology 1990;126:3204.
35. Carroll RS, Corrigan AZ, Gharib SD, Vale W, Chin WW. Inhibin, activin and follistatin-regulation of FSH beta mRNA levels. Mol Endocrinol 1989; 3:1969.
36. Carroll RS, Corrigan AZ, Chin WW. Effect of activin on FSH beta mRNA stability in cultured pituitary cells [Abstract]. Proceedings of the Endocrine Society 72nd annual meeting 1990;219 (abstract #777).
37. Gharib SD, Wierman ME, Shupnik MA, Chin WW. Molecular biology of the pituitary gonadotropins. Endocr Rev 1990;11:177.
38. Savoy-Moore RT, Schwartz NB. Differential control of FSH and LH secretion. In: Greep RO, ed. Reproductive physiology II: International review of physiology. Baltimore: University Park Press, 1980;22:203.
39. Zmeili SM, Papavasiliou SS, Thorner MO, Evans WS, Marshall JC, Landefeld TD. Alpha and LH beta subunit mRNAs during the rat estrous cycle. Endocrinology 1986;119:1867.
40. Ortolano GA, Haisenleder DJ, Dalkin AC, et al. FSH beta subunit mRNA concentrations during the rat estrous cycle. Endocrinology 1988;123:2149.
41. Fox SE, Smith MS. Changes in the pulsatile pattern of LH secretion during the rat estrous cycle. Endocrinology 1985;116:1485.
42. Levine JE, Ramirez VD. LHRH release during the rat estrous cycle and ovariectomy, as estimated with push-pull cannulae. Endocrinology 1982; 111:1439.
43. Savoy-Moore RT, Schwartz NB, Duncan J, Marshall JC. Pituitary GnRH receptors during the rat estrous cycle. Science 1980;209:941.
44. Rivier C, Rivier J, Vale W. Inhibin mediated feedback control of FSH secretion in the female rat. Science 1986;234:205.
45. Mercer JE, Clement JA, Funder JW, Clarke IJ. Rapid and specific lowering of pituitary FSH beta mRNA levels by inhibin. Mol Cell Endocrinol 1987; 53:251.
46. Attardi B, Keeping HS, Winters SJ, Kotsuji F, Maurer RA, Troen P. Rapid and profound suppression of mRNA encoding FSH beta by inhibin from primate Sertoli cells. Mol Endocrinol 1989;3:280.
47. Haisenleder DJ, Ortolano GA, Jolly D, et al. Inhibin secretion during the rat estrous cycle: relationships to FSH secretion and FSH beta subunit mRNA concentrations. Life Sci 1990;47:1769.
48. Haisenleder DJ, Barkan AL, Papavasiliou S, et al. LH subunit mRNA concentrations during the LH surge in ovariectomized estradiol-replaced rats. Am J Physiol 1988;254:E99.

49. Smith MW, Vale WW. Desensitization to GnRH observed in superfused pituitary cells on cytodex beads. Endocrinology 1981;108:752.
50. Hubert JF, Simard J, Gagne B, Barden N, Labrie F. Effect of LHRH and [D-Trp^6, Des-Gly-NH$_2^{10}$] LHRH ethylamide on alpha-subunit and LH beta mRNA levels in rat anterior pituitary cells in culture. Mol Endocrinol 1988; 2:521.
51. Lalloz MRA, Detta A, Clayton RN. GnRH desensitization preferentially inhibits expression of the LH beta-subunit gene in vivo. Endocrinology 1988;122:1689.
52. Shupnik MA. Effects of GnRH on rat gonadotropin gene transcription in vitro: requirement for pulsatile administration of LH beta gene stimulation. Mol Endocrinol 1990;4:1444.
53. Wierman ME, Rivier JE, Wang C. GnRH dependent regulation of gonadotropin subunit mRNA levels in the rat. Endocrinology 1989;124:272.
54. Garcia A, Schiff M, Marshall JC. Regulation of pituitary GnRH receptors by pulsatile GnRH injections in male rats—modulation by testosterone. J Clin Invest 1984;74:920.
55. Steiner RA, Bremner WJ, Clifton DK. Regulation of LH pulse frequency and amplitude by testosterone in the adult male rat. Endocrinology 1982; 111:2055.
56. Haisenleder DJ, Katt JA, Ortolano GA, et al. Influence of GnRH pulse amplitude, frequency and treatment duration on the regulation of LH subunit mRNAs and LH secretion. Mol Endocrinol 1988;2:338.
57. Haisenleder DJ, Ortolano GA, Dalkin AC, Paul SJ, Chin WW, Marshall JC. GnRH regulation of gonadotropin subunit gene expression: studies in T$_3$ suppressed rats. J Endocrinol 1989;122:117.
58. Iliff-Sizemore SA, Ortolano GA, Haisenleder DJ, Dalkin AC, Krueger KA, Marshall JC. Testosterone differentially modulates gonadotropin subunit mRNA responses to GnRH pulse amplitude. Endocrinology 1990;127: 2876–83.
59. Haisenleder DJ, Ortolano GA, Dalkin AC, Ellis TR, Paul SJ, Marshall JC. Differential regulation of gonadotropin subunit gene expression by GnRH pulse amplitude in female rats. Endocrinology 1990;127:2869–75.
60. Carr FE, Ridgway EC, Chin WW. Rapid simultaneous measurement of rat alpha and TSH beta-subunit mRNAs by solution hybridization: regulation of TSH subunit mRNAs by thyroid hormones. Endocrinology 1985;117:1272.
61. Haisenleder DJ, Ortolano GA, Dalkin AC, Paul SJ, Chin WW, Marshall JC. GnRH regulation of gonadotropin subunit gene expression: studies in T$_3$ suppressed rats. J Endocrinol 1989;122:117.
62. Haisenleder DJ, Khoury S, Zmeili SM, et al. The frequency of GnRH secretion regulates expression of alpha and LH beta subunit mRNAs in male rats. Mol Endocrinol 1987;1:834.
63. Katt JA, Duncan JA, Herbon L, Barkan A, Marshall JC. The frequency of GnRH stimulation determines the number of pituitary GnRH receptors. Endocrinology 1985;116:2113.
64. Dalkin AC, Haisenleder DJ, Ortolano GA, Ellis TR, Marshall JC. The frequency of GnRH stimulation differentially regulates gonadotropin subunit mRNA expression. Endocrinology 1989;125:917.

65. Leung K, Kaynard AH, Negrini BP, Kim KE, Maurer RA, Landefeld TD. Differential regulation of gonadotropin subunit mRNAs by GnRH pulse frequency in ewes. Mol Endocrinol 1987;2:724.
66. Haisenleder DJ, Dalkin AC, Ortolano GA, Marshall JC, Shupnik MA. A pulsatile GnRH stimulus is required to increase transcription of the gonadotropin subunit genes: evidence for differential regulation of transcription by pulse frequency. Endocrinology 1991;128.

Part II

Molecular and Developmental Control of GnRH Expression

4

Molecular Studies of GnRH, Part I

Nonresponse of 5′ Flanking Region of Rat GnRH Gene to Estrogen In Vitro or In Vivo

C.T. Bond, R. Seal, R. Simerly, and J.P. Adelman

Control of Reproduction in Vertebrates by a Cascade of Hormonal Events in the Hypothalamic-Pituitary-Gonadal Axis

Reproduction in vertebrates is controlled by the decapeptide gonadotropin releasing hormone (1). Secreted from terminals of preoptic hypothalamic neurons that send projections to the median eminence, GnRH binds to specific receptors on pituitary gonadotrope cells, eliciting synthesis and secretion of the gonadotropins, luteinizing hormone and follicle stimulating hormone. In turn, these hormones travel via the circulation to gonadal tissues, where, acting through specific cell surface receptors, they initiate a metabolic cascade that results in the synthesis and secretion of steroid hormones, such as estrogen. Completing the hypothalamic-pituitary-gonadal (HPG) axis, these steroids feed back to the hypothalamus, where they modulate release of GnRH, and to the pituitary, where they dampen the effects of GnRH binding.

The balance of hormones in the HPG axis is influenced by neural signals to GnRH neuroendocrine cells, transducing information such as circadian timing (2), nutritional or metabolic state (3), and social status (4). Additional complexity of the system is indicated by studies that show that factors not previously recognized as players in the reproductive system have the capability to input directly onto the HPG loop. For example, endothelin, a vasoconstrictive peptide, acting independently of the GnRH receptor, stimulates the release of gonadotropins from pituitary cells (5). The role endothelin might play in the physiology of reproduction is currently unknown. Other releasing factors under neural control in the hypothalamus may also influence levels of pituitary hormones. The existence of a separate FSH releasing factor has been postulated and evidence of its actions reported (6), although molecular characterization of such a factor has not yet been accomplished.

Molecular biology has opened the details of reproductive biology to ever more intricate study. In addition to antisera specific for the GnRH decapeptide, tools employed to examine changes in levels of GnRH include antisera to the prohormone and nucleic acid probes that hybridize to the GnRH mRNA, derivation of these tools made possible by the molecular cloning of genomic and cDNA sequences encoding the GnRH preprohormone (7–9). These tools have been employed in paradigms of normal reproduction, gonadectomy, and gonadectomy followed by steroid replacement to determine when changes in GnRH levels occur and to discern where control is exerted, whether it be transcriptional, translational, posttranslational modification, or control of secretion.

Influence of Gonadal Steroids on Levels of GnRH Expression

Employing quantitative in situ hybridization, Zoeller and Young have shown that GnRH mRNA levels fluctuate more than two-fold in hypothalamic neurons of normal, intact female rats over the course of the 4-day estrous cycle (10). Based on results that show a coincidence in the rise of GnRH mRNA levels and a surge in GnRH decapeptide release on the afternoon of proestrous, the authors postulated that GnRH synthesis and release are coupled. The overall level of GnRH mRNA appeared to be inversely related to changes in plasma estrogen levels occurring during the estrous cycle (11). Previous studies have shown that estrogen influences pituitary secretion of LH (12), as well as secretion of GnRH into portal vessels in either a positive (13) or a negative (14) manner. Removal of the gonads disrupts the interactions of the HPG axis, resulting in elevated mean plasma LH levels (15). King et al. have shown by immunocytochemistry that the number of neurons detectable for GnRH first decreases, then increases differentially between males and females following gonadectomy (16). Further ultrastructural studies by King and Seiler concluded that removal of gonadal steroids results in increased biosynthetic activity in GnRH neurons (17). Estradiol replacement at the time of gonadectomy is effective in preventing the augmented synthesis of GnRH within preoptic-hypothalamic neurons (18). These results are in agreement with studies employing in situ hybridization which suggest that GnRH mRNA levels are lower in ovariectomized/estrogen-replaced females than in ovariectomized females (19, 20). The effect of estrogen in these studies was thought not to be mediated through effects on LH expression, because similar reductions in GnRH mRNA levels in response to estrogen were seen in androgen-sterilized rats (19), a paradigm that has been shown to eliminate the effect of estrogen on LH release (21). These results are in contrast to those of Pfaff (22) and those of

Roberts et al., who employed solution hybridization/nuclease protection assays and RIA and concluded that estrogen replacement following gonadectomy resulted in increased mRNA and prohormone levels (23). Such discrepancies may reflect differences in paradigm, such as timing of estrogen treatment following gonadectomy.

Mechanisms of Steroid Action

Independent studies from many laboratories have produced a coherent picture of how steroids in general affect target cells. Steroids passively diffuse through the lipid bilayer; once they are inside the cell, an intricate interaction with specific cytoplasmic receptor/heat shock protein complexes results in nuclear translocation of the steroid-receptor complex. In the nucleus, this complex binds with high affinity to specific genomic DNA sequences, usually positioned 5' to genes that are affected by the steroid. Through interactions with other parts of the transcriptional control apparatus, this binding influences gene expression at the level of transcription. Structural information from the cloning of steroid hormone receptors has demonstrated that different receptors, with distinct ligands and DNA targets, share an overall architecture, consisting of a steroid hormone-binding domain, a DNA sequence-specific binding domain, and regions involved in mediating protein-protein contacts with other members of the transcription complex. A single class of steroid receptor binds a defined ligand, and this complex usually influences gene expression from more than one locus. Although the DNA sequences recognized by a given class of steroid receptor at individual target sites are usually not identical, examination of many different sequences known to bind a specific class of steroid receptor has provided a consensus binding sequence. Thus, gonadal steroids such as estrogen could, through estrogen-responsive sequences at the GnRH locus and expression of estrogen receptors in GnRH neurons, directly affect levels of expression of GnRH. (For a review of the steroid hormone receptor gene family, mode of action, and consensus sequences, see reference 24.)

At least two other mechanisms by which estrogen might exert influence on GnRH are possible. GnRH neurons, lacking estrogen receptors, may receive synaptic input from neurons that do possess these receptors. The actions of the estrogen within those cells could result in altered neural signals to GnRH neurons, causing changes in GnRH biosynthesis. This pathway would allow integration of estrogen influence from diverse sources. Alternatively, estrogen and other steroids could exert influence on GnRH expression and/or release through direct interaction with cell surface molecules, independently of the classical steroid-hormone receptors. Puia et al. have recently shown that neurosteroids, produced from metabolism of progesterone and deoxycortisone, directly influence GABA receptors and their intrinsic ion channels (25). Changes in ion

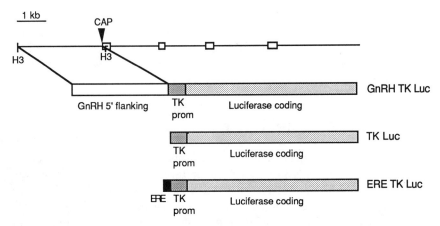

FIGURE 4.I.1. Schematic representation of reporter gene constructs. The top line indicates the rat GnRH gene structure, with boxes showing the positions of exons. A three-kilobase HindIII fragment used in reporter constructs is shown.

channel function could ramify throughout the cell, possibly affecting diverse properties of the cells, including biosynthesis or regulated release of stored products. Whatever the mechanism, a multitude of studies have shown that estrogen affects GnRH levels. Reports of changes in GnRH mRNA levels in response to estrogen treatment necessitate examination of the ability of estrogen to affect transcription of the GnRH gene.

Results

Nonresponse to Estrogen of 5' Flanking Sequences of the Rat GnRH Gene

We have determined the sequence of 10.5 kilobases of rat genomic DNA containing the GnRH gene, including 3 kb of 5' flanking DNA (26). Computer analysis of the rat GnRH gene locus revealed no consensus estrogen response element (ERE). However, a number of variations on the consensus sequence have been shown to confer regulation by estrogen (27). We have directly assayed the ability of three kilobases of 5' flanking sequence of the rat GnRH gene to respond to estrogen by construction of reporter gene plasmids that fuse GnRH sequences to the thymidine kinase (TK) constitutive promoter and luciferase coding sequences (GnRH TK Luc) (Fig. 4.I.1). TK promoter/luciferase gene constructs, either containing (ERE TK Luc) or lacking (TK Luc) a 19-base pair synthetic ERE 5' to the TK promoter served as control plasmids. These constructs were individually transfected into a human breast carcinoma cell line, MCF-7, which has been shown to possess high levels of func-

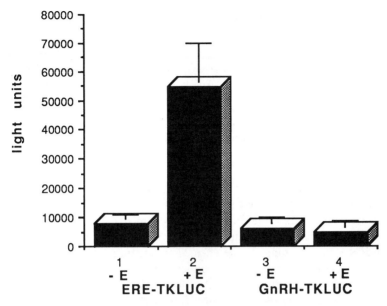

FIGURE 4.I.2. Results of transfections of luciferase constructs into MCF-7 cells in the presence (+E) or absence (−E) of 5×10^{-8}M estrogen. No change from basal levels of luciferase activity resulted in treatment of TK Luc with estrogen (not shown). A separate reporter plasmid, TK CAT, was cotransfected in all experiments, and transfection efficiencies were standardized by levels of CAT expression.

tional estrogen receptors (28). As Figure 4.I.2 shows, transfection of MCF-7 cells with ERE TK Luc followed by treatment with 5×10^{-8}M estrogen resulted in a 7–10-fold increase in luciferase activity. However, estrogen treatment of GnRH TK Luc in MCF-7 cells resulted in no significant change from basal expression.

These studies necessarily employed the TK promoter to achieve basal expression of luciferase activity. No heterologous cell line has been found in which the rat GnRH hypothalamic promoter sequences are active. A GnRH-expressing cell line has recently been derived from hypothalamic tumors in transgenic mice expressing SV-40 T-antigen driven by GnRH 5′ flanking sequences (29). Although these studies have not been repeated using this GnRH-expressing cell line, it has been determined that these cells do not express estrogen receptors (30).

Absence of Estrogen Receptors in GnRH Neurons in the Rat

In order for estrogen to exert transcriptional control on the GnRH gene through the actions of the estrogen receptor, genomic sequences that

TABLE 4.I.1. Localization of GnRH- and estrogen receptor-expressing cells in the rat brain.

GnRH	Estrogen receptor	Areas of overlap
Diagonal band of Broca	Ventral area of lateral	Medial preoptic nucleus
Magnocellular preoptic nucleus	septal nucleus	Rostral part of the
Anteroventral preoptic nucleus	Anteroventral PVN	lateral preoptic area
Medial septal nucleus	Preoptic region of the PVN	Anteroventral preoptic
Medial preoptic nucleus	Medial and central regions	nucleus
OVLT	of medial preoptic nucleus	
Lateral preoptic area		

encode the estrogen receptor must be transcribed and translated within GnRH neurons, resulting in the presence of the estrogen receptor protein in those neurons. Combined immunohistochemistry and in situ hybridization is a very sensitive technique that allows detection of protein products and mRNA on the same tissue slice. This technique has shown that all GnRH mRNA-containing cells produce GnRH peptides (19, 31). Subjecting tissue sections from the rostral forebrain of adult male rats first to antibodies to the estrogen receptor followed by hybridization with an RNA probe complementary to the GnRH mRNA has allowed us to examine the distribution of neurons expressing these two gene products. Although an extensive overlap of anatomical regions containing neurons that express one or the other of these two genes was demonstrated, no neurons were observed that expressed both estrogen receptor proteins and GnRH mRNA (Table 4.I.1). This result is in agreement with studies by Langub, Maley, and Watson employing double-label immunocytochemistry and electron microscopy in the guinea pig (32). Both studies found estrogen receptor-containing cells closely apposed to GnRH-expressing cells. Electron micrographs clearly show GnRH peptide-containing terminals synapsing on estrogen receptor-positive neurons. This may represent a feedback loop in the interplay of GnRH neurons and estrogen responsiveness. Synapses of estrogen receptor-containing neurons onto GnRH-expressing cells have not been unequivocally demonstrated, however, leaving open the question of how an estrogen effect is mediated.

Discussion

Future Studies of GnRH Regulation

The results of the studies presented here provide strong evidence that effects of estrogen on levels of hypothalamic GnRH are not mediated by a direct, transcriptional mechanism of estrogen receptors on the rat GnRH gene. Further support for this conclusion is provided by the observation that the neuronally derived GnRH-expressing cell line does not express estrogen receptors.

The reproductive hormones of the HPG axis function in a complex interplay, where levels of each hormone affect the levels of the others. The complexity is not confined to the mutual effects of the HPG hormones on each other, however. Many other factors feed into the loop, via neural input onto GnRH neurons in the hypothalamus, by actions of additional releasing factors on pituitary cells, and by many physiological influences on the metabolism of the gonads. The neural network that includes the GnRH neurons is not a simple projection of terminals to the median eminence for the release of hormone into portal vessels to influence pituitary hormone secretion. Only a portion of GnRH neurons send terminals to the median eminence (21, 33). GnRH neurons also send projections to regions of the brainstem, amygdala, and cortex (34). GnRH-containing terminals have been shown in synaptic contact with GnRH neurons (35). Studies by Zoeller et al. examining GnRH mRNA levels following estrogen treatment concluded that only a subpopulation of GnRH neurons showed changes in message levels in response to estrogen (19). King et al. demonstrated by three-dimensional modeling of immunocytochemistry results that the population of neurons detectable for GnRH changes upon gonadectomy, indicating recruitment of GnRH-expressing cells (16). All of these studies clearly show that GnRH neurons are not a homogeneous population.

GnRH neurons have been shown to receive catecholaminergic and dopaminergic inputs (36, 37). Molecular cloning of the receptors for these and other neurotransmitters and elucidation of their mode of action (38, 39) have opened the way for more detailed examination of synaptic influence on GnRH expression. Future studies employing approaches such as immunocytochemistry and in situ hybridization, electrophysiology in brain slice preparations, and coculture techniques with GnRH-expressing cells will characterize the different populations of GnRH neurons and begin to define the roles of those subpopulations in the complex physiology and behavior of reproduction.

References

1. Shivers BD, Harlan RE, Pfaff DW. Reproduction: the central nervous system role of luteinizing hormone releasing hormone. In: Krieger D, Brownstein M, Martin J, eds. Brain peptides. New York: John Wiley and Sons, 1983.
2. Turek FW, Swann J, Earnest D. Role of the circadian system in reproductive phenomena. Recent Prog Horm Res 1984;40.
3. Schneider JE, Wade GN. Availability of metabolic fuels controls estrous cyclicity of Syrian hamsters. Science 1989;244:1326–1328.
4. Bediz GM, Whitsett JM. Social inhibition of sexual maturation in male prairie mice. J Comp Physiol Psychol 1974;93:493–500.

5. Staojilkovic SS, Merelli F, Iida T, Krsmanovic LA, Catt K. Endothelin stimulation of cytosolic calcium and gonadotropin secretion in anterior pituitary cells. Science 1990;248:1663–1666.

6. Lumpkin MD, Moltz JH, Yu WH, Samson WK, McCann SM. Purification of FSH-releasing factor: its dissimilarity from LHRH of mammalian, avian, and piscian origin. Brain Res Bull 1987;18:175–178.

7. Seeburg PH, Adelman JP. Characterization of cDNA for precursor of human luteinizing hormone-releasing hormone. Nature 1984;311:666–668.

8. Adelman JP, Mason AJ, Hayflick JS, Seeburg PH. Isolation of the gene and hypothalamic cDNA for the common precursor of gonadotropin-releasing hormone and prolactin release-inhibiting factor in human and rat. Proc Natl Acad Sci USA 1986;83:179–183.

9. Mason AJ, et al. A deletion truncating the gonadotropin-releasing hormone gene is responsible for hypogonadism in the hpg mouse. Science 1986;234: 1366–1371.

10. Zoeller RT, Young S III. Changes in cellular levels of messenger ribonucleic acid encoding gonadotropin-releasing hormone in the anterior hypothalamus of female rats during the estrous cycle. Endocrinology 1988;123:1688–1689.

11. Nequin LG, Alvarez J, Schwarts NB. Measurement of serum steroid and gonadotropin levels and uterine and ovarian variables throughout the 4 day and 5 day estrous cycles in the rat. Biol Reprod 1979;20:659.

12. McCann SM, Ramirez VD. The neuroendocrine regulation of hypophyseal luteinizing hormone secretion. Recent Prog Horm Res 1964;20:131–181.

13. Sherwood NM, Chiappa SA, Sarkar DK, Fink G. Gonadotropin-releasing hormone (GnRH) in pituitary stalk blood from proestrous rats: effects of anesthetics and relationship between stored and released GnRH and luteinizing hormone. Endocrinology 1980;107:1410.

14. Sarkar DK, Fink G. Luteinizing hormone releasing factor in pituitary stalk plasma from long term ovariectomized rats: effects of steroids. J Endocrinol 1980;86:511.

15. Leipheimer RE, Gall RV. Acute and long-term changes in central and pituitary mechanisms regulating pulsatile luteinizing hormone secretion after ovariectomy in the rat. Neuroendocrinology 1983;37:421–426.

16. King JC, Kugel G, Zahniser D, Wooledge K, Damassa DA, Alexsavich B. Changes in population of LHRH-immunopositive cell bodies following gonadectomy. Peptides 1987;8:721–735.

17. King JC, Seiler GR. Ultrastructural evidence suggests variations in biosynthesis and processing within LH-RH neurons as a function of ovariectomy in rats. Brain Res 1988;452:127–140.

18. King JC, Anthony ELP, Damassa DA, Elkin-Hirsch KE. Morphological evidence that luteinizing hormone-releasing hormone neurons participate in the suppression by estradiol of pituitary luteinizing hormone secretion in ovariectomized rats. Neuroendocrinology 1987;45:1–13.

19. Zoeller RT, Seeburg PH, Young WS III. In situ hybridization histochemistry for messenger ribonucleic acid (mRNA) encoding gonadotropin-releasing hormone (GnRH): effect of estrogen on cellular levels of GnRH and mRNA in female rat brain. Endocrinology 1988;122:2570–2577.

20. Toranzo D, Dupont E, Simard J, et al. Regulation of pro-gonadotropin-releasing hormone gene expression by sex steroids in the brain of male and female rats. Mol Endocrinol 1989;3:1748–1756.
21. Jennes L, Stumpf WE. Gonadotropin-releasing hormone immunoreactive neurons with access to fenestrated capillaries in mouse brain. Neuroscience 1986;13:403.
22. Pfaff DW. Gene expression in hypothalamic neurons; luteinizing hormone releasing hormone. J Neurosci Res 1986;16:109.
23. Roberts JL, Dutlow CM, Jakubowski M, Blum M, Millar RP. Estradiol stimulates preoptic area-anterior hypothalamic proGnRH-GAP gene expression in ovariectomized rats. Mol Brain Res 1989;6:127–134.
24. Evans RM. The steroid and thyroid hormone receptor superfamily. Science 1988;240:889–895.
25. Puia G, Santi M, Vicini S, et al. Neurosteroids act on recombinant $GABA_A$ receptors. Neuron 1990;4:759–765.
26. Bond CT, Hayflick JS, Seeburg PH, Adelman JP. The rat gonadotropin-releasing hormone: SH locus: Structure and hypothalamic expression. Mol Endocrinol 1989;3:1257–1262.
27. Slater EP, Redeuihl G, Karin T, Suske G, Beato M. The uteroglobin promoter contains a noncanonical estrogen responsive element. Mol Endocrinol 1990;4:604–610.
28. Brooks SC, Locke ER, Soule HD. Estrogen receptor in a human cell line (MCF-7) from breast carcinoma. J Biol Chem 1973;17:6251–6253.
29. Mellon PL, Windle JJ, Goldsmith PC, Padula CA, Roberts JL, Weiner RI. Immortalization of hypothalamic GnRH neurons by genetically targeted tumorigenesis. Neuron 1990;5:1–10.
30. Mellon PL (personal communication).
31. Ronnekleiv OK, Naylor BR, Bond CT, Adelman JP. Combined immuno-histochemistry for gonadotropin-releasing hormone (GnRH) and pro-GnRH and in situ hybridization for GnRH messenger ribonucleic acid in rat brain. Mol Endocrinol 1989;3:363–371.
32. Langub MC Jr, Maley BE, Watson RE Jr. Ultrastructural evidence for luteinizing hormone-releasing hormone neuronal control of estrogen responsive neurons in the preoptic area. Endocrinology 1991;128:27–35.
33. Silverman AJ, Jhamandas J, Renaud L. Localization of luteinizing hormone-releasing hormone (LHRH) neurons that project to the median eminence. J Neurosci 1987;7:2312.
34. Barry J, Hoffman GE, Wray S. LHRH-containing systems. In: Bjorklund A, Hökfelt T, eds. Handbook of chemical neuroanatomy, part I. Amsterdam: Elsevier/North Holland; vol 4:166.
35. Leranth CS, Segura LMG, Palkovits M, MacLusky NJ, Shanabrough M, Naftolin F. The LH-RH-containing neuronal network in the preoptic area of the rat: demonstration of LH-RH-containing nerve terminals in synaptic contact with LH-RH neurons. Brain Res 1985;345:332–336.
36. Wray S, Hoffman G. Catecholamine innervation of LH-RH neurons: a developmental study. Brain Res 1986;399:327–331.
37. Kuljis RO, Advis JP. Immunocytochemical and physiological evidence of a synapse between dopamine—and luteinizing hormone releasing hormone—

containing neurons in the ewe median eminence. Endocrinology 1989;124: 1579–1581.

38. Dohlman HG, Caron MG, Lefkowitz RJ. A family of receptors coupled to guanine nucleotide regulatory proteins. Biochemistry 1987;26:2657–2664.

39. Bonner TI, Buckley NJ, Young AC, Brann MR. Identification of a family of muscarinic acetylcholine receptor genes. Science 1987;237:527–532.

4

Molecular Studies of GnRH, Part II

Isolation and Characterization of Teleost PreproGnRH Encoding cDNA from the African Cichlid *Haplochromis burtoni*

C.T. BOND, R. FERNALD, R. FRANCIS, AND J.P. ADELMAN

Evolution of the GnRH Decapeptide

During 500 million years of evolution, the primary structure of GnRH has been remarkably conserved. Recently, peptide sequence analysis of GnRH-like immunoreactive material from lamprey brain has shown that five of ten amino acid residues are identical between agnathan and mammalian GnRH. In addition, the pyro-glu amino terminal structure and amidation of the carboxy terminus of the decapeptide are conserved (1). To data, the amino acid sequence has been determined and bioactivity demonstrated for five separate forms of the GnRH decapeptide (2). Two GnRH decapeptide sequences have been found in chickens (3, 4). Immunologic and chromatographic evidence indicates that there may be two decapeptides in other vertebrates, including some species of reptiles and teleost fish. However, amino acid sequences for these putative second GnRH forms have not yet been determined (5).

A Nonmammalian Model for the Study of GnRH

In the teleost, *Haplochromis burtoni*, an African cichlid species, sexual development in males in regulated by social interactions (6, 7). A normal population of *H. burtoni* includes two distinct male types: those which are territorial and those which are not. Territorial males are brightly colored, sexually mature, and are called "machos" because of the aggressive behavior they display in establishing and defending territories for feeding and breeding. In contrast, nonterritorial males, called "wimps," are cryptically colored, sexually immature, and do not reproduce. The social dominance of machos over wimps is correlated with the size of forebrain magnocellular neurons that express GnRH immunoreactivity. Concomitant with the emergence of aggressive behavior and establishment of territory is an increase in the size of specifically those neurons which express GnRH (8). The most significant influence on the development of reproductive capability in wimp males is the proximity of larger, threatening conspecifics. Territorial dominance, breeding capability, and enlargement of GnRH neurons are reversible conditions; in the presence of a larger, more dominant male, a previously macho male will lose its bright coloration, the testes will regress and the GnRH magnocellular neurons shrink to normal size (R. Fernald, personal communication). This amazing plasticity is probably mediated by diverse sensory inputs and may be reflected in the level of expression of the GnRH gene in these neurons. As a first step in understanding the cellular and molecular basis of this aspect of teleost reproduction, we have cloned the cDNA encoding *H. burtoni* preproGnRH.

Results

Conservation of Prohormone Structure Between Teleosts and Mammals

Oligonucleotide pools encompassing all possible coding sequences of the first eight amino acids of the known teleost decapeptide sequence (9) were used as radiolabeled probes on a cDNA library constructed from poly(A+) RNA isolated from the brains of macho male *H. burtoni*. Hybridization specificity was obtained by washing library screen filters in 3 M tetramethylammonium chloride (10). Sequence analysis of the cDNA clone thus isolated shows remarkable conservation of structure relative to the mammalian prohormones (11). This structural conservation is like that seen for other polyprotein precursors that have been characterized from diverse species (12) (Fig. 4.II.1).

Absence of Homology to Mammalian GAP in Teleost GnRH-Associated Peptide

Despite the conservation of overall structure between these evolutionarily distant GnRH prohormones, the amino acid sequences differ considerably. There is significant amino acid homology within the signal sequences; eight of 23 residues are identical, and a basic residue—lysine in the fish, arginine in the mammal—occupies a conserved position. The decapeptide and proteolytic processing site sequences are identical except for the previously known two amino acid substitutions. However, the associated C-terminal peptide of the teleost prohormone has no significant homology to mammalian GAP.

```
                   Signal  Peptide            GnRH

CICHLID     MEAGSRVIMQVLLLALVVQVTLS  QHWSYGWLPG  GKR

MOUSE        MILKLMAGILLLTVCLEGCSS  QHWSYGLRPG  GKR

RAT         METIPKLMAAVVLLTVCLEGCSS  QHWSYGLRPG  GKR

HUMAN       MKPIQKLLAGLILLTWCVEGCSS  QHWSYGLRPG  GKR

                                      GAP

CICHLID     SVGELEATIRMMGTGGVVSLPDEANAQIQERLRPYNIINDDSSHFDRKKRFPNN

MOUSE       NTEHLVESFQEMGKEVDQMAEPQHFECTVHWPRSPLRDLRGALESLIEEEARQKKM

RAT         NTEHLVDSFQEMGKEEDQMAEPQNFECTVHWPRSPLRDLRGALERLIEEEAGQKKM

HUMAN       DAENLIDSFQEIVKEVGQLAETQRFECTTHQPRSPLRDLKGALESLIEEETGQKKI
```

FIGURE 4.II.1. Comparison of preprohormone sequences of teleost and mammalian GnRH. The teleost preproGnRH contains a signal peptide of 23 amino acids immediately preceding the decapeptide sequence. A dibasic proteolytic cleavage site follows the decapeptide and amide-donating glycine, providing a substrate for maturation of the decapeptide and separation from the 54 amino acid-associated C-terminal peptide.

Mammalian GAP has been implicated in the control of prolactin release from pituitary lactotrophs (13). Although the physiological properties mediated by prolactin in mammals (lactation, parturition) are not germane in the fish, human GAP has recently been shown to effect prolactin release from the pituitary of the tilapia *Oreochromis mossambicus* (14). Teleosts express two forms of prolactin that are under control of unknown hypothalamic factors (15, 16), and both forms are thought to function in osmoregulation (17, 18).

Examination of all possible reading frames encoded by the teleost GnRH cDNA revealed that a single base insertion 3' of the decapeptide encoding sequence would yield an incomplete open reading frame that contains a significant block of homology to a region of mammalian GAP that is highly conserved among the three known sequences. In light of the prolactin study cited above, and in spite of the fact that this possible island of homology lay within a reading frame that was not contiguous with that of the decapeptide, it was essential to verify the sequence of the GnRH coding sequence isolated from the *H. burtoni* library. To do so, three independent reverse transcription reactions were performed on *H. burtoni* brain RNA, followed by multiple PCR reactions employing oligonucleotide primers specific for untranslated regions of the *H. burtoni* GnRH sequence. Nucleotide sequence analysis of PCR reaction products, although containing occasional transitions from T to C, probably representing PCR mistakes, verified the reading frame of the original clone. This sequence was further verified by the subsequent isolation of additional cDNA clones from the original library during low-stringency hybridization experiments described below.

Failure of Low-Stringency Hybridization Studies to Detect a Second GnRH Coding Sequence

Immunologic and chromatographic studies have found evidence that a second decapeptide sequence is expressed in some species of teleost (19); however, exact amino acid sequence data have not been reported. Expression of a second decapeptide might be the result of an earlier gene duplication event, in which case the coding sequence should bear significant homology to the characterized teleost cDNA. We examined this possibility by a series of hybridization experiments employing randomly primed DNA probes derived from the full-length *H. burtoni* GnRH cDNA applied to *H. burtoni* brain library filters, genomic Southern blots and Northern blots containing poly(A+) and total RNA from *H. burtoni* macho male brains. None of these experiments yielded any evidence of a related prohormone coding sequence.

The inability to uncover a second GnRH encoding sequence in *H. burtoni* by low-stringency hybridization does not eliminate the possibility that such a gene exists. The alternative GnRH decapeptide might be encoded in an otherwise unrelated DNA milieu, rendering it undetectable by this type of hybridization study. If indeed a GnRH-like decapeptide did arise from gene sequences that are completely nonhomologous, it raises questions about the evolutionary relatedness of the decapeptides. Perhaps the decapeptide motif found in GnRH has occurred twice coincidentally, with the second decapeptide encoded by a distinct locus and subserving unrelated functions. There may be circumstantial evidence for this in the distribution of each decapeptide type in the brains of various species (20). Resolution of this question awaits the cloning of two GnRH-encoding sequences from a single species.

Discussion

Future GnRH Gene Regulation Studies Employing H. burtoni *as a Model System*

The dissimilarity of sequence between mammalian GAP and this teleost GAP, combined with studies indicating prolactin-related bioactivity of mammalian GAP in teleost pituitaries, is at present enigmatic. Studies are currently being initiated to examine the biological role of the teleost GAP peptide in the fish. Divergence of associated peptides concurrent with extreme conservation of the principal peptide hormone within a polyprotein precursor is a common thread in evolution (12). Perhaps this format allows evolutionary experimentation within the structure and function of the associated peptides while preserving essential functions mediated by the principal hormone. In this light it is interesting to note that a frame shift at the appropriate location within the teleost GAP sequence yields a stretch of amino acids with a high degree of homology to a sequence in mammalian GAP that is highly conserved across the three cloned species. Perhaps as prolactin came to serve functions more directly related to reproduction, evolution found a way to tie the regulation of prolactin release to the expression of GnRH.

Haplochromis burtoni, whose reproductive capability is mediated by social factors, offers an exquisite model for the study of regulation of GnRH. The interplay of sensory inputs and development and the combined effect on expression of GnRH can be examined. Also of interest is the role that GnRH might play in mediating the corresponding behaviors of the separate male types. Sexual differences in the regulation of GnRH and subsequent behavioral patterns are also accessible in this model.

References

1. Sherwood NM, Sowers SA, Marshak DR, Fraser BA, Brownstein MJ. Primary structure of gonadotropin-releasing hormone from lamprey brain. J Biol Chem 1986;261:4812–4819.
2. King JA, Millar RP. Genealogy of the GnRH family. Prog Clin Biol Res 1990;342:45–59.
3. King JA, Millar RP. Structure of chicken hypothalamic luteinizing hormone-releasing hormone: II. Isolation and characterization. J Biol Chem 1982;257: 10729–10732.
4. Miyamoto K, Hasegawa Y, Nomura M, Igarashi M, Kangawa K, Matsuo H. Identification of the second gonadotropin-releasing hormone in chicken hypothalamus: evidence that gonadotropin secretion is probably controlled by two distinct gonadotropin-releasing hormones in avian species. Proc Natl Acad Sci USA 1984;81:3874–3878.
5. Sherwood N. The GnRH family of peptides. Trends Neurosci 1987;10: 129–132.
6. Fernald RD, Hirata N. Field study of *Haplochromis burtoni*: quantitative behavioral observations. Animal Behavior 1977;25:964–975.
7. Fraley NB, Fernald RD. Social control of developmental rate in the African cichlid fish *Haplochromis burtoni*. Z Tierpsychol 1982;60:66–82.
8. Davis MR, Fernald RD. Social control of neuronal soma size. J Neurobiol 1990;21:1180–1188.
9. Sherwood N, Eiden L, Brownstein M, Spiess J, Rivier J, Vale W. Characterization of a teleost gonadotropin-releasing hormone. Proc Natl Acad Sci USA 1983;80:2794–2798.
10. Wood WI, Gitzchier J, Lasky LA, Lawn RM. Base composition independent hybridization in tetramethylammonium chloride: a method for oligonucleotide screening of highly complex gene libraries. Proc Natl Acad Sci USA 1985; 82:1585–1588.
11. Adelman JP, Mason AJ, Hayflick JS, Seeburg PH. Isolation of the gene and hypothalamic cDNA for the common precursor of gonadotropin-releasing hormone and prolactin release-inhibiting factor in human and rat. Proc Natl Acad Sci USA 1986;83:179–183.

12. Sherwood NM, Parker DB. Neuropeptide families: an evolutionary perspective. J Exp Zool 1990;4:53–71
13. Nikolics K, Mason AJ, Szónyi E, Ramachandran J, Seeburg PH. A prolactin-inhibiting factor within the precursor for human gondatotropin-releasing hormone. Nature 1985;316:511–517.
14. Planas J, Bern HA, Millar RP. Effects of GnRH-associated peptide and its component peptides on prolactin secretion from the tilapia pituitary in vitro. Gen Comp Endocrinol 1990;77:386–396.
15. Nishioka RA, Kelley KM, Bern HA. Control of prolactin and growth hormone secretion in teleost fishes. Zool Sci 1988;5:267–280.
16. Rivas RJ, Nishioka RS, Bern HA. In vitro effect of somatostatin and urotensin II on prolactin and growth hormone secretion in tilapia: *Oreochromis mossambicus*. Gen Comp Endocrinol 1986;63:245–251.
17. Brown PS, Brown SC. Osmoregulatory actions of prolactin and other adenohypophysial hormones. In: Pan PKT, Schreibman M, eds. Vertebrate endocrinology; vol 2. San Diego: Academic Press: 45–84.
18. Loretz CA, Bern HA. Prolactin and osmoregulation in vertebrates. Neuroendocrinology 1982;35:292–304.
19. Sherwood NM. In: Idler DR, Crim LW, Walsh JM, eds. Reproductive physiology of fish: proceedings of the Third International Symposium on the Reproductive Physiology of Fish, St. Johns, Newfoundland, August 1987.
20. Katz IA, Millar RP, King JA. Differential regional distribution and release of two forms of gonadotropin-releasing hormone in the chicken brain. Peptides 1990;11:443–450.

5

Characterization, Expression, and Estradiol Regulation of the Human GnRH Gene

SALLY RADOVICK, FREDRIC E. WONDISFORD, SUSAN WRAY,
CHRISTINE TICKNOR, YUKO NAKAYAMA, GORDON B. CUTLER, JR.,
BRUCE D. WEINTRAUB, HEINER WESTPHAL, AND ERIC LEE

The molecular mechanisms involved in the control of gonadotropin releasing hormone gene expression are largely unknown in humans. Although it is well recognized that estradiol is a potent regulator of GnRH release from the hypothalamus, the mechanism of this regulation is unknown. Physiologic studies have indicated that estradiol can increase, decrease, or not change GnRH secretion from the hypothalamus (1–4). Apparent contradictions in these studies may be explained by different effects of gonadal steroids on hypothalamic GnRH release, depending on the duration and dosage of hormone exposure, on the method used to measure GnRH secretion, or perhaps on species differences in GnRH regulation.

To examine the effect of estrogen on GnRH expression, several investigators have used in situ hybridization histochemistry to monitor changes in GnRH mRNA. Pfaff (5) reported that estradiol given over 7 days increased GnRH mRNA in ovariectomized rats. Moreover, Rothfeld et al. (6) noted that male rats castrated for 2 weeks had a significant decrease in GnRH mRNA compared with control animals. Similarly, Roberts et al. (7), Rothfeld et al. (8), and most recently, Park et al. (9) reported stimulatory effects of estradiol on GnRH gene expression. However, Zoeller et al. (10) found that 2 days of estradiol treatment to ovariectomized rats significantly inhibited GnRH mRNA expression, and Wray et al. (11) similarly found inhibition of GnRH gene expression by estradiol in select GnRH neuronal populations maintained in vitro. Lastly, Toranzo et al. (12) showed that estradiol replacement decreased proGnRH mRNA accumulation in the brain of ovariectomized rats. Apparent contradictions among these in situ studies point out the difficulties in studying GnRH neuronal regulation where complex neuronal pathways, different populations of GnRH neurons, differences in sensitivity of various techniques, and the physiologic time points studied may be major confounding variables. However, it is clear from these studies that estrogen regulates GnRH mRNA expression.

Estrogen interacts with a specific nuclear receptor that binds to specific DNA sequences, termed estrogen response elements (EREs). Thus, estrogen-responsive cells must contain estrogen receptors. Estrogen receptors are present in brain areas that largely overlap those of GnRH-containing neurons (13). However, whether the GnRH neuron itself contains estrogen receptors is unclear. For instance, Shivers et al. (14) reported that only 0.2% of GnRH neurons concentrate a measurable amount of radiolabeled estradiol. Moreover, Watson et al. (15) reported that only a few GnRH neurons were immunopositive for the estrogen receptor. These studies, though, may lack the sensitivity needed to detect a low abundance of estrogen receptors sufficient to mediate a hormonal response. This was recently demonstrated by Komm et al. (16) and Eriksen et al. (17), who reported the presence of low numbers of estrogen receptors in bone cells previously undetectable by standard methods. Moreover, it is certainly plausible that only certain subpopulations of GnRH neurons contain sufficient estrogen receptors and are directly responsive to estrogen. Thus, whether estrogen affects GnRH expression, directly or indirectly, via other neuronal circuits remains to be determined.

In order to pursue the question of estrogen regulation of the GnRH gene, the human GnRH gene was cloned and sequenced, and its transcriptional start site was determined. This was followed by expression of the GnRH gene in JEG-3 cells, a human choriocarcinoma cell line, and by deletional mutation studies to determine if an estrogen-responsive area was present in the hGnRH gene. This was followed by structural data, including DNase I footprinting and the avidin-biotin DNA-binding (ABCD) assay, to determine if the area identified by functional data bound the estrogen receptor. Finally, a GnRH-secreting neuronal cell line was obtained from central nervous system tumors in transgenic mice expressing a human GnRH-simian virus 40 (SV40) large T antigen fusion gene. An ^{125}I estradiol binding study confirmed the presence of high-affinity nuclear estrogen receptors in this cell line. This gives credence to the theory that estradiol receptors, present in the nucleus of a specific population of GnRH neurons, directly regulate the expression of the GnRH gene via a stimulatory ERE in the 5' flanking region.

The Human GnRH Gene

A 5.2-kilobase DNA fragment was isolated by screening 1×10^6 recombinant bacteriophage clones from a chromosome 8 library with an oligonucleotide probe complementary to the published cDNA sequence

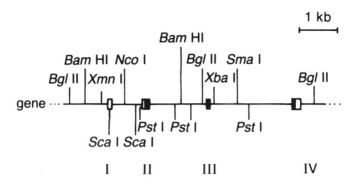

FIGURE 5.1. Structure of the human GnRH gene with selected restriction enzyme sites. The open boxes represent the 5' and 3' untranslated sequence. Darkened boxes represent protein coding regions (18, 22). Reprinted with permission from Ref. 22.

(18). Isolation of this gene from a chromosome 8 library confirmed the location reported by in situ hybridization and Southern blot analysis (19). A restriction map (see Fig. 5.1) was constructed using Southern blots of bacteriophage DNA hybridized to the human GnRH placental cDNA (gift of Genentech, San Francisco, CA). Four exons separated by three introns were observed with a coding sequence identical to the published cDNA sequence (18), except for a polymorphism in the signal peptide sequence that resulted in either a serine or a tryptophan residue at position −8 in the leader peptide (20). Southern blot analysis of normal human DNA under both stringent and moderately stringent hybridization conditions showed a similar pattern and suggested a single gene (data not shown).

Determination of the Transcriptional Start Site in the Hypothalamus

Due to a low abundance of GnRH mRNA in human hypothalamus, the polymerase chain reaction (PCR) technique, as described by Frohman et al. (21), was used to amplify cDNA from human hypothalamic mRNA. First-strand synthesis used an oligo(dT)$_{12-18}$ primer and avian myeloblastosis virus reverse transcriptase followed by tailing with dATP. For specific amplification of the 5' end, a primer with multiple cloning sites and a (dT)$_{20}$ tail was used along with a specific primer complementary to the 5' end of the second exon. The product was size-fractionated on a 2% agarose gel, blotted, and hybridized to the human placental GnRH cDNA. Autoradiography showed a band of approximately 150 basepairs (bp), corresponding to the size of the first exon, part of the second exon, and the oligonucleotides used for amplification. The ampli-

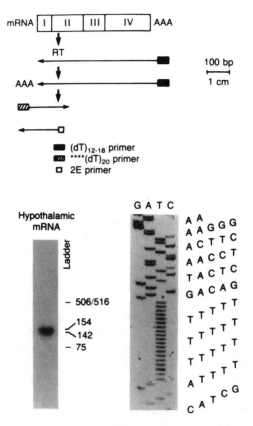

FIGURE 5.2. Mapping of the transcriptional start site of human GnRH in the hypothalamus. The PCR strategy used to generate human hypothalamic cDNA is shown at the top (see text). Using a primer specific for the second exon (2E) and the ****(dT)$_{20}$ primer, a 150-bp product was synthesized that hybridized to a human GnRH cDNA probe (bottom left). This product was subcloned, and its DNA sequence determined (bottom right). Reprinted with permission from Ref. 22.

fication product was digested and cloned into the Sal I and Hind III sites of pGEM-4Z, and after repeat hybridization to the cDNA, the hybridizing clones were sequenced.

Figure 5.2 shows the DNA sequence of one of the eight equivalent clones. Following the polydeoxythymidine tail the next base is a deoxyguanosine residue, which may represent either a thermus aquaticus polymerase artifact or a capping artifact, since it is not found in the genomic sequence. This is followed by a deoxyadenosine residue, the first base of the first exon (see Fig. 5.3). We repeated this amplification in the hypothalamus several times and never obtained longer cDNA clones even with two rounds of amplification (22). This start site is characteristic of

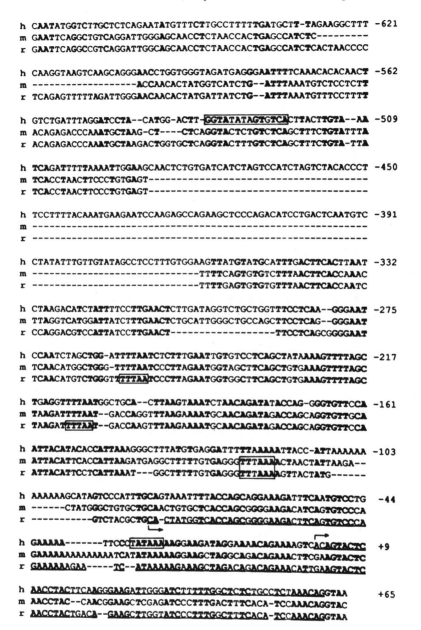

FIGURE 5.3. The DNA sequence of the human GnRH 5' flanking region and its comparison with the mouse and rat GnRH genes. The human (h), mouse (m), and rat (r) 5' flanking regions are aligned to maximize homology. The TATA and CAAT boxes in the human GnRH gene are boxed, as well as a putative TATA box in the mouse and rat (27) genes. The first exon is in bold type, and numbering is relative to the transcriptional start site in the human, shown as a bent arrow. The estrogen response element is boxed at position −521 to −534 bp in the human GnRH gene.

other mammalian genes with the consensus sequence PyCAPy, where the deoxyadenosine residue is the start of transcription (23, 24). Moreover, these data rule out the possibility of other more 5' exons.

Comparison of Human, Mouse, and Rat GnRH Gene Sequences

Interestingly, both the human and mouse genes contain a long stretch of polydeoxyadenosine residues in the 5' flanking region, although in different locations. The significance of these DNA sequences is unknown, but they do occur near the promoter elements in both genes. Moreover, like other eucaryotic genes, the 5' flanking region of the human GnRH gene contains a TATA or Goldberg/Hogness box at position −32/−25 and CAAT boxes at −53/−50 and −162/−159 bp. These sequences are thought to be important in efficient transcription of eucaryotic genes by RNA polymerase II (24) and are in similar positions in the mouse gene, except that the CAAT sequence at position −53/−50 in the mouse is modified to CAGT. The TATA box used in the human gene may differ from that predicted in the mouse (26) and does differ from that in the rat gene, recently reported to be located at −124/−119 (numbering relative to the human sequence) (27). The TATA box at this position is TTTAAA and differs somewhat from the consensus sequence TATA(A/T)A that has been reported (23, 24). The absence of sequence homology 3' to this TATA box among the human, mouse, and rat and the insertion of a deoxycytidine in the rat sequence that changes the TATAAAA box in the human to TCATAAAA in the rat gene may be responsible for the observed differences in transcriptional start sites among species. However, the transcriptional start site in the mouse remains unknown and is approximated in the rat (26, 27). Of great interest is the estrogen response element in the human gene, GGTATATAGTGTCA, which bears high sequence homology to DNA sequences found in both the mouse, GGTACTCTGTCTCA, and the rat, GGTACTTTGTCTCA, GnRH genes. The functional significance of these DNA sequences in the mouse and rat gene are presently unknown.

DNA Transfection Studies to Localize an Estrogen-Responsive Region in the Human GnRH Gene

To determine whether the human GnRH gene contains DNA sequences that may mediate estrogen responsiveness, chloramphenicol acetyl transferase (CAT) expression vectors using the native promoter were initially constructed but gave very low basal activity. Therefore, three 5' flanking regions, -1131 to -546 bp, -551 to $+5$ bp, and -551 to -459 bp of the human GnRH gene were placed upstream of the herpes thymidine kinase (TK) promoter fused to the CAT reporter gene (pTKCAT). These constructs were transfected into JEG-3 cells, and CAT activity was determined. We have previously demonstrated low levels of estrogen receptor mRNA by Northern blot analysis in JEG-3 cells (data not shown); but to augment ER levels, an expression vector containing the SV40 early promoter and the human ER cDNA (pKCR2ER, gift of P. Chambon) was cotransfected in some experiments. Figure 5.4A shows that in the absence of cotransfected ER, 0.1 nM or 10 nM estradiol did not stimulate CAT activity from pTKCAT, p-1131/−546TKCAT, or p-551/+5TKCAT. However, when 1 µg of pKCR2ER was cotransfected, the constructs

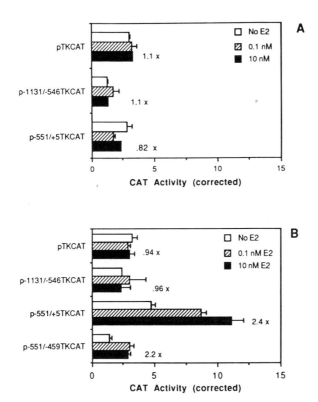

FIGURE 5.4. 5′ flanking regions of the human GnRH gene were ligated upstream of the TK promoter in pTKCAT. The regions placed upstream of TK are indicated by the numbers that precede TKCAT. These constructs were transfected into JEG-3 cells with or without a human ER cDNA (pKCR2ER) expression vector; and CAT activity was measured 48 h after either no treatment or treatment with 0.1 nM or 10 nM estradiol (E_2). CAT activity is expressed as percentage of acetylation in 16 h per mg of protein.

p-551/+5TKCAT and p-551/−459TKCAT but not p-1131/−546TKCAT or pTKCAT displayed a 2.4 and 2.2-fold increase, respectively, in CAT activity when exposed to 10 nM estradiol (Fig. 5.4B). This figure also demonstrates a concentration-dependence of this estrogen effect over a range of 0.1 nM to 10 nM estradiol for the p-551/+5TKCAT construct. These data indicate that, in the presence of cotransfected ER, estrogen-responsiveness could be conferred to the heterologous TK promoter in JEG-3 cells by using DNA sequences located between −551 and −459 bp of the human GnRH gene.

To study estrogen regulation of the native promoter, we initially utilized only the 5′ flanking region of the gene (−1131 to +5 bp) fused to the luciferase (LUC) gene; but again this construct displayed low basal LUC activity. Thus, we constructed several human GnRH LUC expression vectors containing DNA sequences downstream from the transcription initiation site. As shown in Figure 5.5, pGnRH.3E contains −1131 to +2684 bp (end of the third exon) of GnRH; pGnRH.2E contains −1131 to +1073 bp (end of the second exon) of GnRH; and pGnRH.2E/−82 contains −82 to +1073 bp of GnRH. To prevent read-through translation from GnRH coding sequences, translation stop codons were introduced into each of these constructs in the appropriate reading frame. To control for nonspecific effects, a construct containing the Rous sarcoma virus promoter, pRSVL, was utilized. Figure 5.5 shows the results of an experiment done in JEG-3 cells with all constructs cotransfected with pRSVCAT (to correct for transfection efficiency) and pKCRZEZ (to maximize the estradiol response). Cell cultures trans-fected with pGnRH.2E and pGnRH.3E displayed a significant 3–5-fold increase in LUC activity upon treatment with 10 nM estradiol. Since there was somewhat of a reduction in estrogen-responsiveness when the second intron and third exon were deleted (pGnRH.3E versus pGnRH.2E), we cannot exclude that an additional ERE is located in this region. However, a 5′ deletion of pGnRH.2E, pGnRH.2E/−82, displayed no signifi-cant increase in activity. As expected, LUC activity from pRSVL was unaltered by estradiol treatment. These results provide additional evi-dence that an ERE is located between −1131 and −82 bp of the human GnRH gene; and when these results are combined with previous CAT data, this ERE can be localized to −551 to −459 bp.

DNase I Footprinting of the Human GnRH Gene Using Purified Estrogen Receptor

To determine whether ER binds to the human GnRH gene, a DNA fragment from −661 to −82 bp was radiolabeled at the 5′ end, incubated with various concentrations of purified ER derived from calf uterus (gift of A. Notides), and partially digested with DNase I. Figure 5.6 demon-

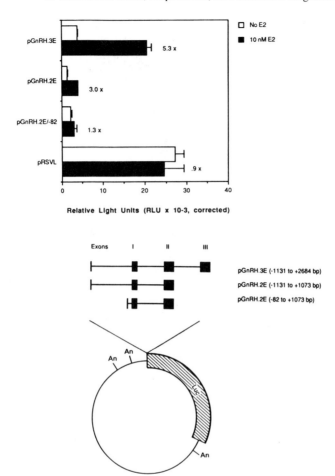

FIGURE 5.5. Human GnRH-LUC expression constructs were cotransfected into JEG-3 cells with pKCRZER. Constructs are shown diagrammatically in this figure and are described in the text. Shown is the relative light unit production corrected for transfection efficiency from cell cultures receiving either no treatment or treatment with 10 nM estradiol (E_2). Activity of pRSVL (RSV) was determined from 0.1% of the cell lysate used for human GnRH construct determinations.

strates that increasing concentrations of ER from 0.17 nM to 17 nM resulted in a strong footprint between −514 and −567 bp at 17 nM. These results are consistent with previous data from other investigators (28), who have determined that the dissociation constant (K_d) of ER binding to an estrogen response element was 2–5 nM. The footprinted region is somewhat larger than expected. This may be due to the pattern of DNase I digestion and the location of the radiolabel near the 5′ border of the footprint. Other investigators have also had difficulty establishing clear

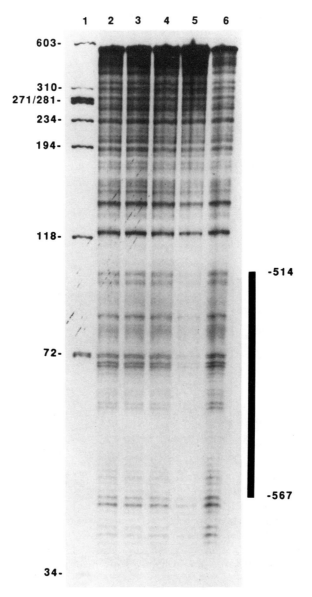

FIGURE 5.6. DNase I footprinting of the human GnRH gene using purified ER. A radiolabeled human GnRH probe (−611 to −82 bp) was incubated with either no receptor (lanes 2 and 6) or 0.17 nM, 1.7 nM, or 17 nM purified calf uterine ER (lanes 3, 4, and 5, respectively) in 50 μl of a buffer containing 50 nM KCl, 10% glycerol, 20 mM Tris pH 9.0, 1 mM DTT, 1 mM MgCl₂, 1 mM EDTA, 100 nM 17-β-estradiol, 100 μg/ml bovine serum albumin, and 4 μg of poly dI-dC for 30 min at 25°C. The binding reactions were partially digested with DNase I (0.6 μg, 2 min 25°C) and separated on an 8% denaturing polyacrylamide gel. Lane 1 contains a radiolabeled molecular weight marker.

borders of ER binding using a modification of the DNase I footprinting technique (29).

Avidin-Biotin DNA-Binding Assay to Confirm ER Binding to the Human GnRH Gene

We employed the avidin-biotin DNA-binding assay to confirm the results of ER binding to sequences identified by DNase I footprinting. A biotinylated DNA fragment containing −551 to −512 bp of the human GnRH gene (GnRH.ERE) was utilized in the avidin-biotin DNA-binding assay. As a positive control, a well defined ERE from the Xenopus vitellogenin gene (VIT.ERE) was utilized; and as a negative control, we employed the same DNA fragment used by other investigators (30) studying ER binding to biotinylated DNA fragments in this assay, a region of the long terminal repeat of adenovirus 5 (AD5). Figure 5.7 demonstrates that both GnRH.ERE and VIT.ERE bound approximately

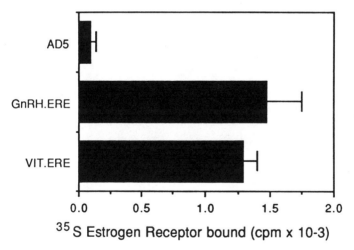

FIGURE 5.7. ER binding to human GnRH gene utilizing the avidin-biotin DNA-binding assay. Double-stranded oligonucleotides from the long terminal repeat of adenovirus 5, the Xenopus vitellogenin ERE, and the human GnRH gene (−551 to −512 bp) were synthesized with identical 5' overhangs and filled in with biotin-11 dUTP. Radiolabeled (^{35}S met) human ER was prepared using an in vitro transcription-translation system. Each binding reaction contained 1 pm of the respective biotinylated DNA fragment (20 nM) and 1×10^{-4} cpm of ^{35}S-labeled human ER as determined by trichloroacetic acid precipitation. Data represent the mean ± SE of triplicate determinations.

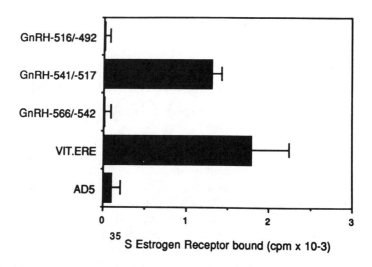

FIGURE 5.8. ER binding to hGnRH gene fragments utilizing the avidin-biotin DNA-binding assay, as above. Double-stranded oligonucleotides from the long terminal repeat of the hGnRH gene -516 to -492 bp, -541 to -517 bp, and -566 to -542 bp were synthesized and filled in as above. Data represent the mean $\pm$ SE of triplicate determinations.

15-fold more ^{35}S-labeled ER than the negative control fragment (AD5) at a DNA concentration of 20 nM.

To define further the limits of the ERE, three biotinylated DNA fragments containing -516 to -492 bp, -541 to -517 bp, and -566 to -542 bp of the human GnRH gene were utilized in the avidin-biotin DNA-binding assay. Again these studies were done using the Xenopus vitellogenin gene as a positive control and AD5 as the negative control. Figure 5.8 demonstrates that the DNA region between -541 and -517 bound the estrogen receptor nearly as well as the vitellogenin ERE. In contrast, the -566 to -542 bp fragment and the -516 to -492 bp fragment did not bind significant amounts of ^{35}S-labeled ER.

These results confirm that the ER binds to the hGnRH gene, and localize the region of binding from -541 to -517 bp. To determine the affinity of ER binding to the GnRH ERE and the vitellogenin ERE, the avidin-biotin DNA-binding assay was again employed with various concentrations of biotinylated DNA fragments. Figure 5.9 demonstrates that both the hGnRH ERE (-551 to -512 bp) and the vitellogenin ERE bound ^{35}S-labeled ER with high affinity ($K_d \sim 1$ nM), while AD5 bound estrogen receptor at considerably lower affinity.

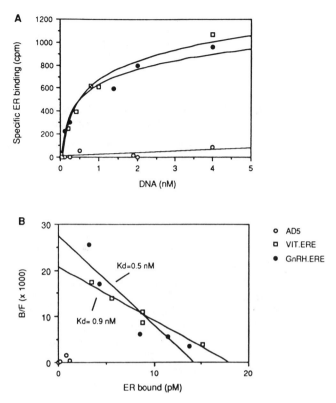

FIGURE 5.9. Affinity of ER binding to the GnRH and vitellogenin ERE. The avidin-biotin DNA-binding assay was performed with various concentrations of biotinylated DNA fragments as described in the legend of Figure 5.4. Specific ER (ER) binding in cpm versus the concentration of biotinylated DNA fragments is displayed. Data points are the mean of duplicate determinations from three separate experiments. (B) Scatchard analysis of DNA binding was performed. The dissociation constants (Kd) were calculated from the Scatchard plots.

Localization by Sequence Homology, DNase I Footprinting, and Avidin-Biotin DNA-Binding Assay

Although a consensus palindromic estrogen response element was not found upon sequencing the 1.2 kb of 5' flanking GnRH DNA, one area with high homology to known EREs was found. As shown in Figure 5.10, between −534 and −521 in the human GnRH gene (boxed) is a DNA sequence that is 80% homologous to EREs in the rat prolactin, Xenopus vitellogenin, and rat LHβ genes (28, 31, 32). Figure 5.10 also demonstrates that both functional and structural assays used in this study localize a stimulatory ERE to this region of DNA sequence homology.

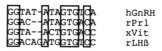

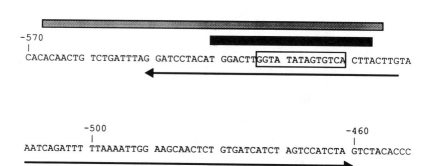

FIGURE 5.10. Summary of functional and structural assays used to determine an estrogen response element in the human GnRH 5′ flanking region. Localization by functional assays (line with arrowheads) of estrogen-responsiveness, and structural assays, DNase I footprint (stippled box) and avidin-biotin DNA-binding assays (black-stippled box), of ER binding. At the top of the figure, comparison of the putative ERE sequence in the human GnRH gene, between −534 and −521 bp (boxed), with that of the EREs in the rat prolactin, Xenopus vitellogenin, and rat LHβ genes is shown.

Functional assays indicate that a stimulatory ERE is localized between −551 and −459 bp (line with arrowheads), while DNase I footprinting (stippled box) and the avidin-biotin DNA-binding assay (black-stippled box) indicate that the ER binds to −567 to −514 bp and −541 to −517 bp, respectively, of the human GnRH gene. These regions overlap between −541 and −517 bp—which, as noted above, contains a DNA sequence homologous to that of other reported EREs between −534 and −521 bp.

Comparisons among the EREs indicate that the EREs from the rLHβ and hGnRH genes contain one and two base pair insertions, respectively, between putative half-sites of ER binding (33). The relatively modest stimulatory response to estrogen (3-fold) noted in the rLHβ and hGnRH genes versus the dramatic stimulatory response to estrogen noted in the vitellogenin gene (60-fold) may be due to differences in ER binding among these elements. Moreover, differences among EREs may have physiological importance where either a modest or dramatic stimulatory response to estrogen may be required to elicit the appropriate biological response.

Establishment of a GnRH-Secreting Cell Line

In order to examine the ability of the human GnRH promoter to direct cell-specific expression and establish stable cell lines expressing the GnRH gene from this low-abundance neuron, we inserted the human GnRH gene promoter from -1131 to $+5$ bp (22) upstream of the simian virus 40 T antigen (Tag) coding region in the pEMP construct (34) at the BamH 1 site. A 4 kb DNA fragment containing the human GnRH/Tag hybrid gene, and devoid of vector sequences, was injected into fertilized one-cell embryos as described. A similar strategy was used by Mellon et al. to develop a mouse GnRH-secreting cell line, using the rat GnRH promoter (35). Transgenic animals were identified by using Southern blot analysis and a human GnRH cDNA probe. An F1 male had a large mass visible directly over the olfactory bulbs, which extended rostrally into the nasal region. This mass contained an abnormal collection of Tag- and GnRH-immunopositive neurons. Figure 5.11 shows low magnification of serial parasagittal sections (rostral is to the right) through the brain of a transgenic mouse showing cells immunostaining for (A) Tag and (B) GnRH. Cells expressing the construct infiltrated the olfactory bulb but did not cross into the forebrain proper (arrows). C–E show serial parasagittal sections of the same mouse brain at the level of the anterior hypothalamus/preoptic area (ah/poa) immunostained (C and E) for Tag and (D) for GnRH. No GnRH cells were detected within the brain at their normal locations. Cells expressing the construct were caudal to the major cell mass shown in A and B ventrally, along, but outside the brain (arrows). F is a schematic representation of anterior brain, adapted from Wray et al. (36), showing the normal location, left, of GnRH neurons in the anterior hypothalamus and preoptic area (ah/poa), compared with the location in transgenic animals (right). Note the abnormal collection in the boxed area representing neurons shown in A and B and the absence of cells in the ah/poa in the lower boxed area representing C–E. The star represents the point at which the migrating GnRH neurons enter the forebrain during development. PCR analysis of this male and several other F1 progeny revealed expression of Tag mRNA in the brain but not in the liver, heart, bowel, or spleen of these animals (data not shown). Thus as little as 1100 bp of human GnRH 5′ flanking DNA was sufficient to direct Tag expression to the GnRH neuron. Since hypothalamic depletion of GnRH neurons was associated with an abnormal collection of Tag-positive GnRH neurons along the migratory pathway from the olfactory placode to the hypothalamus (36, 37) in some animals, it seems likely that Tag expression during a critical phase of development resulted in a migratory arrest of these neurons before they entered the forebrain.

Tumors were dispersed with collagenase by using standard methods (38), and cultured. The cells were found to grow in clusters and were

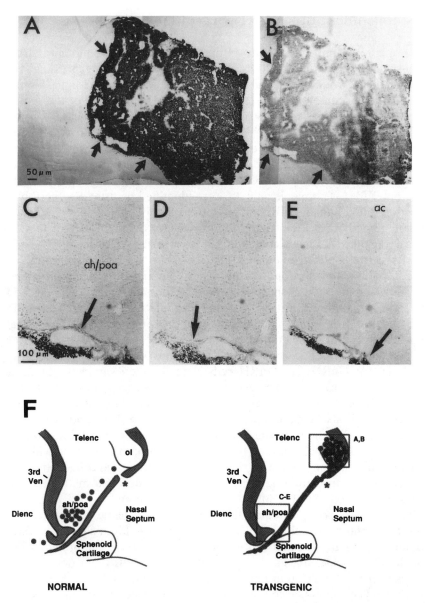

FIGURE 5.11. Low magnification of serial parasagittal sections (rostral is to the right) through the brain of a transgenic mouse, showing cells immunostaining for (A) T-antigen and (B) GnRH. Cells expressing the construct infiltrated the olfactory bulb but did not cross into the forebrain proper (arrows). (C–E) Serial parasagittal sections of the same mouse brain at the level of the anterior hypothalamus/preoptic area (ah/poa) immunostained (C and E) for T antigen and (D) for GnRH. (F) Schematic representation of anterior brain, adapted from Wray et al. (36), showing the normal location, left, of GnRH neurons in the

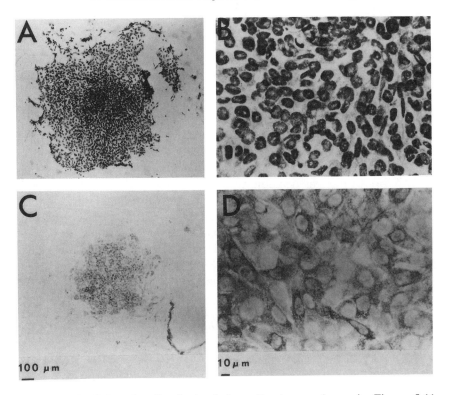

FIGURE 5.12. Cultured cells obtained from the tumor shown in Figure 5.11 dispersed with collagenase using standard methods (38). (A) low magnification and (B) high magnification: cultured cells stained with SV40 T antigen, showing extensive nuclear staining. (C) low magnification and (D) high magnification: cells stained with GnRH, showing staining in the cytoplasm.

relatively large compared with GnRH neurons normally found in the brain. Figure 5.12 shows (A) low magnification and (B) high magnification of cultured cells stained with SV40 T antigen, showing extensive nuclear staining, and (C) low magnification and (D) high magnification of cells stained with GnRH, showing staining in the cytoplasm. Double labeling indicated Tag and GnRH within the same cells. PCR analysis of these dispersed cell cultures confirmed that they contained Tag and GnRH mRNA (data not shown).

◄──

anterior hypothalamus and preoptic area (ah/poa), compared with the location in transgenic animals. Note the abnormal collection in the boxed area representing neurons shown in A and B and the absence of cells in the ah/poa in the lower boxed area representing C–E. The star represents the point at which the migrating GnRH neurons enter the forebrain during development.

Estrogen Binding in the GnRH Neuron

For estradiol to have a direct effect on a cell, high-affinity ERs are necessary. Although we have demonstrated that the ER complex interacts
with a specific sequence on the GnRH gene, the physiologic implications
of this finding are unclear, because ERs in the GnRH neuron have not
been demonstrated. The GnRH neuronal cell line described above was
used to determine the existence of nuclear ERs. Cells were grown in
phenol red-free media (39) containing 10% fetal calf serum devoid of
steroid hormones. An ^{125}I estradiol-binding study revealed binding sites
(Fig. 5.13) with a dissociation constant (K_d) of 0.4 nM. This value is
consistent with the calculated value for the ER in uterine or breast
tumor cells (40–43) and the recently described ER in osteosarcoma cells
(16, 17). This GnRH neuronal cell population contains about 3000 high-
affinity ER binding sites per nucleus. This mean concentration was higher
than that required to induce transcription in experimental animals (42,
43), and was in the range of that found in estrogen-responsive endometrial
tissue.

Thus, these data suggest that the hGnRH gene contains an ERE
between −541 and −517 bp, providing evidence for direct estradiol

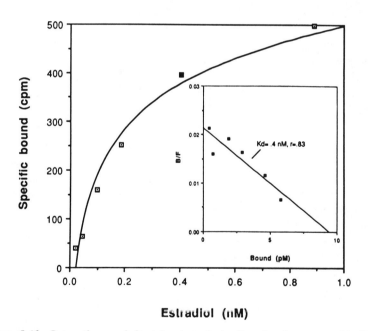

FIGURE 5.13. Saturation and Scatchard analysis (inset) of estrogen binding in
nuclear extracts of a GnRH neuronal cell line described above. Kd ≈ 0.4 nM and
Nmax ≈ 3000 sites per nucleus.

regulation of the GnRH neuron. Moreover, at least one population of GnRH neurons contains a significant number of high-affinity ERs. However, these data would not exclude indirect estrogen regulation of hGnRH expression by other neuropeptides.

Acknowledgment. The authors thank Michelle E. Hall for her careful preparation of this manuscript.

References

1. Carmel PW, Araki S, Ferin M. Pituitary stalk portal blood collection in rhesus monkeys: evidence for pulsatile release of gonadotropin-releasing hormone (GnRH). Endocrinology 1975;99:243–248.
2. Gross DS. Effect of castration and steroid replacement on immunoreactive gonadotropin-releasing hormone in the hypothalamus and preoptic area. Endocrinology 1980;106:1442–1450.
3. Rudenstein RS, Bigdeli H, McDonald MH, Snyder PJ. Administration of gonadal steroids to the castrated male rat prevents a decrease in the release of gonadotropin-releasing hormone from the incubated hypothalamus. J Clin Invest 1979;63:262–267.
4. Reame N, Sauder SE, Kelch RP, Marshall JC. Pulsatile gonadotropin secretion during the human menstrual cycle: evidence for altered frequency of gonadotropin-releasing hormone secretion. J Clin Endocrinol Metab 1984;59:328–337.
5. Pfaff DW. Gene expression in hypothalamic neurons: luteinizing hormone releasing hormone. J Neurosci Res 1986;16:109–115.
6. Rothfeld JM, Hejtmancik JF, Conn PM, Pfaff DW. LHRH messenger RNA in neurons in the intact castrate male rat forebrain, studied by in situ hybridization. Exp Brain Res 1987;67:113–118.
7. Roberts JL, Dutlow CM, Jakubowski M, Blum M, Millar RP. Estradiol stimulates preoptic area-anterior hypothalamic pro-GnRH-GAP gene expression in ovariectomized rats. Mol Brain Res 1989;6:127–134.
8. Rothfeld J, Hejtmancik JF, Conn PM, Pfaff DW. In situ hybridization for LHRH mRNA following estrogen treatment. Mol Brain Res 1989;6:121–125.
9. Park O, Gugneja S, Mayo KE. Gonadotropin-releasing hormone gene expression during the rat estrous cycle: effects of pentobarbital and ovarian steroids. Endocrinology 1990;127:365–372.
10. Zoeller RT, Seeburg PH, Young WS III. In situ hybridization histochemistry for messenger ribonucleic acid (mRNA) encoding gonadotropin-releasing hormone (GnRH): effect of estrogen on cellular levels of GnRH mRNA in female rat brain. Endocrinology 1988;122:2570–2577.
11. Wray S, Zoeller RT, Gainer H. Differential effects of estrogen on luteinizing hormone-releasing hormone gene expression in slice explant cultures prepared from specific rat forebrain regions. Mol Endocrinol 1989;3:1197–1206.
12. Toranzo D, Dupont E, Simardt J, et al. Regulation of pro-gonadotropin-releasing hormone gene expression by sex steroids in the brain of male and female rats. Mol Endocrinol 1989;3:1748–1756.

13. Marshall JC, Kelch RP. Gonadotropin-releasing hormone: role of pulsatile secretion in the regulation of reproduction. N Engl J Med 1986;315:1459–1468.

14. Shivers BD, Harlan RE, Morrell JI, Pfaff DW. Absence of oestradiol concentration in cell nuclei of LHRH-immunoreactive neurones. Nature 1983;304:345–347.

15. Watson RE, Langub MC, Landis JW. Further evidence that LHRH neurons are not directly estrogen responsive: LHRH and estrogen receptor immunoreactivity in the guinea pig brain [Abstract]. Neuroscience 1990:495.

16. Komm BS, Terpening CM, Benz DK, et al. Estrogen binding, receptor mRNA, and biologic response in osteoblast-like osteosarcoma cells. Science 1988;241:81–84.

17. Eriksen EF, Colcard DS, Berg NJ, et al. Evidence of estrogen receptors in normal human osteoblast-like cells. Science 1988;304:84–86.

18. Adelman JP, Mason AJ, Hayflick JS, Seeburg PH. Isolation of the gene and hypothalamic cDNA for the common precursor of gonadotropin-releasing hormone and prolactin-inhibiting factor in human and rat. Proc Natl Acad Sci USA 1986;83:179–183.

19. Yang-Feng TL, Seeburg PH, Francke U. Human luteinizing hormone-releasing hormone gene (LHRH) is located on the short arm of chromosome 8 (region 8p11.2>p21). Somatic Cell Genet 1986;12:95–100.

20. Nakayama Y, Wondisford FE, Lash RW, et al. Analysis of gonadotropin-releasing hormone gene structure in families with familial central precocious puberty (FCPP) and idiopathic hypogonadotropic hypogonadism (IHH). J Clin Endocrinol Metab 1990;70:1233–1238.

21. Frohman MA, Dush MK, Martin GR. Rapid production of full length cDNAs from rare transcripts: amplification using a single gene-specific oligonucleotide primer. Proc Natl Acad Sci USA 1988;85:8998–9002.

22. Radovick S, Wondisford FE, Nakayama Y, Yamada M, Cutler GB Jr, Weintraub BD. Isolation and characterization of the human gonadotropin-releasing hormone gene in the hypothalamus and placenta. Mol Endocrinol 1990;4:476–480.

23. Corden J, Wasylyk B, Buchwalder A, Sassone-Corsi P, Kedinger C, Chambon P. Promoter sequences of eukaryotic protein-coding genes. Science 1980;209:1406–1414.

24. Bucher P, Trifonov EN. Compilation and analysis of eukaryotic POL II promoter sequences. Nucleic Acids Res 1986;14:10009–10026.

25. Breathnach R, Chambon P. Organization and expression of eucaryotic split genes coding for proteins. Annu Rev Biochem 1981;50:349–383.

26. Mason AJ, Hayflick JS, Zoeller T, et al. A deletion truncating the gonadotropin-releasing hormone gene is responsible for hypogonadism in the hpg mouse. Science 1986;234:1366–1371.

27. Bond CT, Hayflick JS, Seeburg PH, Adelman JP. The rat gonadotropin-releasing hormone: SH locus: structure and hypothalamic expression. Mol Endocrinol 1989;3:1257–1262.

28. Maurer RA, Notides AC. Identification of an estrogen-responsive element from the 5' flanking region of the rat prolactin gene. Mol Cell Biol 1987; 7:4247–4254.

29. Cridland NA, Wright CVE, McKenzie EA, Knowland J. Selective photochemical treatment of oestrogen receptor in a Xenopus liver extract destroys hormone binding and transcriptional activation but not DNA binding. EMBO J 1990;9:1859–1866.

30. Glass CK, Holloway JM, Devary OY, Rosenfeld MG. The thyroid hormone receptor binds with opposite transcriptional effects to a common sequence motif in thyroid hormone and estrogen response elements. Cell 1988;54:313–323.

31. Klein-Hitpass L, Schorpp M, Wagner U, Ryffel GU. An estrogen-responsive element derived from the 5′ flanking region of the Xenopus vitellogenin A2 gene functions in transfected human cells. Cell 1986;46:1053–1061.

32. Shupnik MA, Weinmann CMN, Notides AC, Chin WW. An upstream region of the rat luteinizing hormone β gene binds estrogen receptor and confers estrogen responsiveness. J Biol Chem 1989;264:80–86.

33. Kumar V, Chambon P. The estrogen receptor binds tightly to its responsive element as a ligand-induced homodimer. Cell 1988;55:145–156.

34. Benoist C, Chambon P. Deletions covering the putative promoter region of early mRNAs of simian virus 40 do not abolish T-antigen expression. Proc Natl Acad Sci USA 1980;77:3365–3369.

35. Mellon PL, Windle JJ, Goldsmith PC, Padula CA, Roberts JL, Weiner RI. Neuron 1990;5:1–10.

36. Wray S, Grant P, Gainer H. Evidence that cells expressing luteinizing hormone-releasing hormone mRNA in the mouse are derived from progenitor cells in the olfactory placode. Proc Natl Acad Sci USA 1989;86:8132–8136.

37. Schwanzel-Fukuda M, Pfaff DW. Origin of luteinizing hormone-releasing hormone neurons. Nature 1989;338:161–164.

38. Ben-Jonathan N, Pelig E, Hoefer MT. Optimization of culture conditions for short-term pituitary cell culture. Methods Enzymol 1983:249–251.

39. Berthois Y, Katzenellenbogen JA, Katzenellenbogen BS. Phenol red in tissue culture media is a weak estrogen: implications concerning the study of estrogen-responsive cells in culture. Proc Natl Acad Sci USA 1986;83:2496–2500.

40. Jensen EV, DeSombre ER. Mechanism of action of the female sex hormones. Annu Rev Biochem 1972;41:203–222.

41. Brooks SC, Locke ER, Soule HD. Estrogen receptor in a human cell line (MCF-7) from breast carcinoma. J Biol Chem 1973;248:6251–6253.

42. Spelsberg TC, Graham ML, Berg NJ, et al. A nuclear binding assay to assess the biological activity of steroid receptors in isolated animal and human tissues. Endocrinology 1987;121:631–644.

43. Mulvihill ER, Palmiter RD. Relationship of nuclear estrogen receptor levels to induction of ovalbumin and conalbumin mRNA in chick oviduct. J Biol Chem 1977;252:2060–2068.

6

Control of Rat Gonadotropin Releasing Hormone Promoter Activity in Placental Cells

Margaret E. Wierman, Wei Sun, Chun Wang,
David F. Gordon, and William W. Wood

Gonadotropin releasing hormone is a hypothalamic releasing factor that controls gonadotropin subunit gene expression and ultimately both gametogenesis and gonadal steroid synthesis and biosynthesis and thus ensures reproductive competence (1) (Fig. 6.1). Many hormones, including gonadal steroids and other hypothalamic releasing factors and neurotransmitters, are thought to impact on GnRH production. An understanding of the regulation of the expression of the GnRH gene would thus allow for the study of the basic mechanisms that underlie the control of sexual maturation and infertility.

In addition to the hypothalamus, the other major tissue where the GnRH gene is expressed is the placenta of many species (2–9), where it may play a role in controlling hCG production (10–17) (Fig. 6.2). Other potential GnRH regulators such as peptide and steroid hormones are also produced by the placenta. Although the genes encoding GnRH have been cloned for several species (18–24), little is known about the architecture of the GnRH promoter. Thus we cloned the rat GnRH to begin to examine the *cis*-acting elements important for rGnRH promoter activity in the placenta. These initial studies attempt to identify specific sequences in the 5′ flanking region that mediate basal activity in placental cells and estrogen regulation of GnRH expression.

Cloning of the Rat GnRH Gene

The rat GnRH gene was cloned from a rat genomic library by using a human placental cDNA probe (18). Structural features are as published by Adelman and coworkers (21, 23) (Fig. 6.3). There are 4 exons and

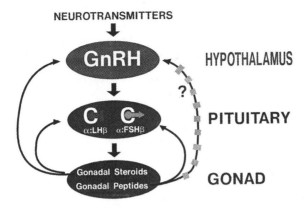

FIGURE 6.1. The organization of the hypothalamic-pituitary-gonadal axis: Gonadotropin releasing hormone, follicle stimulating hormone beta, luteinizing hormone
beta, and free alpha subunit.

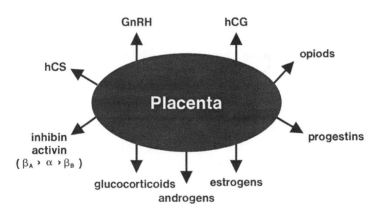

FIGURE 6.2. Steroid and peptide hormones produced by the placenta. Human
chorionic gonadotropin (hCG), β_A, β_B, the gonadal peptides—dimers compris-
ing either $\alpha\beta_A$, $\alpha\beta_B$ (inhibin) or $\beta_A\beta_B$, $\beta_A\beta_A$ (activin), human chorionic
somatomammotropin (hCS).

3 introns and the gene is approximately 4.5 kb in size. The first exon
encodes 5′ untranslated sequences. The second exon codes for the
signal peptide, the decapeptide GnRH, and the amino portion of the
GnRH-associated peptide (GAP). The third and fourth exons encode
the remainder of the GAP sequences, and the fourth exon encodes the
3′ untranslated region.

It has been demonstrated in the human placenta, in contrast to the
hypothalamus, that the first intron is not spliced, resulting in different

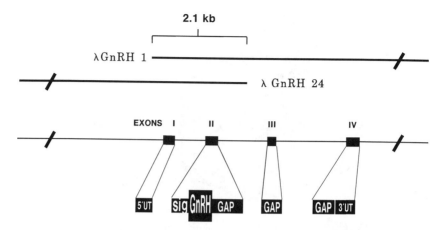

FIGURE 6.3. Genomic map of the rat GnRH gene. Two recombinant lambda phage clones containing 8–10 kb inserts, including one 2.1-kb overlapping region, were isolated from a rat liver EMBL-3 genomic DNA library. The GnRH gene spans approximately 4.5 kb of DNA and consists of 4 exons separated by 3 introns. Exon 1 encodes the 5' untranslated region (UT), exon 2 the signal peptide (sig), the decapeptide GnRH, and the aminoterminal portion of the GnRH-associated peptide (GAP). Exons 3 and 4 encode the remainder of GAP, and exon 4 encodes the 3' untranslated region.

messenger ribonucleic acid sizes in the two tissues and tissue-specific alternative sliced mRNA species (19, 23). Figure 6.4 is a Northern blot analysis of 10 μg of polyA$^+$ RNA, demonstrating a single mRNA species of 5–600 nucleotides in hypothalamic RNA, which hybridizes to a 2.1-kb genomic fragment encoding exon 1 and exon 2 of the GnRH sequence. We, like others, have been unable to demonstrate placental mRNAs in the human or rat placenta by Northern blot analysis. Polymerase chain reaction studies are under way in the laboratory.

Optimization of a Transient Transfection Assay

After cloning and sequencing the rat GnRH gene, we then fused fragments of the 5' flanking region to the firefly luciferase gene in an expression plasmid that contains a trimerized simian virus 40 (SV40) polyadenylation signal placed upstream of inserted promoter sequences, resulting in minimal background luciferase activity (pA$_3$LUC) (25, 26). Resultant luciferase activity was standardized to a neutral promoter derived from the long terminal repeat of the Rous sarcoma virus transfected in parallel (pRSVLUC). In the absence of a GnRH-producing placental cell line or hypothalamic cell line when these studies were initiated, the placenta-derived choriocarcinoma cell line JEG-3 was used in transient transfection assays.

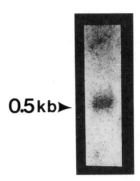

FIGURE 6.4. Northern blot analysis of rGnRH. Rat hypothalamic polyA$^+$ RNA (20 μg) was electrophoresed in a 1.4% agarose gel, transferred to nitrocellulose, and hybridized with a radiolabeled 2.1 genomic fragment specific for exons 1 and 2 of rGnRH. The blot was washed and exposed to autoradiography for 1 day at −70°C. A single mRNA species of 5–600 nucleotides is observed.

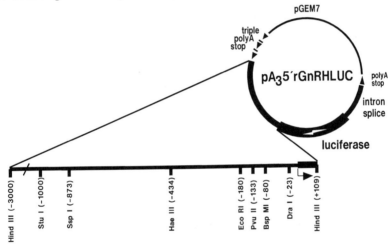

FIGURE 6.5. Deletions of the rGnRH promoter in a luciferase expression vector. Constructs (5′ deletional) were prepared by using convenient restriction sites to examine areas important for basal promoter activity and estrogen regulation in placental cells. The 3′ extent of all inserts was to the HindIII site at +109. Fragments were inserted into the SmaI-HindIII site in pA$_3$LUC.

Figure 6.5 demonstrates promoter deletions inserted into the luciferase expression vector. Convenient restriction enzyme sites were used to construct the promoter deletions from −3000 to −23 bp. The 3′ extent of all inserts was to the HindIII site at +109. Initial efforts in the laboratory determined that electroporation rather than calcium phosphate or lipofection methods provided more sensitive and more reproducible rat GnRH promoter expression. Additional experiments determined the optimal conditions for transfection, including the linearity of amount of DNA transfected and the time of incubation after transfection before harvest of the cells. Experiments demonstrated that 10 or 20 μg of DNA transfected produced a linear increment in promoter activity of the p-180GnRHLUC as expressed in relative light units per 10^7 light units of RSV, with little effect on the promoterless vector pA₃LUC. We harvested cells at 4, 6, 9, or 22 h after transfection, and observed optimal activity of the rat GnRH promoter at 6 to 9 h. Thus, in further studies cells were harvested at 6 to 9 h.

rGnRH Basal Promoter Activity in Placental Cells

After optimizing the conditions of the transfection, we then examined promoter activities in various rat GnRH deletional constructs (Fig. 6.6). To our surprise, large fragments of the rat GnRH promoter exhibited low levels of luciferase activity, suggesting the presence of repressor sequences. Deletion to −434 bp increased basal activity 8–10-fold. Luciferase activity persisted and increased an additional 2-fold with deletion to −80 bp. Further deletion to −23 bp resulted in significant loss

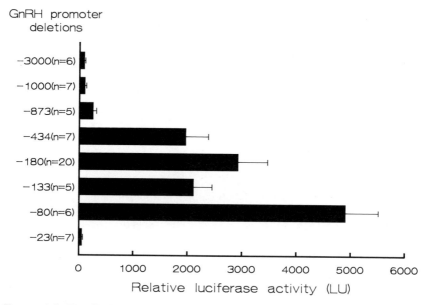

FIGURE 6.6. Rat GnRH promoter activity in placental cells. Deletional constructs were prepared by using convenient restriction sites. All constructs shown extend to +109 bp in their 3′ extent. Twenty μg of DNA was electroporated into JEG-3 cells, and cells were harvested after 6–9 h. Lysates were assayed for luciferase activity. Data are expressed relative to 10^7 LU of pRSVLUC transfected in parallel. N refers to the number of experiments performed for each construct.

of basal promoter activity, possibly through interference with TATA sequences.

Effects of Estrogen on rGnRH Promoter Activity

After demonstrating basal activity of promoter deletions, we then assessed whether estrogen had a direct effect on rat GnRH promoter activity in placental cells. Since JEG-3 cells are deficient in estrogen receptor (MEW, unpublished observations), cotransfection of an expression vector containing the human estrogen receptor coding region provided by Andrew Baker in the $pCDL_2$ expression vector created a receptor-positive cell line (data not shown).

In all experiments examining the effects of estrogen on rat GnRH promoter activity, cells were first incubated for 48 h in E-stripped media before transfection and the addition of $5 \times 10^{-8}M$ estradiol. Figure 6.7 demonstrates the inhibitory effects of estrogen on rat GnRH promoter activity. Data are expressed as percentages of control cells grown in the absence of estrogen. Cotransfection of the promoterless vector, pA_3LUC, with the human ER had low basal activity and was not affected by E. Cotransfection of pRSVLUC and the ER construct resulted in high basal

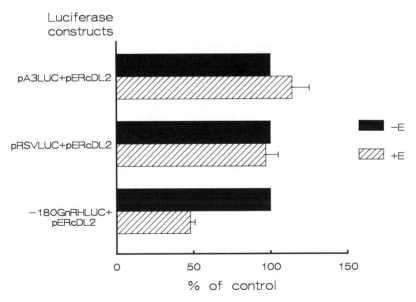

FIGURE 6.7. Estrogen inhibition of rGnRH promoter activity. JEG-3 cells were placed in E-depleted media 48 h prior to transfection. Twenty μg of plasmid DNA and 0.5–20 μg of ER was cotransfected with GnRH DNA. Data are expressed as percentages of luciferase activity in control cells grown in the absence of E.

activity but was also unchanged by estrogen. However, cotransfection of
p-180GnRHLUC + ER resulted in significant basal activity and a consistent 50–60% inhibition of rat GnRH promoter activity in the presence
of E.

In addition, the negative regulation of the rat GnRH promoter by E
was dependent on coexpression of the estrogen receptor (Fig. 6.8). In
these studies as before, pA$_3$LUC with ER was not affected by E, while
p-180GnRHLUC with ER was consistently inhibited in the presence of E.
However, cotransfection of p-180GnRHLUC with the plasmid containing
the plasmid pCDL$_2$ but lacking the ER coding region sequences resulted
in no E response. Subsequent studies utilized the positive ERE of the
vitellogenin gene, which was linked to the thymidine kinase promoter in
the luciferase plasmid (pEREtKLUC). These experiments demonstrated
that estrogen positively regulated the pEREtKLUC, and this effect was
also dependent on cotransfection of the ER. When the EREtKLUC was
cotransfected with pCDL$_2$ lacking the ER coding region sequences, the
positive regulation by estrogen was lost.

We then examined the extent of negative regulation by estrogen. Large
fragments of the rat GnRH promoter that had exhibited low basal activity
were variably affected by E (data not shown). Deletion to −434 bp

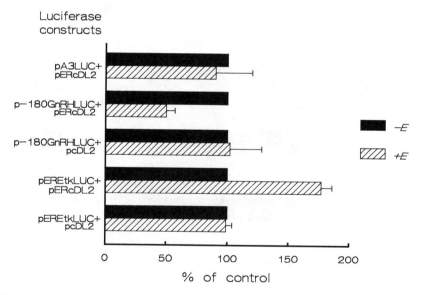

FIGURE 6.8. Negative regulation of the rGnRH promoter and positive regulation
of the EREtK promoter by E are dependent on cotransfection of estrogen
receptor. JEG-3 cells were grown in E-depleted media for 48 h prior to
transfection. Cells were harvested after 6–9 h of incubation. Data are expressed
as percentages of control cells in the absence of E.

increased basal activity and revealed the prominent negative regulation by estrogen. This response was maintained in further deletional constructs until deletion reached −23 bp, where again the low basal activity made interpretation of the estrogen response somewhat difficult.

Summary and Conclusions

In summary, *cis*-acting elements responsible for rat GnRH promoter activity in placental cells appear to lie within a proximal region of the rat GnRH promoter between −80 and −23 bp. Suppressor sequences in the rat GnRH promoter are localized primarily to the region −876 to −434 bp. A smaller region of suppressor sequences may be important in the area −133 to −80 bp. In contrast to the human gene, where estrogen positively regulates rat GnRH promoter activity (27, 28), in the rat gene estrogen negatively regulates rat GnRH promoter activity in placental cells. The sequences that mediate this effect lie within the region −80 to −23 bp of the promoter. Of interest, the sequences that Radovick and colleagues have demonstrated confer a positive response to estrogen (27, 28) are not conserved in the flanking region of the rat (21, 23) or the mouse (20) GnRH gene.

In conclusion, specific DNA regions are associated with both repression and enhancement of rat GnRH promoter activity in placental cells. Estrogen negatively regulates rat GnRH promoter activity in placental cells, and this effect is dependent on the presence of functional estrogen receptor. Future studies in the laboratory are examining the specific *trans*-acting factors that mediate basal expression of rat GnRH promoter activity in placental cells and the newly derived hypothalamic neuronal cell lines (29). We also plan to dissect the potential mechanisms by which estrogen suppresses rat GnRH promoter activity in an area proximal to the transcription initiation site.

Acknowledgments. We thank Peter Seeberg for the human placental cDNA, Andrew Baker for the hER, and DNAX Research Institute for the pCDL$_2$ vector. We also thank Ms. Gloria Smith for her careful preparation of the manuscript. These studies were supported by VA Merit Review 001 and HD 25275. MEW is the recipient of a Research Associate Award.

References

1. Seeburg PH, Mason AJ, Stewart TA, Nikolics K. The mammalian GnRH gene and its pivotal role in reproduction. Recent Prog Horm Res 1987;43: 69–98.

2. Siler-Khodr TM, Khodr GS. Content of luteinizing hormone-releasing factor in the human placenta. Am J Obstet Gynecol 1978;130:216–219.

3. Gibbons JM Jr, Mitnick M, Chieffo V. In vitro biosynthesis of TSH and LH-releasing factors by the human placenta. Am J Obstet Gynecol 1975;121:127–131.

4. Khodr GS, Siler-Khodr TM. Localization of luteinizing hormone-releasing factor in the human placenta. Fertil Steril 1978;29:523–526.

5. Lee J-N, Seppälä M, Chard T. Characterization of placental luteinizing hormone-releasing factor-like material. Acta Endocrinol 1981;96:394–397.

6. Khodr GS, Siler-Khodr TM. Placental luteinizing hormone-releasing factor and its synthesis. Science 1980;207:315–317.

7. Nowak RA, Bahr JM. Secretion of a gonadotrophin-releasing hormone (GnRH)-like factor by the rabbit fetal placenta in vitro. Placenta 1987;8:299–304.

8. Rice GE, Smirnis M. Identification of luteinizing hormone releasing hormone-like immunoactivity in ovine cotyledons. Regulatory Peptides 1990;27:51–59.

9. Sarkar DK. Gonadotropin-releasing hormone-like immunoreactivity in rat placenta. Neuroendocrinology 1986;44:397–400.

10. Belisle S, Lehoux J-G, Bellabarba D, Gallo-Payet N, Guévin J-F. Dynamics of LHRH binding to human term placental cells from normal and anencephalic gestations. Mol Cell Endocrinol 1987;49:195–202.

11. Haning RV Jr, Choi L, Kiggens AJ, Kuzma DL. Effects of prostaglandins, dibutyryl cAMP, LHRH, estrogens, progesterone, and potassium on output of prostaglandin $F_{2\alpha}$ 13,14-dihydro-15-keto-prostaglandin $F_{2\alpha}$, hCG, estradiol, and progesterone by placental minces. Prostaglandins 1982;24:495–506.

12. Haning RV Jr, Choi L, Kiggens AJ, Kuzma DL, Summerville JW. Effects of dibutyryl adenosine 3'5'-monophosphate, luteinizing hormone-releasing hormone, and aromatase inhibitor on simultaneous outputs of progesterone, 17β-estradiol, and human chorionic gonadotropin by term placental explants. J Clin Endocrinol Metab 1982;55:213–218.

13. Siler-Khodr TM, Khodr GS, Valenzuela G, Rhode J. Gonadotropin-releasing hormone effects on placental hormones during gestation: I. Alpha-human chorionic gonadotropin, human chorionic gonadotropin and human chorionic somatomammotropin. Biol Reprod 1986;34:245–254.

14. Barnea ER, Kaplan M. Spontaneous, gonadotropin-releasing hormone-induced, and progesterone-inhibited pulsatile secretion of human chorionic gonadotropin the first trimester placenta in vitro. J Clin Endocrinol Metab 1989;69:215–217.

15. Iwashita M, Watanabe M, Adachi T, et al. Effect of gonadal steroids on gonadotropin-releasing hormones stimulated human chorionic gonadotropin release by trophoblast cells. Placenta 1989;10:103–112.

16. Siler-Khodr TM, Khodr GS, Rhode J, Vickery BH, Nestor JJ Jr. Gestational age-related inhibition of placental hCG, αhCG and steroid hormone release in vitro by a GnRH antagonist. Placenta 1987;8:1–14.

17. Kim SJ, Namkoong SE, Lee JW, Jung JK, Kang BC, Park JS. Response of human chorionic gonadotrophin to luteinizing hormone-releasing hormone stimulation in the culture media of normal human placenta, choriocarcinoma

cell lines, and in the serum of patients with gestational trophoblastic disease. Placenta 1987;8:257–264.

18. Seeburg PH, Adelman JP. Characterization of cDNA for precursor of human luteinizing hormone releasing hormone. Nature 1984;311:666–668.

19. Adelman JP, Mason AJ, Hayflick JS, Seeburg PH. Isolation of the gene and hypothalamic cDNA for the common precursor of gonadotropin-releasing hormone and prolactin release-inhibiting factor in human and rat. Proc Natl Acad Sci USA 1986;83:179–183.

20. Mason AJ, Hayflick JS, Zoeller RT, et al. A deletion truncating the gonadotropin-releasing hormone gene is responsible for hypogonadism in the hpg mouse. Science 1986;234:1366–1371.

21. Adelman JP, Bond CT, Douglass J, Herbert E. Two mammalian genes transcribed from opposite strands of the same DNA locus. Science 1987; 235:1514–1517.

22. Hayflick JS, Adelman JP, Seeburg PH. The complete nucleotide sequence of the human gonadotropin-releasing hormone gene. Nucleic Acids Res 1989; 17:6403–6404.

23. Bond CT, Hayflick JS, Seeburg PH, Adelman JP. The rat gonadotropin-releasing hormone: SH locus: structure and hypothalamic expression. Mol Endocrinol 1989;3:1257–1262.

24. Radovick S, Wondisford FE, Nakayama Y, Yamada M, Cutler GB Jr, Weintraub BD. Isolation and characterization of the human gonadotropin-releasing hormone gene in the hypothalamus and placenta. Mol Endocrinol 1990;4:476–480.

25. Wood WM, Kao MY, Gordon DF, Ridgway EC. Thyroid hormone regulates the mouse thyrotropin β-subunit gene promoter in transfected primary thyrotropes. J Biol Chem 1989;264:14840–14847.

26. Maxwell JH, Harrison GS, Wood WM, Maxwell F. A DNA cassette containing a trimerized SV40 polyadenylation signal which efficiently blocks spurious plasmid-initiated transcription. Biotechniques 1989;7:276–280.

27. Radovick S, Nakayama Y, Cutler GB Jr. Control of human gonadotropin-releasing hormone gene expression by estrogen [Abstract]. Clin Res 1989; 37:831A.

28. Radovick S, Wondisford FE, Wray S, et al. Characterization, expression, and estradiol regulation of the human gonadotropin-releasing hormone (GnRH) gene. Symposium on Modes of Action of GnRH and GnRH Analogs, 1991. (See Chapter 5, this volume.)

29. Mellon PL, Windle JJ, Goldsmith PC, Padula CA, Roberts JL, Weiner RI. Immortalization of hypothalamic GnRH neurons by genetically targeted tumorigenesis. Neuron 1990;5:1–10.

7

Cellular and Molecular Aspects of LHRH Secretion and Bioactivity

ANDRÉS NEGRO-VILAR, WILLIAM WETSEL, MARCELO VALENÇA, ISTVAN MERCHENTHALER, FRANCISCO LÓPEZ, ZSOLT LIPOSITS, MELVIN CHING, RICHARD WEINER, AND PAMELA MELLON

It is now well established that the central nervous system controls reproductive functions by way of specific brain messengers that provide the neurochemical link between the brain and the pituitary-gonadal axis. The primary hypothalamic hormonal messenger regulating gonadotropin secretion and, hence, gonadal function, is the decapeptide luteinizing hormone releasing hormone. Indeed, LHRH has been shown to control, directly or indirectly, every aspect of reproduction. In its absence, gonadal development is arrested (1), and disorders of LHRH secretion and function result in advanced or delayed puberty, hypogonadism, infertility, and other reproductive dysfunctions (2).

Unique Characteristics of the LHRH Neuronal System

An outstanding feature of the LHRH neuronal system is its ability to control gonadal function by periodic, pulsatile regulatory signals that encode messages regulating gonadotropin biosynthesis and secretion (3–6). Alterations in pulsatile LHRH signals lead to distinct changes in gonadotropin secretion and these, in turn, modify gonadal activity (2–4, 7).

Several unique characteristics of the LHRH neuronal system are worth noting, because of the implications regarding our understanding of the physiology, pharmacology, and pathophysiology of this system. These characteristics are described in Table 7.1 and will be discussed below in some detail.

Anatomical/Functional Characteristics

LHRH neurons have a particular fusiform structure, are either bipolar or unipolar, and present with few dendrites and long, beaded axons (8, 9).

116

TABLE 7.1. Unique characteristics of the LHRH neuronal system.

Characteristics	Comments/significance
Small number of neurons (ca. 1500).	Redundancy still present since few neurons are needed to establish gonadal function.
Neurons are scattered, not arranged in a nucleus.	Peculiar arrangement for neurons that need to be synchronized.
Neurons originate and migrate from outside the brain.	Lack of migration leads to dysfunction (Kallmann).
Limited colocalization with other neurotransmitters.	Galanin is colocalized, and cosecreted with LHRH, modulating its action.
Absence of steroid receptors.	Steroids profoundly affect function. Actions on interneurons. Nongenomic effects?
Recurrent collateral innervation and connectivity.	Autoregulation of secretion and rhythmic activity.
Neuronal subpopulations may exist.	Specialized or distinct functions, endocrine and neural.

The total number of LHRH neurons in the rodent or primate brain is very small (ca. 1500 in the rat). Although small, this number may still be sufficient to maintain the principle of redundancy, which is a common feature in central neuronal systems. Evidence for this principle is afforded by the experiments involving transplantation of fetal hypothalamic neurons into the brains of hypogonadal mice that have a truncated LHRH gene and, consequently, do not express LHRH. In some cases in which some recovery of gonadal function was observed after neuronal transplantation, a very small number of LHRH-positive neurons (<10) was detected by immunocytochemistry, suggesting that a few neurons can provide adequate input to the pituitary (10). Another interesting anatomical feature is the fact that the LHRH neurons are not located in a single nucleus but, rather, are dispersed over the mediobasal hypothalamus (primate) or septal-preoptic (rodent) regions of the brain. Since physiological considerations suggest that these neurons must have synchronous activity (11), it is peculiar that they are not arranged in an anatomically restricted area, as is the case for other hypophysiotropic or magnocellular neuronal systems. Nevertheless, the fact that there is anatomical evidence for direct innervation of LHRH neurons by other (or even the same) LHRH neurons suggests that it is still feasible that the LHRH neuronal system is arranged in a syncytium-like structure, supporting the notion of synchronized activity. As discussed below, we have presented clear evidence indicating that LHRH can regulate its own secretion both in vivo and in vitro (12). Evidence has recently been presented to indicate that LHRH neurons originate outside of the brain and migrate, during the fetal period, to their final location in the brain (13). It has been reported that disorders in this migration process may

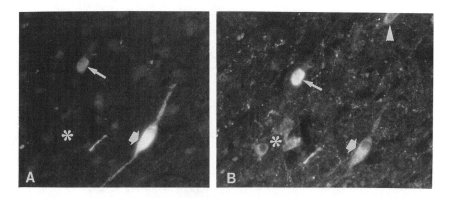

FIGURE 7.1. Colocalization of LHRH (A) and galanin (B) in the rat hypo-thalamus, using the indirect immunofluorescence technique. Identical arrows in A and B indicate perikarya immunoreactive for both peptides. Note that not every galanin-immunoreactive perikaryon is immunopositive for LHRH. Perikarya around asterisk and the perikaryon labeled with an arrowhead in B are immuno-positive for galanin but not for LHRH.

lead to hypothalamic hypogonadism, as is the case in patients with Kallmann syndrome. These aspects are discussed in detail elsewhere in this volume.

Galanin Colocalization with LHRH

Many hypophysiotropic peptidergic neurons have been shown to have a fair degree of colocalization with other neurotransmitters. LHRH neurons, on the other hand, have only recently been shown to contain galanin (14). The colocalization of galanin and LHRH (Fig. 7.1) appears to occur in a subpopulation of LHRH neurons, located mainly in the preoptic region. This colocalization appears to have important functional significance, since galanin can (a) enhance LHRH secretion (15), (b) be cosecreted with LHRH into the hypophyseal portal circulation (16), and (c) interact with LHRH to enhance its gonadotropin-releasing activity at the level of the anterior pituitary (16).

Is Regulation of LHRH by Steroids Receptor-Mediated?

Gonadal factors, both steroidal and peptide, have long been known to be important regulators of pituitary gonadotropin secretion. At least a portion of the gonadal influence over the gonadotropins is manifested through the brain and is expressed as alterations in the function of the LHRH system. In both sexes, gonadectomy induces a gradual reduction in the LHRH content of the median eminence (ME) and hypothalamus, while the levels of gonadotropins in plasma increase dramatically (17, 18).

A very important question regarding the effects of estrogens and androgens on LHRH mRNA levels, biosynthesis, processing, and secretion relates to the site of action where those effects may occur. The evidence presented so far indicates that LHRH neurons neither contain estrogen or other steroid receptors nor have the ability to take up labeled steroids (19). So how are steroids affecting the LHRH neuron? Several possible alternative explanations can be invoked. First, steroids are known to affect the neuronal activity of a number of peptidergic and aminergic neuronal systems which, in turn, are linked morphologically and/or functionally to the LHRH neurons. Second, it is still possible, albeit unlikely, that very low levels of steroid receptors, below the sensitivity of current assay systems, are present in the LHRH neurons. Nevertheless, if this postulate is correct, this very low level of receptors must be sufficient to convey the signal of the circulating steroids to affect LHRH gene expression. Third, steroids could exert their actions through nongenomic effects, interacting at the membrane level to modify neuronal activity and/or sensitivity to other neuronal input. Enhanced responsiveness to neurotransmitters may lead to second messenger stimulation of LHRH biosynthesis.

Recurrent Collateral Innervation: Possible Role in Autoregulation of LHRH Secretion

The presence of recurrent collateral innervation and synaptic-like contacts of LHRH within its own neuronal network provides an anatomical substrate supporting the concept that LHRH can modulate its own neuronal activity. This concept, which for neuroendocrine systems has been defined as "ultrashort loop feedback" mechanism, was first introduced as a hypothesis by Hÿppä et al. (20) to suggest that hypophysiotropic hormones may regulate their own secretion. Since then, direct evidence in support of this mechanism has been reported for somatostatin (21, 22), for growth hormone releasing hormone (23), and, more recently, for LHRH (12, 24), with both in vivo and in vitro paradigms. In the study of Valença et al. (12), daily, systemic administration of a potent LHRH agonist inhibited endogenous LHRH release into the hypophyseal portal circulation, both in intact and in orchidectomized animals. Similarly, LHRH-agonist-treated animals released less LHRH in vitro after membrane depolarization than untreated controls (12, 24). Significantly, addition of a potent LHRH antagonist to ME nerve terminals incubated in vitro enhanced basal secretion of LHRH, suggesting that binding of the antagonist to LHRH receptor sites blocked the inhibitory effect of endogenous LHRH on the secretory activity of the LHRH neuronal system. These observations strongly suggest that LHRH may modulate the neuronal activity of its own neuronal system and, further, point to a presynaptic regulatory mechanism for this system similar to that seen in classical monoaminergic neurotransmitter systems. The implications of these observations are numerous and, in particular, indicate that a recurrent inhibitory system may reside within the LHRH neuron, a characteristic shared by other neuronal systems with intrinsic, rhythmic activity. Since the LHRH neuronal network is thought to represent, or be part of, the "pulse generator" system responsible for the control of pulsatile gonadotropin secretion, it is plausible that the ultrashort loop-feedback system described above may play an important role in the pulse-generating capacity of this system.

Neuronal Subpopulations and Differential Activity Within the LHRH System

Some LHRH projections that originate from perikarya in the septal, preoptic, and suprachiasmatic regions do not form terminals in the median eminence and OVLT but reach diencephalic (via the stria medullaris thalami), telencephalic (via the stria terminalis), and lower brainstem regions (via the periventricular pathway and fasciculus retroflexus) (8). The functional significance of these projections is largely unknown. Since many of these pathways and their sites of projections are known to influence LH secretion, it is possible that they may operate as an intracerebral feedback circuit for LHRH. Some of these pathways may also be involved in behavioral aspects of reproduction. Through these pathways, LHRH neurons could interact with such distant and diverse structures as the olfactory system, cortex, hippocampus, and the mesencephalic central gray and raphe nuclei, all of which belong to the limbic system.

One important question regarding the functional anatomy of the LHRH neuronal system is related to how many of the LHRH neurons actually project to the median eminence, i.e., do all neurons project to the ME, including those that also project to extrahypothalamic regions, as discussed in the preceding paragraph, or are there specialized LHRH neurons subserving selective neuroendocrine or neuromodulatory roles? We addressed these questions in a recent study (25) in which the LHRH neurons projecting to the ME were identified by in vivo injection of a retrograde tracer, the lectin wheat germ agglutinin (WGA), into the external zone of the ME. Approximately 24 h after WGA injection, colchicine was given to interrupt axonal transport and enhance neuropeptide staining in the perikarya. Twenty-four hours later, the animals were sacrificed and the brains removed and stained for both WGA and LHRH using a dual immunocytochemical technique. The validation of the WGA technique has been presented earlier by Lechan et al. (26).

The data indicate that approximately 70% of the LHRH neurons in the telencephalon innervate the ME. These are the hypophysiotropic neurons whose function is regulation of the activity of the anterior pituitary. The remaining 30% of the LHRH cells project to brain regions other than the ME, where LHRH is likely to play a role as neurotransmitter or neuromodulator.

The results of this study (25) are in agreement with those of Silverman et al. (27) and Jennes and Stumpf (28), and suggest that LHRH neurons can be classified into two major functional groups: (1) those that project to the ME (hypophysiotropic neurons), and (2) those that project to other regions of the brain. The major function of the LHRH neurons that project to the ME is the regulation of LH and FSH release from the anterior pituitary. In those neurons that form axon terminals in other regions of the brain (8, 25) LHRH may function as a neurotransmitter and/or neuromodulator.

In addition to the two major groups of LHRH neurons (i.e., hypophysiotropic and nonhypophysiotropic), it is likely that certain hypophysiotropic LHRH neurons may give rise to axon collaterals and simultaneously innervate both the ME and other regions within the central nervous system (8). This possibility has not yet been explored experimentally, although branching of LHRH-containing axons has been observed (8). Studies currently under way in our laboratory address this question and will complete the characterization of hypophysiotropic LHRH neurons by identifying their collateral terminal fields with double retrograde labeling in combination with LHRH immunocytochemistry.

A distinct subpopulation of LHRH neurons has been uncovered recently in our studies of the colocalization of galanin and LHRH. As reported (14, 16), we observed that the neurons colocalizing LHRH and galanin are located primarily in a distinct area of the preoptic-anterior hypothalamic region, caudal to the OVLT (Fig. 7.2). Using fluorogold and double staining for LHRH and galanin, we were able to show that many of these neurons project to the median eminence and are functionally linked to the portal vasculature. These neurons are, therefore, "hypophysiotropic" (16). We have also observed a sex difference in the number of neurons coexpressing LHRH and galanin, with females having a 2–4-fold higher number than males. This difference appears to be estrogen-dependent. Thus, a distinct subpopulation of LHRH neurons is present, and "recruitment" of LHRH neurons into this subpopulation can be achieved by appropriate steroid priming. Although the full functional significance of these observations is still undetermined, the fact that galanin and LHRH are cosecreted into the portal vasculature and that both peptides show a cooperative interaction to stimulate gonadotropin secretion suggests an important functional role for this subset of LHRH neurons.

Studies Using an Immortalized LHRH Neuronal Cell Line

Recently, Mellon and coworkers developed the first neuroendocrine clonal cell line (29). These cells were derived from immortalized, hypothalamic LHRH cells that had been genetically targeted for tumorigenesis.

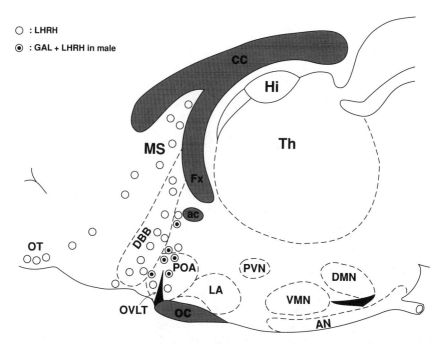

○ : LHRH

◉ : GAL + LHRH in male

FIGURE 7.2. Schematic representation of the distribution of neurons immuno-reactive for LHRH (open circles) or LHRH and galanin (closed circles) in a sagittal section of the male rat brain. Note that the perikarya containing both peptides are located in areas close to the organum vasculosum of the lamina terminalis (OVLT), such as the diagonal band of Broca (DBB) and medial preoptic area (POA). (ac: anterior commissure; AN: arcuate nucleus; CC: corpus callosum; DMN: dorsomedial nucleus; Fx: fornix; Hi: hippocampus; LA: lateral hypothalamus; MS: medial septum; OC: optic chiasm; OT: olfactory tubercle; PVN: paraventricular nucleus; VMN: ventromedial nucleus.)

Briefly, a gene construct, composed of the LHRH promoter coupled to the coding region of the simian virus 40 T antigen, was made. This construct was introduced into transgenic mice. Dispersed cells taken from an anterior hypothalamic tumor that had developed in one of the mice (GT-1) were purified and cloned. The cloned cells lines (GT1-1, GT1-3, GT1-7) have been reported: (1) to exhibit a neuronal phenotype and synthesize neuronal but not glial markers (29), (2) to express the LHRH mRNA (29), (3) to synthesize and release GnRH and GAP-immunoreactive (IR) materials (29, 30), and (4) to process the LHRH prohormone in a fashion similar to that described in the rat (30, 31).

Morphological Studies

Immortalized cells secreting LHRH from the GT1-7 subclone were charac-terized at the light (Fig. 7.3) and electron microscopic levels (29, 32).

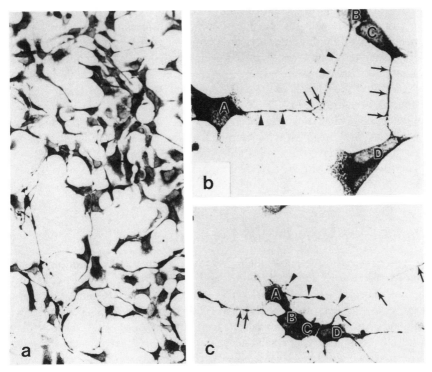

FIGURE 7.3. GT1-7 cells immunostained for GAP. (a) The cells are organized in clusters and contact each other by processes. (b) Thin processes (arrowheads) arising from neurons A and B seem to establish connections (double arrow). Cells C and D are interconnected by a single process (arrows). (c) Cell cluster consists of four neurons (A, B, C, D), all immunoreactive for GAP. The thin, axon-like fiber (arrows), originating from neuron D, gives rise to an axon-collateral (arrowheads) that contacts the perikaryon of neuron A. A beaded process (double arrow) also arises from neuron B.

The cells were fixed 18–36 h after their plating onto slides. LHRH and gonadotropin releasing hormone-associated peptide immunoreactivities were detected by immunocytochemistry using colloidal gold labeling (32). At the light microscopic level, these cultured cells exhibited such neuronal features as growing dendrites, varicose axons, and axon-collaterals. The cells formed clusters and presented a wide variety of contacts with each other. All of the cells showed both GAP and LHRH immunoreactivities in their cell bodies and processes. At the ultra-structural level, the nondividing cells possessed indented nuclei, well-developed Golgi complexes, a large number of ribosomes and secretory granules. Clathrin-coated vesicles were found in fusion with the plasma membrane. Neighboring neurons were coupled by tight junctions, while some of the cells with distinct locations were interconnected by neuronal processes. Colloidal gold particles, indicating GAP immunoreactivity, were associated with neurosecretory granules that were frequently situated beneath the plasma membrane (32). Ultrastructural double-labeling revealed that the same secretory vesicles contained both LHRH and GAP immunoreactivities (32). These data indicate that the cultured GT1-7 cells possess a neuronal phenotype, express LHRH and GAP immuno-reactivities, and establish morphological connections with each other, and thus that they may offer a suitable model for studying the subcellular regulatory mechanisms of LHRH production, processing and secretion in vitro (29, 32, 33).

Studies on LHRH Prohormone Processing

Recently, we conducted studies to biochemically and immunologically characterize the IR materials within and secreted from the GT1 cells and their 3 subclones (33). Both LHRH- and GAP-like IR materials were present in and secreted from these 4 cell lines. Up to 3% of the total cellular protein was composed of LHRH and GAP materials. When materials from the cell lysate and media were separated according to molecular weight (M_r), at least 3 different pro-LHRH species were detected. The GAP and LHRH antisera both recognized materials in the void volume, and at approximately 10,000 to 12,000 M_r and 8,300 M_r (Fig. 7.4). Materials that contained GAP-like IR eluted at approximately 6,600 M_r. This material is probably mouse GAP-(1-56), because it eluted on a reversed-phase column in the approximate position of rat GAP-(1-56). Two additional GAP-like forms were also found in media at approximately 3,500 and 2,800 M_r; however, these species were present in very low quantities. Cell lysates contained a single LHRH-like IR form that coeluted with synthetic LHRH. This material stimulated LH from anterior pituitary cells in a dose-response manner. By comparison, two different molecular forms of LHRH were detected in media at approximately 1,500 and 540 M_r. HPLC analyses revealed these peaks to be heterogeneous and to contain at least (Gln^1)-LHRH-$(Gly^{11}, Lys^{12}, Arg^{13})$, (Gln^1)-LHRH-(Gly^{11}, Lys^{12}), LHRH, and LHRH-(Gly^{11}). These experiments demonstrate that the GT1-derived cells contain and secrete multiple molecular forms of the pro-LHRH and that processing of the prohormone must involve (1) cleavage by an endopeptidase to give GAP-(1-56) and a C-terminally extended LHRH, (2) removal of C-terminal basic amino acids by a carboxypeptidase, (3) amidation of LHRH-(Gly^{11}) to LHRH, and (4) cyclization of glutamine to pyroglutamate at the N-terminal of LHRH. These results provide the first evidence for intermediates in the metabolic pathway of pro-LHRH to LHRH (33).

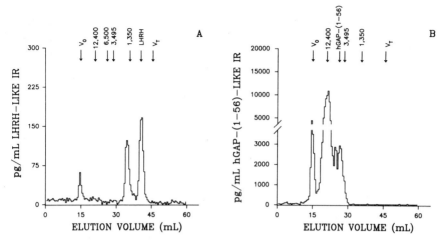

FIGURE 7.4. A chromatographic profile of LHRH- and GAP-like immunoreactive materials from media separated according to molecular weight. (A) Materials in media from GT1 cells were separated according to size and the fractions were screened with an LHRH (A772) antiserum. At the top of the figure the molecular weight markers can be found. V_0 refers to the void volume, while V_T represents the total volume. The elution position of synthetic LHRH is shown. The data are corrected for recovery of LHRH-like immunoreactivity, which was 83% from the GT1 media. (B) The fractions were further screened with a GAP (MC-2) antiserum. The elution position of synthetic hGAP-(1–56) is shown. The chromatogram is corrected for recovery of GAP-like immunoreactivity, which was 75.1% from the GT1 media.

Coupling Between Processing and Secretion of Pro-LHRH Peptides: Evidence for Spontaneous Pulsatile Activity

In more recent studies (34), we have examined processing of the LHRH precursor in media secreted from cells grown either on tissue culture plates or on cytodex beads and placed in a perifusion system. When grown on cytodex beads, the cells establish clear contacts with each other within the same bead and develop bridges across beads, creating a true syncytium, as ascertained by scanning electron microscopy analysis. The cells appear to be electrically coupled, since injection of the dye Lucifer Yellow in a single cell resulted, within minutes, in the spread of the dye to multiple perikarya and processes in the neighboring area (Armstrong, Wetsel, and Negro-Vilar, unpublished). When cells cultured in the cytodex beads matrix are placed in a perifusion system, and spontaneous release of LHRH and GAP is measured at frequent (5–10-min) intervals, it can be observed that secretion of LHRH, as well as GAP, is pulsatile

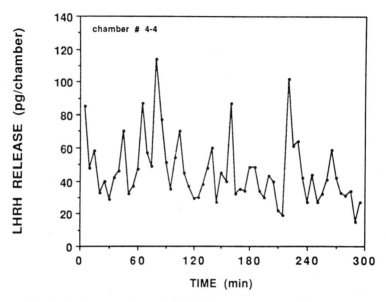

FIGURE 7.5. Pulsatile secretion of LHRH-like immunoreactivity from perifused GT1-7 cells grown on cytodex beads, loaded into a plastic syringe, and perifused with Krebs-Ringer bicarbonate glucose buffer. Perifusate was collected at 5-min intervals over a 5-h period under basal conditions. LHRH-like immunoreactivity was measured by RIA using A772 antiserum.

in nature (Fig. 7.5). Statistically defined pulses are detected using the algorithm "Detect." This observation strongly indicates that the LHRH neuronal system appears to have the intrinsic capacity to generate pulsatile secretory activity. Another important observation in using this system is that the GAP/LHRH ratio secreted in the perifusion system is much lower than that seen in static cultures, and it approaches the ratio (1 to 2) normally seen with hypothalamic tissue fragments.

Secretagogue-Induced LHRH and GAP Release: Novel Observations

Recently (35) we have perifused cells from the GT1-7 subclone and quantitated secretion of LHRH and GAP into the media in response to $[K^+]$-depolarization, phorbol 12,13-dibutyrate (PDBu), phospholipase C (PLC), and prostaglandin E_2 (PGE$_2$) stimulation. We have previously shown that all of these secretagogues can increase LHRH and GAP secretion in vitro from median eminence tissue fragments (4). A 4-fold stimulation of LHRH and GAP secretion from the cells was elicited with

56 mM $[K^+]$. Removal of the stimulus resulted in a rapid return to baseline for LHRH release, while the GAP return was slower. A similar magnitude of LHRH and GAP secretion was accomplished with 200 nM PDBu and 500 mU/ml PLC. As with $[K^+]$ depolarization, peak LHRH and GAP secretion was not necessarily coincident. Therefore, GAP to LHRH molar ratios differed during these secretory events. These data indicate that LHRH and GAP secretion from GT1-7 cells is regulated and that PDBu and PLC can stimulate release of these peptides to an extent similar to that seen with in vitro ME incubations. When 25 μM PGE_2 was added to the perifusate, LHRH secretion was significantly stimulated over baseline. The magnitude of LHRH secretion in response to PGE_2 in GT1-7 cells and ME nerve terminals is similar. Quantitation of PGE_2 levels in the perifusate of GT1-7 cells during basal or stimulated secretion with $[K^+]$, PDBu, or PLC revealed very low to undetectable levels. It appears that despite the well-known effect of $[K^+]$, PDBu, and PLC on PGE_2 secretion from ME tissue fragments in vitro, no PGE_2 is released by GT1-7 cells in response to these agents. This finding suggests that, under the above conditions, GT1-7 cells neither biosynthesize nor secrete PGE_2, although they are able to respond to exogenous PGE_2 as do LHRH neurons in situ. These results raise the possibility that neurotransmitters enhancing LHRH release through a PGE_2-mediated step actually act on an interneuron or cell and that the prostaglandin, therefore, activates LHRH secretion by an extracellular mechanism. In addition, the results also emphasize the importance of the use of this cell line, because it permits the mechanisms underlying basal and stimulated secretion of pro-LHRH-derived peptides to be studied in detail.

Concluding Remarks

As discussed above, the application of morphological, molecular biology, and cell biology techniques to the study of the LHRH neuronal system and its interaction(s) with the internal and external environment has greatly enhanced our understanding of the intrinsic mechanisms that play a key role in the developmental and regulatory aspects of reproductive functions. As is usually the case, each innovative approach has helped to answer some outstanding questions while, simultaneously, originating new questions addressing issues of increased complexity. Some of the fundamental questions in this field that have remained largely unanswered are: (1) how do steroids regulate LHRH and LH release? (2) what is the nature of the LHRH "pulse generator"? and (3) what is the relative contribution of each level of integration (hypothalamic, pituitary) to the overall response? However, the powerful approach of molecular biology combined with a judicious mix of other new or established techniques and, importantly, with the use of well-known and controlled reproductive models should greatly increase our understanding of the function of this key neural regulatory system. Indeed, the recently developed LHRH neuronal cell line appears to provide a unique opportunity to study the biosynthesis, processing, and secretion of LHRH, the intrinsic rhythmic activity of these cells, and the mechanisms that contribute to the establishment of coordinated pulsatile secretory activity in the LHRH neuronal system.

References

1. Mason AJ, Hayflick JS, Zoeller RT, et al. A deletion truncating the GnRH gene is responsible for hypogonadism in the hpg mouse. Science 1986;234: 1366–1371.
2. Crowley WF, Filicori M, Sratt DI, Santoro NF. The physiology of gonadotropin-releasing hormone (GnRH) secretion in men and women. Recent Prog Horm Res 1985;41:473–531.
3. Knobil E. The neuroendocrine control of the menstrual cycle. In: Recent Prog Horm Res 1980:53–88.
4. Negro-Vilar A. LHRH: physiology, pharmacology, and its role in fertility regulation. In: Paulson JD, Negro-Vilar A, Lucena E, Martini L, eds. Male fertility and sterility. New York: Academic Press, 1986:3–14.
5. Haisenleder DJ, Katt JA, Ortolano GA, et al. Influence of GnRH pulse amplitude, frequency and treatment duration on the regulation of LH subunit mRNAs and LH secretion. Mol Endocrinol 1988;2:338–343.
6. Conn PM. The molecular basis of gonadotropin releasing hormone action. Endocr Rev 1986;7:3–10.
7. Negro-Vilar A, Culler MD, Valença MM, Flack TB, Wisniewski G. Pulsatile peptide secretion: encoding of brain messages regulating endocrine and reproductive functions. Environ Health Perspect 1987;75:37–43.
8. Merchenthaler I, Görcs T, Sétáló G, Petrusz P, Flerkó B. Gonadotropin-releasing hormone (GnRH) neurons and pathways in the rat brain. Cell Tissue Res 1984;237:15–29.
9. Silverman AJ, Silverman R, Lehman MN, Witkin JW, Millar RP. Localization of a peptide sequence contained in the precursor to gonadotropin releasing hormone (GnRH). Brain Res 1987;402:346–350.
10. Gibson MJ, Krieger DT, Charlton HM, Zimmerman EA, Silverman AJ, Perlow MJ. Mating and pregnancy can occur in genetically hypogonadal mice with preoptic area brain grafts. Science 1984;225:949–951.
11. Knobil E. GNRH pulse generator. In: Delemarre-van de Waal HA, Plant TM, van Rees GP, Schoemaker J, eds. The control of the onset of puberty, III. Amsterdam: Elsevier, 1989.
12. Valença MM, Johnston CA, Ching M, Negro-Vilar A. Evidence for a negative ultrashort loop feedback mechanism operating on the LHRH neuronal system. Endocrinology 1987;121:2256–2259.
13. Schwanzel-Fukuda M, Pfaff DW. Origin of luteinizing hormone-releasing hormone neurons. Nature 1988;338:161–164.
14. Merchenthaler I, López FJ, Negro-Vilar A. Co-localization of galanin and luteinizing hormone-releasing hormone in a subset of preoptic-hypothalamic

neurons: anatomical and functional correlates. Proc Natl Acad Sci USA 1990;87:6326–6330.

15. López FJ, Negro-Vilar A. Galanin stimulates LHRH secretion from arcuate nucleus-median eminence fragments in vitro: involvement of an alpha-adrenergic mechanism. Endocrinology 1990;127:2431–2436.

16. López FJ, Merchenthaler I, Ching M, Wisniewski G, Negro-Vilar A. Galanin: a hypothalamic peptide with neuromodulatory and hypophysiotropic functions. Proc Natl Acad Sci USA 1991.

17. Kalra SP. Neural circuitry involved in the control of LHRH secretion: model for preovulatory LH release. In: Ganong WF, Martini L, eds. Frontiers in neuroendocrinology. New York: Raven Press, 1986:31–75.

18. Advis JP, McCann SM, Negro-Vilar A. Evidence that catecholaminergic and peptidergic (LHRH) neurons in suprachiasmatic-medial preoptic, medial basal hypothalamus and median eminence are involved in estrogen negative feedback. Endocrinology 1980;107:892–901.

19. Shivers BD, Harlen RE, Morrel JI, Pfaff DW. Absence of estradiol concentration in cell nuclei of LHRH immunoreactive neurons. Nature 1983; 304:345–347.

20. Hÿppä M, Motta M, Martini L. "Ultrashort" feedback control of follicle-stimulating hormone-releasing factor secretion. Neuroendocrinology 1971; 7:227–235.

21. Lumpkin MD, Negro-Vilar A, McCann SM. Paradoxical elevation of growth hormone by intraventricular somatostatin: possible ultrashort-loop feedback. Science 1981;211:1072–1074.

22. Abe H, Kato Y, Chihara K, Imura H. Central effect of somatostatin on the secretion of growth hormone in the anesthetized rat. Proc Soc Exp Biol Med 1978;159:346–349.

23. Lumpkin MD, Samson WK, McCann SM. Effects of intraventricular growth hormone-releasing factor on growth hormone release: further evidence for ultrashort loop feedback. Endocrinology 1985;116:2070–2074.

24. Zanisi M, Messi E, Proverbio MC, Motta M. Control of LHRH release: evidence for an "ultra-short" feedback mechanism [Abstract]. In: 67th annual meeting of the Endocrine Society. Baltimore, MD, 1985:271.

25. Merchenthaler I, Setalo G, Csontos C, Petrusz P, Flérko B, Negro-Vilar A. Combined retrograde tracing and immunocytochemical LHRH and somatostatin-containing neurons projecting to the median eminence of the rat. Endocrinology 1989;125:2812–2821.

26. Lechan RM, Nestler JL, Jacobson S. The tuberoinfundibular system of the rat as demonstrated by immunohistochemical localization of retrogradely transported wheat germ agglutinin (WGA) from the median eminence. Brain Res 1982;245:1–15.

27. Silverman AJ, Jhamandas J, Renaud LP. Localization of luteinizing hormone-releasing hormone (LHRH) neurons that project to the median eminence. J Neurosci 1987;7:2312–2319.

28. Jennes L, Stumpf WE. Gonadotropin-releasing hormone immunoreactive neurons with access to fenestrated capillaries in mouse brain. Neuroscience 1986;18:403–416.

29. Mellon PL, Windle JJ, Goldsmith PC, Padula CA, Roberts JL, Weiner RI. Immortalization of hypothalamic GnRH neurons by genetically targeted tumorigenesis. Neuron 1990;5:1–10.

30. Wetsel WC, Mellon PL, Weiner RI, Negro-Vilar A. Processing of the LHRH precursor in the GT1 cell lines derived from transgenic mice [Abstract]. Soc Neurosci Abstr 1990;16:284.
31. Wetsel WC, Culler MD, Johnston CA, Negro-Vilar A. Processing of the LHRH precursor in the preoptic area and hypothalamus of the rat. Mol Endocrinol 1988;2:22–31.
32. Liposits Z, Merchenthaler I, Wetsel WC, Mellon PM, Weiner R, Negro-Vilar A. Light and electron microscopic evaluation of immortalized hypothalamic luteinizing hormone-releasing hormone neurons. (Submitted for publication.)
33. Wetsel WC, Mellon PM, Weiner RI, Negro-Vilar A. Metabolism of pro-LHRH in immortalized hypothalamic neurons. (Submitted for publication.)
34. Wetsel WC, Valença MM, Mellon PM, Negro-Vilar A. Pro-LHRH processing in static and dynamic cultures of immortalized hypothalamic neuronal cells [Abstract]. In: Endocrine Society 1991.
35. Negro-Vilar A, Wetsel WC, Mellon PM, Valença MM. Secretagogue-stimulated secretion of LHRH and GAP elicited from a perifused, immortalized LHRH neuronal cell line [Abstract]. In: Endocrine Society 1991.

8

Theories of Luteinizing Hormone Releasing Hormone Neuronal Migration: Mechanisms and Biological Importance

MARLENE SCHWANZEL-FUKUDA AND DONALD W. PFAFF

Demonstration and Generality

Details of LHRH Cell Migration

LHRH in the Adult Vertebrate Brain

Luteinizing hormone releasing hormone (also called gonadotropin hormone releasing hormone) is a decapeptide present in the brain and nose of all species of vertebrates, including humans. Essential for reproductive functions, it has been shown to regulate the release of both luteinizing hormone and follicle stimulating hormone from gonadotropes of the anterior pituitary gland (1) and to facilitate reproductive behavior (2, 3).

In the brain, the cells that synthesize and release LHRH have been localized, by immunocytochemical procedures, in specific areas, including the accessory olfactory bulb, the olfactory tubercle, the nucleus and tract of the diagonal band, the septal and the preoptic areas, the organum vasculosum of the lamina terminalis, the hypothalamus, and the median eminence (4, 5). In adult animals, these LHRH neurons are not restricted to a discrete nuclear group. Instead, they appear to form a loosely organized continuum that can be traced through the specific brain regions described above, from the ventromedial forebrain to the hypothalamus. On the other hand, the axons of the LHRH cells, either side of the midline, converge in large numbers on the organum vasculosum of the lamina terminalis and the median eminence (6) and to a lesser extent on the subfornical organ (7), terminating on the capillary plexuses in these circumventricular organs.

LHRH in the Adult Vertebrate Terminalis Nerve

In the nose, LHRH has been localized in a population of ganglion cells and axons of the terminalis nerve (nervus terminalis), a cranial nerve found in all vertebrates that courses from the epithelium of the vomeronasal organ to the septal and preoptic areas of the brain (8, 9). The terminalis nerve, like the vomeronasal organ and nerve, develops from the medial part of the olfactory placode. Although there are some species-specific variations in the pattern of distribution of LHRH cells and axons in the brain, the distribution of this hormone in the ganglion cells and fascicles of the terminalis nerve is very similar across vertebrate species, as seen in guinea pigs (10, 11), rats (12–14), hamsters (15), opossums (16, 17), primates (18, 19), dolphins (20, 21), amphibians (22, 23), teleosts (24), and platyfish (25).

Studies of the Development of LHRH Neurons

Those studies that focused on the development of LHRH neurons, in guinea pigs (10, 11), rats (13), teleost fish (24, 26), and platyfish (25) showed that LHRH immunoreactivity was initially detected in ganglion cells of the terminalis nerve, before it was seen in any area of the brain. The striking association between LHRH neurons and the terminalis nerve in amphibians (22, 23) and teleosts (24) led these investigators to speculate that all LHRH cells are embryologically derived from the terminalis nerve and, in turn, the olfactory placode. However, LHRH cells were rarely seen in the epithelium of the olfactory pit in these animals. The majority of LHRH-immunoreactive cells were observed with branches of the terminalis nerve on the nasal septum, or coursing into the brain with the central roots of this nerve. Under these circumstances, a migration of cells, including LHRH cells, from the brain into the ganglia of the terminalis nerve was equally plausible. In fact, Pearson (27), in his study of the development of the terminalis nerve in humans, concluded that the ganglion terminale, the major ganglion of the terminalis nerve (28), received an influx of cells from the forebrain.

Origin and Migration of LHRH Neurons from the Olfactory Placode

Investigation into the origin of LHRH neurons in mice, using antisera to LHRH and immunocytochemical procedures, led to the discovery that LHRH neurons originate in the epithelium of the medial olfactory pit and migrate into the brain along branches of the terminalis and vomeronasal nerves (29–33). In mice, LHRH-immunoreactive neurons were first detected in the epithelium of the medial olfactory pit at about 11 days of gestation (the first day of pregnancy counted as "day 0"). At about 11.5 days they were seen turning out of the epithelium into the nasal mesenchyme, in company with axons of the terminalis and vomeronasal nerves, and by day 12 and 13 of embryonic life, cords of LHRH-immunoreactive cells were seen migrating across the nasal septum, toward the forebrain. By day 14 most of the LHRH neurons were observed in the anlage of the ganglion terminale, medial and caudal to the developing olfactory bulb, and in the central roots of the terminalis nerve as they entered the forebrain. The 16-day-old fetal mouse brain showed most LHRH-immunoreactive neurons arching through the forebrain into the preoptic area and the hypothalamus, and the migration of these cells was essentially over. From days 16 to 20 of gestation and in the newborn mouse, an increase in the number of LHRH-immunoreactive cells was seen in the septum, the preoptic area, and the hypothalamus, while a concomitant decrease was found in the epithelium of the medial olfactory pit and on the nasal septum. In contrast, we have not seen LHRH cells migrating from the ventricles of the brain, nor late-dividing LHRH cells in POA. Thus, increase in the number of LHRH-immunoreactive cells seen in the brain appears to be due to the migration of LHRH cells into the brain from the nose rather than to cell division within the brain.

Characteristics of Migrating LHRH Neurons

Combined Immunocytochemistry and Thymidine Autoradiography

Studies carried out in this laboratory using tritiated thymidine autoradiography in combination with LHRH immunocytochemistry showed that the uptake of radioactive precursor in the nuclei of LHRH-immunoreactive neurons was greatest in mice whose mothers were injected with tritiated thymidine on day 10 of pregnancy. No evidence of LHRH cell division was seen in the brain. Our finding of this brief period (days 10–11) in which LHRH neurons are generated is in agreement with that reported by Wray and coworkers (33).

In Situ Hybridization

Could the immunocytochemical product have originated outside the olfactory apparatus? In situ hybridization studies of the epithelium of the medial olfactory pit and adjacent nasal mesenchyme of 10-, 11-, 12-, and 13-day-old embryonic mice (33–35) demonstrated gene expression for LHRH by cells in the placode and their migration into the nasal mesenchyme. Wray and coworkers (33) saw cells expressing LHRH mRNA in the epithelium of the olfactory pit on embryonic day 11.5, and in greater numbers on the nasal septum on day 12.5, a developmental pattern identical to that seen by immunocytochemical procedures and antiserum to LHRH. Similar observations were made by Zheng et al. (34, 35) in 12- and 13-day-old embryonic mice; they also noticed the tendency of LHRH-expressing cells to form clumps.

Electron Microscopy

Examination of the ultrastructure of the migrating neurons from the epithelium of the olfactory pit (36, 37) showed two populations of cells with similar morphology, only one of which contained LHRH immuno-reactivity. Before and during migration, no LHRH immunoreactivity was seen in Golgi bodies or in neurosecretory granules. Zheng and coworkers surmised that these neurons do not have a secretory function before they attain their target organs. In support of this notion, a recent study, in rats, by Daikoku-Ishido et al. (38), presented evidence, based on intra-ventricular transplants of nasal placode and specific brain tissues, that LHRH neurons acquire secretory behavior in the presence of the medial basal hypothalamus.

Generality of the Phenomenon of LHRH Cell Migration

Since the original reports of the origin of LHRH cells from the olfactory placode and the migration of these cells into the brain (29–33), several studies have been carried out to test this hypothesis and/or to extend the generality of the phenomenon to other vertebrates.

Kallmann's Syndrome in Humans

By immunocytochemical procedures, we examined the brain and nasal regions of a 19-week-old male fetus that had Kallmann syndrome (hypogonadotropic hypogonadism with anosmia) (39). We compared the distribution of LHRH-immunoreactive cells and fibers in the Kallmann fetus with those obtained from the brain and nasal regions of three normal 19-week-old male fetuses. The results of our study (40) showed LHRH immunoreactivity to be present in cells and fibers in the brain and a few LHRH-immunoreactive cells in ganglia and axons of the terminalis nerve in each of the normal fetuses. The distribution of LHRH cells and fibers was in agreement with that described in the human fetus by other investigators (41–43). In the Kallmann fetus, no LHRH immunoreactivity was seen in any part of the brain. In striking contrast, in the nose of the Kallmann fetus, on either side, just lateral to midline, thick fascicles of LHRH-immunoreactive fibers and clumps of LHRH-immunoreactive cells were seen coursing up through the cribriform plate of the ethmoid bone, ending within the meninges on the dorsal surface of the cribriform plate, below the forebrain. The LHRH-immunoreactive neurons and fibers seen in the Kallmann fetus were entirely within the nose, in a pattern of distribution fitting that of the terminalis nerve, an important component of the migration route. The olfactory bulbs were absent in the Kallmann fetus, and neither the olfactory, vomeronasal, nor terminalis nerves were in contact with the forebrain, ending instead in neuromas within the meninges, either side of midline, below the forebrain. The symptoms of Kallmann's syndrome apparently can be ascribed to a failure of LHRH cells to migrate into the brain. In turn, these data support our hypothesis that LHRH cells originate from the olfactory placode, and they extend the generality of our findings from mice to humans.

Other Species

A recent study of the development of LHRH neurons in rhesus macaques, using immunocytochemistry and in situ hybridization procedures (19), presented convincing evidence, in this species, that LHRH cells originate from the olfactory placode and migrate into the brain along branches of the terminalis nerve. The neurons containing LHRH were first detected in the nasal epithelium, and then with nerve fibers on the developing nasal septum. Examination of the embryonic chick brain, by immunocytochemical procedures, revealed LHRH-immunoreactive neurons in the epithelium of the olfactory pit and showed the migration of these cells into the brain along fibers of the olfactory nerve (44). The localization of LHRH-immunoreactive cells in the epithelium of the olfactory placode in chicks and monkeys is similar to that seen in mice. In guinea pigs (10, 11), rats (13, 14), and opossums (16, 17), it may be that the LHRH neurons originate in the olfactory placode but do not begin synthesis of the hormone (detectable by specific antibodies to LHRH) until they have migrated out of the placode. A more recent study of the ontogenesis of LHRH neurons in rats (38) localized precursor molecules of LHRH in the epithelium of the newly formed vomeronasal organ at 13.5 days of gestation with antiserum to rat gonadotropic hormone releasing hormone-associated peptide 28–56 (rGAP) but not with antiserum to LHRH. They concluded that LHRH neurons originate in the epithelium of the nasal placode and migrate into the forebrain along the terminalis nerve (25, 34).

Specificity Among Neuroendocrine Peptides

In order to determine if other neurohormones originate in olfactory placode-derived tissues, Zheng and coworkers (34, 35) examined the nasal regions, including the epithelium of the medial olfactory pit, of 11-, 12-, and 13-day-old fetal mice, by immunocytochemical procedures using antisera to thyrotropin releasing hormone, corticotropin releasing hormone, oxytocin, vasopressin, neuropeptide Y, and somatostatin. This study confirmed the origin and migration of LHRH neurons, but none of the other antisera detected immunoreactive cells in the epithelia of the olfactory pit under the conditions tested. Thus it appears that LHRH neurons are unique among the neuroendocrine cells in their peripheral origin and migration into the brain.

Experiments Related to LHRH Cell Migration

An interesting study, recently undertaken by Livne and coworkers (45), transplanted nasal tissues from normal embryonic mice into the anterior hypothalamus or preoptic area of hypogonadal mice. These investigators found that the LHRH neurons retained some of their migratory potential after being transplanted into the brain; they were able to elaborate axonal projections to the median eminence, sufficient to induce gonadal recovery in the hypogonadal mice.

Cell culture of LHRH neurons, which would facilitate study of synthesis and secretion, has been hampered by the difficulty in obtaining sufficient numbers of these cells to grow in culture. In the adult vertebrate brain, LHRH neurons are rarely found in a compact group. However, Jorgenson and Pfaff (46) report that the tissues of the embryonic olfactory pit and adjacent nasal mesenchyme offer a source of LHRH neurons for successful tissue culture. The possibility of obtaining enough embryonic LHRH neurons for cell culture opens up a rich field for experimental manipulation, and further confirms the olfactory pit origin of LHRH-expressing cells.

Mechanisms

Association of LHRH Neurons with NCAM

In order to learn more about compounds that might guide the migration of LHRH neurons, we used immunocytochemical procedures with antisera to possible components of the migration route: cytotactin, CTB proteoglycan, fibronectin, laminin, and neural cell adhesion molecule (NCAM). In addition, we used antiserum to LHRH, to localize LHRH neurons along the course from the olfactory pit to the forebrain and to determine if any of these possible components were colocalized with LHRH in these neurons. The results of this study (47, 48) showed only neural cell adhesion molecule (of the components tested) to be present along the migration course of the LHRH cells.

Neural cell adhesion molecule is a cell surface glycoprotein produced by all nerve cells early in development. An integral membrane protein, it mediates cell-to-cell adhesion and it is present on the cell body, the neurites, and the tips of growing axons (49).

Pioneer Cells

Soon after the olfactory placode invaginates to form the olfactory pit, around day 10 of embryonic life, a few cells, showing NCAM immunoreactivity, begin to migrate out of the epithelium of the olfactory pit into the mesenchyme of the developing nose. The number of these "pioneer" NCAM-reactive cells increases and forms an aggregate between the olfactory pit and the anlage of the forebrain. Axons of the olfactory nerves (which also show NCAM immunoreactivity) grow into this cellular aggregate which, by late day 10, is in contact with the rostral tip of the ventromedial forebrain, the site of the future olfactory bulb. At about this same time, a secondary recess forms in the medial wall of the olfactory pit, giving rise to the anlage of the vomeronasal organ. Cords of the NCAM-immunoreactive cells and the axons of the developing vomeronasal and terminalis nerves (which also show NCAM immuno-reactivity) emerge from the epithelium of the medial olfactory pit and join the cellular aggregate below the forebrain.

Initial Appearance and Migration of LHRH Neurons

The events described above are soon followed by the appearance of LHRH-immunoreactive neurons in the epithelium of the medial part of the olfactory pit, and the migration of these cells into the forebrain along NCAM-immunoreactive branches of the terminalis and vomeronasal nerves that cannot be distinguished one from the other at this age.

The following four observations concerning the "pioneer" NCAM-immunoreactive cells and the migrating LHRH neurons were consistent for all the litters of mice we examined: (1) LHRH-immunoreactive cells are detected in the epithelium of the olfactory pit only after the forma-tion of the anlage of the vomeronasal organ; (2) the migrating LHRH neurons, in the nasal mesenchyme, are never seen independently of the NCAM-immunoreactive fascicles; (3) no LHRH-immunoreactive neurons are observed in the brain before the "bridge" of NCAM-immunoreactive cells and fibers is in place between the olfactory pit and the forebrain; and (4) NCAM and LHRH immunoreactivities do not appear to be colocalized in the migrating LHRH neurons.

In transverse sections through the head of an embryonic mouse, begin-ning about day 12, two parts of the NCAM-immunoreactive cellular aggregate can be distinguished: a lateral part that receives the axons of the developing olfactory nerves from the dorsal and lateral parts of the olfactory pit, and a medial part that receives the axons of the vomeronasal and terminalis nerves, and the cords of migrating LHRH neurons. The lateral part will develop into the olfactory nerve layer of the olfactory bulb, while the medial part, which serves as the entrance for LHRH cells into the brain, will form the ganglion terminale, the major ganglion of the terminalis nerve.

Perturbation Studies

Embryonic chick retinal tissues cultured in the presence of antibodies to NCAM (A-NCAM) show a disruption in the normal pattern of histio-genesis (50). Similarly, antibodies to Xenopus NCAM, incorporated into agarose gel spikes and implanted into the optic tecta of juvenile frogs that were undergoing regeneration of their retinotectal projections, resulted in the distortion of normal projections and a decrease in the precision of the projection pattern from the optic nerve (51). In the light of these findings, we were curious about the possible effects of A-NCAM on the migration of LHRH neurons from the epithelium of the olfactory pit into the forebrain, since NCAM appears to be a major component of the nerve fascicles that make up the migration route.

If *all* LHRH cells originate from the olfactory placode, then interruption of the migration route should result in an absence of LHRH cells in the brain. The following account summarizes our findings, so far (52).

Time-mated Swiss mice, on day 10 of pregnancy, were anesthetized with Metofane; the abdominal cavities were opened, the uterine horns were exposed, and 1 μl of A-NCAM (10 mg/ml) was injected by means of a glass micropipette and microliter syringe into the olfactory pit of each embryo of one uterine horn. Each embryo of one uterine horn of control animals received 1-μl injections of rabbit IgG (10 mg/ml) into the olfactory pit, or mechanical damage to the olfactory pit. The uninjected embryos of the second uterine horn, in each case, served as untreated controls. The pregnant mice were sacrificed on either day 11 or day 12; the embryos were collected, fixed in Bouin's solution, and embedded in paraffin. Serial 8-μm sections were prepared, and the tissues were examined by immunocytochemistry for the presence LHRH, NCAM, or IgG.

We determined that injection into the olfactory pit was successful when uptake of either the A-NCAM or the IgG was detected in the epithelium of the olfactory pit by the secondary antibody in our procedure, a goat antirabbit IgG. In most of these cases, immunoreactivity for either A-NCAM or IgG was also seen in the anterior pituitary. This was probably due to the fact that Rathke's pouch, just caudal to the olfactory pit, was still open at 10 days of embryonic life, and the injected substance flowed into and became incorporated into the epithelium as it closed off to form the anterior pituitary gland.

Those animals that showed an uptake of A-NCAM in the epithelium of the olfactory pit showed few or no LHRH-immunoreactive cells along the migration route on the nasal septum, and no LHRH cells in the brain. Untreated control animals, or those which were injected with A-NCAM but did not show uptake of the antibody, showed a normal distribution of LHRH-immunoreactive cells in the forebrain and among the NCAM-immunoreactive fascicles on the nasal septum. If any disruption of the NCAM "scaffolding" resulted from the single 1-μl injection of A-NCAM on day 10 of embryonic life, it was not readily apparent in our histologic preparations. It may be that the 1-μl injection of A-NCAM, while not sufficient at 10 E to disrupt the migration route itself, was sufficient to retard (or prevent) the migration of LHRH cells out of the epithelium of the olfactory pit.

There are undoubtedly complex forces and multiple signals involved in the orchestration of LHRH cell migration from the nose into the forebrain. The studies described above represent the beginning of our attempts to understand this interesting phenomenon. Mechanical forces might act either by excluding LHRH cells—for example, they cannot travel medially because of the septum, nor laterally because of the epithelial surface—or by propulsion. Similarly, chemical cues might act by attraction and by facilitating migration, as NCAM seems to do, or by halting migrating neurons, as we would expect from cytolactin (53, 54). The tendency of LHRH cells to cluster while migrating, their grouping as seen from in situ hybridization results, and their improved survival in culture when contacting each other all bring to mind the large body of work on yeast alpha mating factor (55). This peptide has interesting homology with LHRH and may offer clues as to mode of action and migration. In particular, these yeasts reproduce through a process of cellular aggregation that depends on cell surface agglutinins, which in turn are induced by the appropriate mating factors (56). A G-protein whose gene is expressed in the yeast, *S. cerevisiae*, has been implicated in the mating pheromone response pathway (57). Mechanisms of the mating response and its desensitization are being explored (58). It may be hoped that peptide homologies and cell behavior similarities portend some opportunities to use insights from yeast molecular biology for understanding LHRH neurons.

Biological Perspectives

Under what circumstances would there have evolved this situation in which LHRH neurons—already not a very large population of cells, considering that they control reproduction—must migrate from the olfactory placode to reach their functional positions in the basal forebrain? Basically, the answer to this question is unknown. One attempt in understanding offers an evolutionary perspective. Since the hypophyseal placode develops near the olfactory placodes, there may have been (before the evolution of hagfish, or lampreys) opportunities for LHRH neurons to control gonadotropes through paracrine mechanisms. After that period, as Rathke's pouch evolved to form the anterior pituitary gland, LHRH cells had to migrate and establish axonal connections in order to retain their influence over gonadotropes in the anterior pituitary gland. A second type of perspective depends on the reproductive physiology of aquatic animals. The activation of reproductive processes in such animals can depend on plant and animal pheromones, whose impact could rationalize the olfactory relations of LHRH neurons. Less obviously, physical changes in the nasal epithelium could mediate the environmental signals, such as water temperature, salinity, and hydrostatic pressure, all of which can regulate reproduction. In turn, depolarization of LHRH neurons by such signals could, through stimulus-secretion coupling, allow LHRH release.

References

1. Schally AV, Arimura A, Kastin AJ, et al. Gonadotropin-releasing hormone: one polypeptide regulates secretion of luteinizing hormone and follicle-stimulating hormone. Science 1971;173:1036-1038.
2. Pfaff DW. Luteinizing hormone-releasing factor potentiates lordosis behavior in hypophysectomized ovariectomized female rats. Science 1973;182: 1148-1149.
3. Moss RL, McCann SM. Induction of mating behavior in rats by luteinizing hormone-releasing factor. Science 1973;181:177-179.
4. Silverman A-J. The gonadotropin-releasing hormone (GnRH) neuronal systems: immunocytochemistry. In: Knobil E, Neill J, eds. The physiology of reproduction. New York: Raven Press, 1988:1283-1304.
5. Shivers BD, Harlan RE, Morrell JI, Pfaff DW. Immunocytochemical localization of luteinizing hormone-releasing hormone in male and female rat brains. Neuroendocrinology 1983;36:1-12.
6. Silverman A-J, Krey LC, Zimmerman EA. A comparative study of the luteinizing hormone-releasing hormone (LHRH) neuronal networks in mammals. Biol Reprod 1979;20:98-110.
7. Zheng L-M, Pfaff DW, Schwanzel-Fukuda M. Terminations of LHRH-immunoreactive fibers in the subfornical organ of the opossum: an ultrastructural study. Neuroendocrinology 1990;51:413-424.
8. Larsell O. The nervus terminalis. Ann Otol Rhinol Laryngol 1950;59: 414-435.
9. Bojsen-Moller F. Demonstration of the terminalis, olfactory, trigeminal and perivascular nerves in the rat nasal septum. J Comp Neurol 1975;159: 245-256.
10. Schwanzel-Fukuda M, Silverman A-J. The nervus terminalis of the guinea pig: a new luteinizing hormone-releasing hormone (LHRH) neuronal system. J Comp Neurol 1980;191:213-225.
11. Schwanzel-Fukuda M, Robinson JA, Silverman A-J. The fetal development of the luteinizing hormone-releasing hormone (LHRH) neuronal systems of the guinea pig brain. Brain Res Bull 1981;7:293-315.
12. Witkin JW, Silverman A-J. Luteinizing hormone-releasing hormone (LHRH) in rat olfactory systems. J Comp Neurol 1983;218:426-432.
13. Schwanzel-Fukuda M, Morrell JI, Pfaff DW. Ontogenesis of neurons producing luteinizing hormone-releasing hormone (LHRH) in the rat. J Comp Neurol 1985;238:348-364.
14. Jennes L. Prenatal development of the gonadotropin-releasing hormone-containing systems in rat brain. Brain Res 1989;482:97-108.
15. Jennes L, Stumpf WE. Luteinizing hormone-releasing hormone (LHRH) systems in the brain of the golden hamster. Cell Tissue Res 1980;209: 239-256.
16. Schwanzel-Fukuda M, Fadem BH, Garcia MS, Pfaff DW. Immuno-cytochemical localization of luteinizing hormone-releasing hormone (LHRH) in the brain and nervus terminalis of the adult and early neonatal gray short-tailed opossum (*Monodelphis domestica*). J Comp Neurol 1988;276:44-60.

17. Abraham S, Pfaff DW, Schwanzel-Fukuda M. Ontogenesis of neurons producing luteinizing hormone-releasing hormone (LHRH) in the brain and nervus terminalis and luteinizing hormone (LH) in the anterior pituitary of the gray short-tailed opossium (*Monodelphis domestica*). (Submitted for publication.)

18. Witkin JW. Luteinizing hormone-releasing hormone (LHRH) in olfactory systems in primates. In: Demski LS, Schwanzel-Fukuda M, eds. The terminal nerve (nervus terminalis): structure, function and evolution. Ann NY Acad Sci 1987;519:174–183.

19. Ronnekleiv O, Resco JA. Ontogeny of gonadotropin-releasing hormone-containing neurons in early fetal development of rhesus macaques. Endocrinology 1990;126:498–511.

20. Demski LS, Ridgway S, Schwanzel-Fukuda M. The terminal nerve of dolphins: gross structure, histology and luteinizing hormone-releasing hormone immunocytochemistry. Brain Behav Evol 1990;36:249–261.

21. Ridgway SH, Demski LS, Bullock TH, Schwanzel-Fukuda M. The terminal nerve in odeontocete cetaceans. In: Demski LS, Schwanzel-Fukuda M, eds. The terminal nerve (nervus terminalis): structure, function and evolution. Ann NY Acad Sci 1987;519:102–212.

22. Muske L, Moore FL. Luteinizing hormone-releasing hormone immunoreactive neurons in the amphibian brain are distributed along the course of the nervus terminalis. In: Demski LS, Schwanzel-Fukuda M, eds. The terminal nerve (nervus terminalis): structure, function and evolution. Ann NY Acad Sci 1987;519:433–446.

23. Muske L, Moore FL. The nervus terminalis in amphibians: anatomy, chemistry and relationship with the hypothalamic gonadotropin-releasing hormone system. Brain Behav Evol 1988;32:141–148.

24. Munz H, Class B. The terminal nerve and its development in teleost fishes. In: Demski LS, Schwanzel-Fukuda M, eds. The terminal nerve (nervus terminalis): structure, function and evolution. Ann NY Acad Sci 1987;519:50–59.

25. Halpern-Sebold LR, Schreibman MP. Ontogeny of centers containing luteinizing hormone-releasing hormone in the brain of the platyfish (*Xiphophorus masculatus*) as determined by immunocytochemistry. Cell Tissue Res 1983;229:75–84.

26. Stell WK, Walker SE, Ball AK. Functional-anatomical studies on the terminal nerve projection to the retina of bony fishes. In: Demski LS, Schwanzel-Fukuda M, eds. The terminal nerve (nervus terminalis): structure, function and evolution. Ann NY Acad Sci 1987;519:80–96.

27. Pearson AA. The development of the nervus terminalis in man. J Comp Neurol 1941;75:39–66.

28. Locy WA. On a newly recognized nerve connected with the forebrain of the selachian. Anat Anz 1905;26:33–63.

29. Schwanzel-Fukuda M, Pfaff DW. A proposed migratory route for luteinizing hormone-releasing hormone (LHRH) neurons from the medial olfactory placode to the forebrain in the mouse [Abstract]. Soc Neurosci Abstr 1988; 14:984.

30. Schwanzel-Fukuda M, Pfaff DW. Origin of luteinizing hormone-releasing hormone neurons. Nature 1989;338:161–164.

31. Schwanzel-Fukuda M, Pfaff DW. The migration of luteinizing hormone-releasing hormone (LHRH) neurons from the medial olfactory placode into the medial basal forebrain. Experientia 1990;46:956–962.
32. Wray S, Nieburgs A, Elkabes S. Spatiotemporal cell expression of luteinizing hormone-releasing hormone in the prenatal mouse: evidence for an embryonic origin in the olfactory placode. Dev Brain Res 1989;46:309–318.
33. Wray S, Grant P, Grainer H. Evidence that cells expressing luteinizing hormone-releasing hormone mRNA in the mouse are derived from progenitor cells in the olfactory placode. Proc Natl Acad Sci USA 1989;86: 8132–8136.
34. Zheng L-M, Schwanzel-Fukuda M, Hejtmancik JF, Gibbs RB, Pfaff DW. Properties of neuroendocrine cells migrating from the olfactory placode into the basal forebrain [Abstract]. Soc Neurosci Abstr 1990;16:953.
35. Zheng L-M, Schwanzel-Fukuda M, Gibbs RB, Pfaff DW. Properties of neuroendocrine cells migrating from the olfactory placode into the basal forebrain. (Submitted for publication.)
36. Zheng L-M, Pfaff DW, Schwanzel-Fukuda M. Electron microscopic identification of luteinizing hormone-releasing hormone (LHRH) immunoreactivity in olfactory placode-derived neurons [Abstract]. Soc Neurosci Abstr 1989;15: 1015.
37. Zheng L-M, Pfaff DW, Schwanzel-Fukuda M. Luteinizing hormone-releasing hormone (LHRH)-expressing cells in the medial olfactory placode and basal forebrain of mice during embryonic development. (Submitted for publication.)
38. Daikoku-Ishido H, Okamura Y, Yanaihara N, Daikoku S. Development of the hypothalamic luteinizing hormone-releasing hormone-containing neuron system in the rat: in vivo and in transplantation studies. Dev Biol 1990;140: 374–387.
39. Kallmann F, Schoenfeld WA, Barrera SE. The genetic aspects of primary eunuchoidism. Am J Ment Defic 1944;48:203–236.
40. Schwanzel-Fukuda M, Bick D, Pfaff DW. Luteinizing hormone-releasing hormone (LHRH)-expressing cells do not migrate normally in an inherited hypogonadal (Kallmann) syndrome. Mol Brain Res 1989;6:311–326.
41. Barry J. Characterization and topography of LHRH neurons in the human brain. Neurosci Lett 1976;3:287–291.
42. Paulin C, Dubois MP, Barry J, Dubois PM. Immunofluorescence study of LH-RH producing cells in the human fetal hypothalamus. Cell Tissue Res 1977;182:341–345.
43. Bugnon C, Bloch B, Fellman D. Cyto-immunological study of the ontogenesis of the gonadotropic hypothalamic-pituitary axis in the human fetus. J Steroid Biochem 1977;8:565–575.
44. Norgren RB, Lehman MN. Migration of LHRH neurons from the olfactory placode to the brain in the chick [Abstract]. Soc Neurosci Abstr 1990;16:649.
45. Livne I, Gibson MJ, Silverman A-J. Transplants of migratory GnRH cells into the brain are capable of inducing gonadal recovery in hypogonadal (HPG) mice [Abstract]. Soc Neurosci Abstr 1990;16:1284.
46. Jorgenson KL, Pfaff DW. Cell cultures of luteinizing hormone-releasing hormone neurons from embryonic mouse olfactory placode and nasal septum. (In preparation.)

47. Schwanzel-Fukuda M, Abraham S, Crossin KL, Edelman GM, Pfaff DW. Immunocytochemical demonstration of neural cell adhesion molecule (NCAM) along the migration route of luteinizing hormone-releasing hormone (LHRH) neurons in mice [Abstract]. Soc Neurosci Abstr 1990;16:398.

48. Schwanzel-Fukuda M, Abraham S, Crossin KL, Edelman GM, Pfaff DW. Immunocytochemical localization of neural cell adhesion molecule (NCAM) along the migration route of luteinizing hormone-releasing hormone (LHRH) neurons in mice. (Submitted for publication.)

49. Edelman GM. Cell adhesion molecules in the regulation of animal form and tissue pattern. Annu Rev Cell Biol 1986;2:81–116.

50. Buskirk DE, Theiry J-P, Rutishauser U, Edelman GM. Antibodies to a neural cell adhesion molecule disrupt histogenesis in cultured chick retinae. Nature 1980;285:488–489.

51. Fraser SE, Murray BA, Chuong C-M, Edelman GM. Alteration of the retinotectal map in *Xenopus* by antibodies to neural cell adhesion molecules. Proc Natl Acad Sci USA 1984;81:4222–4226.

52. Schwanzel-Fukuda M, Reinhard G, Abraham S, Crossin KL, Edelman GM, Pfaff DW. Antibodies to neural cell adhesion molecule (NCAM) disrupt the migration of luteinizing hormone-releasing hormone (LHRH) neurons into the brain in mice. (Submitted for publication.)

53. Tan S, Crossin K, Hoffman S, Edelman GM. Asymmetric expression in somites of cytotactin and its proteoglycan ligand is correlated with neural crest cell distribution. Proc Natl Acad Sci USA 1987;84:7977–7981.

54. Crossin K, Prieto A, Hoffman S, Jones F, Friedlander D. Expression of adhesion molecules and the establishment of boundaries during embryonic and neural development. Exp Neurol 1990;109:6–18.

55. Thorner J. Pheromonal regulation of development in *Saccharomyces cerevisiae*. In: Strathern JN, Jones EW, Broach JR, eds. The molecular biology of the yeast saccharomyces: life cycle and inheritance. Cold Spring Harbor, NY: Cold Spring Harbor Laboratory 1981:143–180.

56. Lipke PN, Wojciechowicz D, Kurjan J. A G α1 is the structural gene for the *Saccharomyces cerevisiae* α agglutinin, a cell surface glycoprotein involved in cell-cell interactions during mating. Mol Cell Biol 1989;9:3155–3165.

57. Dietzel C, Kurjan J. The yeast SCG1 gene: A G-like protein implicated in the a- and α-factor response pathway. Cell 1987a;50:1001–1010.

58. Dietzel C, Kurjan J. Pheromonal regulation and sequence of the *Saccharomyces cerevisiae* SST2 gene: a model for desensitization to pheromone. Mol Cell Biol 1987b;7:4169–4177.

9

Functional GnRH Neuronal Transplants in the Hypogonadal Mouse

Marie J. Gibson, Youichi Saitoh, Gregory M. Miller, and Ann-Judith Silverman

Transplantation of neuronal tissue containing GnRH cells into the brain of the mutant hypogonadal mouse has provided us with an important tool to study mechanisms of GnRH secretion. Lacking GnRH because of a deletion in the GnRH gene (1), the adult hpg mouse has an undeveloped reproductive system (2), but responds to implantation of normal fetal or neonatal preoptic area tissue grafts into the third ventricle of the brain with reproductive development. GnRH cells survive within the grafts (Fig. 9.1a) and innervate the median eminence of the host brains (Fig. 9.1b). Both male (3, 4) and female (5) hpg mice with grafts (hpg/POA) increase pituitary gonadotropin production, which results in gonadal development.

Our studies have revealed some remarkable capabilities in individual hpg/POA mice, and some "failures" of reproductive function, that together may prove important in elucidating basic mechanisms in the neuroendocrine regulation of reproduction. As there is only a small and discrete population of GnRH neurons supporting the components of reproductive activity in the hpg/POA, we may study integration of those cells in relation to the observed reproductive abilities in individuals. In this chapter we shall review our findings regarding the range of reproductive abilities in hpg/POA mice, and describe some of our recent approaches, using anatomical and pharmacological methods, to identify some of the connectivity that may underlie such capabilities.

Pulsatile LH Secretion in hpg/POA Male and Female Mice

Reproductive development is dependent on pulsatile secretion of GnRH (6), which stimulates the phasic release of pituitary LH; indeed, tonic

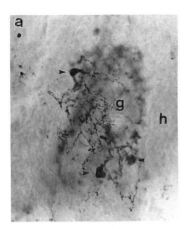 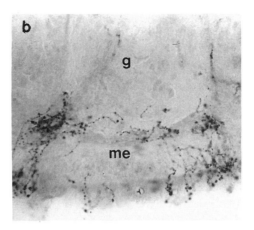

FIGURE 9.1. GnRH immunocytochemistry in an hpg mouse with a POA graft. (a) GnRH neurons (arrowheads) are present within the graft in the third ventricle of the host (h). (b) GnRH fibers exit the graft and primarily innervate the lateral median eminence (me) of the host animal.

GnRH administration results in decreased gonadotropin secretion (7). Therefore a basic question was to evaluate the presence of pulsatile LH secretion in hpg/POA mice. In male mice we demonstrated LH pulses in 11 of 19 castrated hpg/POA, and the characteristics of these pulses did not differ from those in castrated normal males (8). Similarly, significant LH pulses were detected in 9 of 13 hpg/POA ovariectomized female mice and in 9 of 10 normal ovariectomized female mice (9). This suggests a high degree of coordination among the grafted cells and/or between graft and host. Although LH pulse frequency did not differ between normal and hpg/POA female mice (Table 9.1), mean plasma LH and pulse amplitude were higher in the normal ovariectomized animals. There was a similar but insignificant tendency to higher LH levels in normal castrated males. This will be discussed later in regard to negative feedback. Hpg/POA animals in which we detected LH pulsatility were similar in gonadal development (8, 9) to those in which pulses were not apparent, and numbers of GnRH neurons within the grafts and innervation of the host brains were not predictive (8). Although it may be that grafts failed to support pulsatility in a few cases, it is more likely, in view of the reproductive development present in some of the "nonpulsers," that pulses occurred outside of the 4-h sampling period, or were below the limits of the LH assay. That POA grafts support episodic LH release in the majority of hpg/POA mice tested suggests the presence of a functional GnRH pulse generator in these animals.

TABLE 9.1 Measures of pulsatile LH secretion in ovariectomized normal and ovariectomized hypogonadal mice with preoptic area brain grafts (hpg/POA).

	Normal		hpg/POA	
	Pulsing	Nonpulsing	Pulsing	Nonpulsing
Plasma LH (ng/ml)	1.07 ± 0.16 (9)	0.61 (1)	0.49 ± 0.08** (9)	0.34 ± 0.03 (4)
Pulse amplitude (ng/ml)	1.92 ± 0.53 (9)		0.63 ± 0.28 * (9)	
Pulse frequency (per hour)	0.86 ± 0.13 (9)		0.61 ± 0.13 (9)	
Interpeak interval (min)	81.7 ± 20.3 (8)		93.2 ± 24.0 (6)	

Note: Values are expressed as the mean ± SEM. The numbers of animals are in parentheses.
*P < 0.05, **P < 0.005, vs. normals.
Source: Reprinted with permission from Ref. 9, © by The Endocrine Society, 1989.

Ovulation in the Female hpg/POA Mouse

In the adult female hpg/POA mouse the first sign of a successful POA graft is vaginal opening, which occurs at puberty in normal female mice and may be seen as soon as 8 days after graft surgery. This is followed by initiation of persistent vaginal estrus. The absence of corpora lutea in the stimulated ovaries confirms the absence of normal spontaneous ovulatory cycles. However, if hpg/POA females in persistent estrus are mated with normal males, reflex ovulation often occurs (10), with an LH surge evident within minutes of mating (11), implying neural regulation of the grafted GnRH cells and/or their fiber outgrowth by the host animal. These hpg/POA females display sexual behavior that is comparable to that seen in normal mice during the receptive period of the ovulatory cycle (12).

Positive Feedback in hpg/POA Mice

Despite the interesting implications of the ability of hpg/POA mice to show reflex ovulation, we also wished to evaluate why we did not see the more species-typical spontaneous ovulation, which is related to responsivity to changes in gonadal steroids. When we tested such sensitivity by challenge with progesterone, we found that approximately 30% of hpg/POA mice in persistent estrus respond to this steroid administration with an LH surge and ovulation (13). This indicates the ability of grafted GnRH cells (at least in these individuals) to respond to alterations in the hormonal milieu with a "positive feedback" response. In the course of the progesterone challenge studies, some animals were subsequently paired with males, to determine whether both reflex and steroid-induced ovulation is present in the same individuals. (The answer was sometimes, but not always.) After delivering her litter, one animal (who had shown the greatest LH response to progesterone challenge) mated again during the immediate postpartum period and delivered a second litter. Following weaning of all offspring, this hpg/POA mouse displayed spontaneous ovarian cyclicity, confirmed by ovarian histology (13). This first proven example of spontaneous ovulation in a mutant mouse with a brain graft alerted us to look more closely at postpartum females, and we have since identified additional mice that began spontaneously cycling after weaning their young. The results show that some hpg/POA mice are capable of positive feedback responses, and, rarely, of becoming spontaneous ovulators.

Effect of Interruption of Persistent Estrus on Capacity for Positive Feedback

We detected evidence of spontaneous ovulation only in mice that previously had persistent estrus (with its chronic exposure to estrogen) interrupted by pregnancy and lactation. Defects in positive feedback responsivity are described in many models of prolonged persistent estrus, including aged mice in which the ratio of circulating estrogen to progesterone is substantially greater than in younger, cycling mice (14). Positive feedback to a steroid challenge after acute ovariectomy is severely impaired in aged mice, but is present if long-term ovariectomy has prevented chronic exposure to the inappropriate steroid ratio (15). Therefore we tested the hypothesis that interruption of prolonged persistent estrus by long-term ovariectomy would enhance the likelihood of positive feedback in hpg/POA mice. Hpg/POA females were ovariectomized 6 weeks after graft surgery (about 3 weeks after persistent estrus began) and were tested 3 months later. While normal females ovariectomized at 6 weeks of age had significantly enhanced positive feedback to sequential administration of estradiol benzoate and progesterone, hpg/POA mice had minimal LH secretion after long-term ovariectomy (16). These findings indicate that whether or not prolonged exposure to estrogen has a deleterious effect, its absence is not sufficient to reveal positive feedback capability in hpg/POA mice.

The finding of spontaneous cyclicity occurring in some hpg/POA mice after bearing and weaning litters suggested that perhaps induced pseudopregnancy would reveal the capacity for spontaneous ovulation in these animals. Vaginal cytology was followed in hpg/POA females (n = 12) after graft surgery. When the mice had been in persistent estrus for 5 weeks, they were given progesterone capsules for 3 weeks. Vaginal smears were almost entirely leukocytic during this period. Four of the mice had 1 or 2 apparent cycles, and then returned to persistent vaginal estrus. Eight mice returned to persistent estrus after progesterone removal, and 2 mice continued to show leukocytic smears indefinitely. The results suggest that although prolonged progesterone exposure as in pregnancy is not in itself sufficient to induce spontaneous cyclicity in most hpg/POA mice, it may be a factor.

The evolutionary explanations for the two types of ovulation, reflex and spontaneous, are discussed by Ramirez and Beyer (17). It has been suggested that reflex ovulation may be the "earlier" form and that the capacity for it coexists with spontaneous ovulation in those species that are normally spontaneous ovulators (see 18, also); in contrast, positive feedback is deficient in reflex ovulators. That we see reflex ovulation more readily in hpg/POA mice may support the concept that it is a more simply induced form of ovulation, in that less specific afferents to GnRH are required.

Negative Feedback in hpg/POA Mice

It was surprising, in view of the reproductive accomplishments such as reflex ovulation and spontaneous ovulatory cyclicity described above, to discover that "classical" negative feedback is largely absent in both male and female hpg/POA mice. Neither castration nor testosterone administration affects pituitary LH or FSH content (19) or plasma LH levels (16) in male hpg/POA mice. Most hpg/POA female mice also failed to show negative feedback (16). Among the mice that did not increase LH secretion after ovariectomy were some that were capable of a positive LH response to steroid challenge or had previously ovulated (Fig. 9.2). Of 24 hpg/POA females studied in three experiments, just 2 animals had increased plasma LH levels after gonadectomy (not shown) and in only 1 of these was plasma LH suppressed by estradiol treatment. Neither of these animals had shown positive feedback to a steroid challenge. Thus the ability of an individual hpg/POA mouse to show the positive feedback response of increased LH secretion after acute steroid challenge does not predict the ability to show the negative feedback response of increased LH secretion in the chronic absence of steroids. These findings clearly demonstrate that separate components of neuroendocrine function may be dissociated in the hpg mouse bearing a POA graft. As such a large proportion of hpg/POA mice show pulsatile LH secretion in contrast to the very rare ability for negative feedback, for example, it is evident that different degrees of integration of the grafted GnRH neurons are necessary for each neuroendocrine capability. Future studies may permit us to correlate specific anatomical connectivity with particular neuroendocrine constituents.

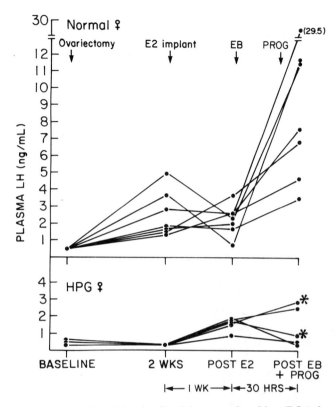

FIGURE 9.2. Negative and positive feedback in normal and hpg/POA female mice. Normal females showed the negative feedback response of increased LH secretion after ovariectomy and suppression after E2 implant, and the positive LH response to sequential challenge with estradiol benzoate (EB) and progesterone (PROG). No hpg/POA mice in this group showed negative feedback, including 2 (*) that had previously mated and borne litters. Reprinted with permission from Ref. 16, © by The Endocrine Society, 1989.

Modulators of GnRH Release in hpg Mice with POA Grafts

In the normal animal, GnRH secretion is influenced by many neuro-modulators. Important among these are the catecholamines, whose effect on LH secretion through stimulation or inhibition of GnRH release is widely reported (20, 21) and the neurotransmitter GABA, which is primarily inhibitory (22, 23). Several peptide hormones have also been implicated in regulation of LH release, with inhibitory actions seen with β-endorphin (24) and CRF (25). A primary candidate as an important stimulus to LH release in steroid-primed animals is neuropeptide Y (26).

We have identified many of these neuromodulators within POA grafts in hpg mice (Fig. 9.3; 27, 28). It should be noted that cell bodies of several of these candidates may often be localized within the graft, including dopamine, GABA, neuropeptide Y, and vasoactive intestinal polypeptide (11). We have identified innervation of grafts by other neuro-modulators that clearly enter the graft from the host brain, including adrenergic (identified by the rate-limiting enzyme phenylethanolamine N-methyltransferase [28]) and beta-endorphin (Fig. 9.3) fibers.

There is considerable evidence in the normal animal that the ovulatory LH surge follows increased GnRH neuronal activity (29–31). As GnRH neurons do not concentrate steroids (32), it is widely accepted that some neuromodulator(s) convey(s) information regarding the steroid milieu. It is not known whether these are identical to or different from the mediator(s) of the sensory input that results in reflex ovulation. We have shown that there is a population of estradiol-concentrating cells in POA grafts in hpg female mice (33) that may be able to relay information to

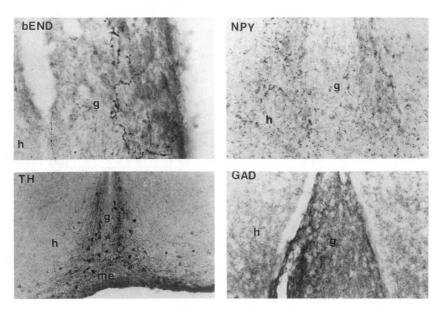

FIGURE 9.3. Representative neurotransmitter systems present in POA grafts within the third ventricle of hpg mice. (A) Beta-endorphin (bEND) fibers enter the graft (g). The cells of origin are the arcuate nucleus of the host (h). (B) Neuropeptide Y (NPY) fibers are present within most grafts and may originate from grafted cells or from the host. (C) Tyrosine hydroxylase (TH)-positive cells concentrate at the level of the medial basal hypothalamus, continuous with TH+ cells in the arcuate nucleus. (me: median eminence.) (D) Glutamic acid decarboxylase (GAD)-immunoreactive terminals ramify throughout the entire graft. GAD is the enzyme marker for GABA. Reprinted with permission from Ref. 27, © by Harwood Academic Publishers.

grafted GnRH neurons. There is also a normal distribution of estradiol-concentrating cells within the hpg brain, but we do not yet know which, if any, of these neurons are carrying out this function.

As noted above, many of these neuromodulators are endogenous to the POA grafts. Therefore we are employing various tracing techniques to identify specific afferents to intragraft GnRH neurons. Ultrastructural studies have established the presence of synapses on GnRH dendrites and soma within POA grafts (34), but associated tracing studies are necessary to establish the host origin of these afferents. Attempts to inject retrograde tracers into the intraventricular grafts in animals after physiological testing have been difficult to accomplish. Even when the graft is localized accurately, the fine glass micropipette often appears to be deflected, apparently by gliosis around the graft. We have recently employed a more effective technique. The carbocyanine dye DiI (35) may be used in fixed tissue to trace both afferents and efferents. The first and most striking observation was that graft outgrowth was almost exclusively directed to the median eminence (36). Only a few examples of fibers entering the arcuate nucleus (Fig. 9.4a) or leaving the median eminence and projecting more laterally were noted. In addition, retrogradely labeled cells were within the host arcuate nucleus (Fig. 9.4b), indicating that this cell group in turn innervates the graft. This is consistent with the immunocytochemical studies that often show beta-endorphin innervation. Systematic tracing studies in animals that have or have not shown particular neuroendocrine capabilities may help us to clarify the role of specific neuronal pathways in mediating certain responses.

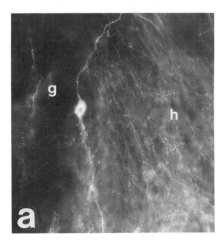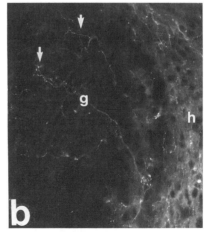

FIGURE 9.4. The tracer, DiI, was applied to the hypothalamus of an hpg/POA host. (a) A retrogradely labeled neuron within the graft projects to the arcuate nucleus of the host brain. (b) Anterogradely labeled fibers enter the graft (g) from the host (h).

Role of Excitatory Amino Acids in Normal and hpg/POA Mice

In addition to the anatomical studies described above, we have initiated a series of experiments using pharmacologic tools to analyze the influence of various modulators on GnRH release in both normal and hpg/POA mice. Numerous studies have implicated endogenous excitatory amino acids as important regulators of GnRH secretion. Peripheral or central administration of glutamate (37), aspartate (38), NMDA or kainic acid (39), and quinolinic acid (40) increases plasma LH levels in male and female rodents and primates. The effect appears to be suprapituitary, since neither NMDA nor glutamate stimulates pituitary LH secretion in vitro (41, 42), and NMDA-induced LH release is abolished by prior treatment with a GnRH receptor antagonist (43). Studies using specific blockers suggest a physiological role for endogenous excitatory amino acids in the onset of puberty (44), in the postovariectomy increase in LH, in the E_2-induced LH surge in the peripubertal (45) and mature ovariectomized rat (46), and in pulsatile LH release in the male rat (47).

We examined the effect of NMDA of LH release in normal and hpg/POA intact and castrated male mice and in normal and hpg/POA ovariectomized and ovariectomized/estrogen-primed female mice (48). Additional groups of normal cycling and hpg/POA female mice that were spontaneously cycling after reflex ovulation-induced pregnancies were tested on the day of estrus. To assess whether pituitary responsivity was a factor in the level of LH release to NMDA, we also challenged selected mice in each group with exogenously administered GNRH. None of the mice increased LH secretion to control injections of saline.

There were significant increases in plasma LH in all normal intact and castrated males. The response to NMDA was higher in castrates, but GnRH challenge tests indicated that this was due to increased pituitary responsivity in this group, rather than a central effect of testicular hormones on GnRH sensitivity to NMDA. In contrast to the significant responses in all normal males tested, only 3 of 17 hpg/POA males tested, whether intact or castrated, increased LH secretion in response to NMDA. Interestingly, pituitary sensitivity to GnRH was heightened in the hpg/POA males as compared with the normal males, and thus was not a factor in the absence of response to NMDA.

In normal female mice there was a greater LH response to NMDA in ovariectomized than in ovariectomized/estrogen-primed animals, that was not correlated to pituitary sensitivity to GnRH, suggesting that estrogen modulates GnRH sensitivity to NMDA. On the other hand, in hpg/POA female mice there was a significant correlation between increases in plasma LH in response to NMDA and plasma LH responses to GnRH challenge. Thus, although most ovariectomized and ovariectomized/

estrogen-primed hpg/POA mice responded to NMDA (in contrast to hpg/POA male mice), the effect of estrogen appeared to be at the level of the pituitary, rather than in the CNS, as it appeared to be in normal female mice. To our surprise, neither the normal intact females tested in estrus nor the hpg/POA females tested in estrus (who had previously shown the important reproductive responses of *both* reflex and spontaneous ovulation!) increased LH secretion after NMDA treatment. This appeared to be due to low gonadotrope sensitivity to GnRH in this stage of the cycle.

It is not established whether NMDA acts directly on GnRH cell bodies or on terminals in the median eminence, or whether its effect is via interneurons that synapse on GnRH cell bodies or axons. There are contradictory reports of a dose-dependent stimulation of GnRH release from the medial basal hypothalamus by kainic acid and NMDA, with one study reporting NMDA twice as effective as kainic acid and its action blocked by addition of AP5 (49), a specific antagonist. Another study found kainic acid and glutamate to be more effective than NMDA (50) and in this case the effects of glutamate were blocked by the non-NMDA antagonist DNQX, but not by the NMDA antagonist AP7, providing evidence that non-NMDA receptors primarily mediate the excitatory actions of glutamate on GnRH release from nerve terminals in the arcuate-median eminence region. Thus, as suggested (50), NMDA action may be primarily in the preoptic area, consistent with the report that direct injection of 50 pmol NMDA in the MPOA but not the VMH or arcuate nucleus of adult male rats (51) stimulates LH release.

From our results it is apparent that NMDA is not acting directly on GnRH terminals in the median eminence, since in that case a much higher number of hpg/POA males would have been expected to respond. We have consistently shown that GnRH innervation of the host's median eminence (Fig. 9.1) is a hallmark of grafts that support gonadal development in hpg mice. Studies using peripheral injections of the tracer, fluorogold, showed that in intact normal males approximately two thirds of GnRH neurons contained FG and therefore both projected outside of the blood brain barrier and were sufficiently active to capture tracer. Hpg males with testicular development were examined 90 days after grafting, and the percentage of GnRH neurons with fluorogold varied from 17% to 75%, indicating that at least that many GnRH neurons within the graft sent their axons into the host (52). It is thus more likely that GnRH release in response to NMDA is being modulated by some other neuronal input that is directly affected by NMDA. The afferents of such a proposed intermediary could act either at the GnRH cell body or on GnRH terminals in the median eminence. Similar or different modulation of the effects of NMDA may be involved in the central role of estradiol in modifying GnRH responsivity that we observed in female mice. We have begun studies to evaluate possible intermediaries in these effects.

Conclusion

Separate facets of reproductive function may be supported to varying degree in individual hpg recipients of POA grafts, ranging from a high percentage of hosts displaying pulsatile LH secretion to almost none able to show classical negative feedback. Since all these components are driven by GnRH secretion from the grafted neurons, it is clear that the grafts—and the extent to which they are integrated with the host brain— are able to provide us with clues as to the regulatory site/mechanism of GnRH secretion that supports a given neuroendocrine response.

Acknowledgment. This research was supported by NIH Grants NS20335 and HD19077.

References

1. Mason AJ, Hayflick JS, Zoeller RT, et al. A deletion truncating the gonadotropin-releasing hormone gene is responsible for hypogonadism in the hpg mouse. Science 1986;234:1366–71.
2. Cattanach BM, Iddon CA, Charlton HM, Chiappa SA, Fink G. Gonadotropin-releasing hormone deficiency in a mutant mouse with hypogonadism. Nature 1977;269:338–40.
3. Krieger DT, Perlow MJ, Gibson MJ, et al. Brain grafts reverse hypogonadism of gonadotropin releasing hormone deficiency. Nature 1982;298:468–71.
4. Silverman AJ, Zimmerman EA, Gibson MJ, et al. Implantation of normal fetal preoptic area into hypogonadal (hpg) mutant mice: temporal relationships of the growth of GnRH neurons and the development of the pituitary/testicular axis. Neuroscience 1985;16:69–84.
5. Gibson MJ, Charlton HM, Perlow MJ, Zimmerman EA, Davies TF, Krieger DT. Preoptic area brain grafts in hypogonadal (hpg) female mice abolish effects of congenital hypothalamic gonadotropin-releasing hormone (GnRH) deficiency. Endocrinology 1984;114:1938–40.
6. Carmel PW, Araki S, Ferin M. Pituitary stalk portal blood collection in rhesus monkeys: evidence for pulsatile release of gonadotropin-releasing hormone (GnRH). Endocrinology 1976;99:243–8.
7. Belchetz PE, Plant TM, Nakai Y, Keogh EJ, Knobil E. Hypophysial responses to continuous and intermittent delivery of hypothalamic gonadotropin-releasing hormone. Science 1978;202:631–3.
8. Kokoris GJ, Lam NY, Ferin M, Silverman A-J, Gibson MJ. Transplanted gonadotropin-releasing hormone neurons promote pulsatile luteinizing hormone secretion in congenitally hypogonadal (hpg) male mice. Neuroendocrinology 1988;48:45–52.
9. Gibson, MJ, Miller GM, Silverman AJ. Pulsatile LH secretion in normal female mice and in hypogonadal female mice with preoptic area implants. Endocrinology 1991.
10. Gibson MJ, Krieger DT, Charlton HM, Zimmerman EA, Silverman AJ,

Perlow MJ. Mating and pregnancy can occur in genetically hypogonadal mice with preoptic area brain grafts. Science 1984;225:949–51.

11. Gibson MJ, Moscovitz HC, Kokoris GJ, Silverman A-J. Plasma LH rises rapidly following mating in hypogonadal female mice with preoptic area (POA) brain grafts. Brain Res 1987;424:133–8.

12. Gibson MJ, Moscovitz HC, Kokoris GJ, Silverman AJ. Female sexual behavior in hypogonadal mice with GnRH-containing brain grafts. Horm Behav 1987;21:211–22.

13. Gibson MJ, Kokoris GJ, Silverman A-J. Positive feedback in hypogonadal female mice with preoptic area brain transplants. Neuroendocrinology 1988; 48:112–9.

14. Nelson JF, Felicio LS, Osterburg HH, Finch CE. Altered profiles of estradiol and progesterone associated with prolonged estrous cycles and persistent vaginal cornification in aging C57BL/6J mice. Biol Reprod 1981;24:784–91.

15. Mobbs CV, Flurkey K, Gee DM, Yamamoto K, Sinha YN, Finch CE. Estradiol-induced adult anovulatory syndrome in female C57BL/6J mice: age-like neuroendocrine, but not ovarian impairments. Biol Reprod 1984;30: 556–63.

16. Gibson MJ, Silverman A-J. Effects of gonadectomy and treatment with gonadal steroids on luteinizing hormone secretion in hypogonadal male and female mice with preoptic area implants. Endocrinology 1989;125:1525–32.

17. Ramirez VD, Beyer C. The ovarian cycle of the rabbit: its neuroendocrine control. In: Knobil E, Neill J, eds. The physiology of reproduction. New York: Raven Press, 1988:1873–92.

18. Jochle W. Coitus-induced ovulation. Cotraception 1973;7:523–64.

19. Charlton HM, Jones AJ, Ward BJ, Detta A, Clayton RN. Effects of castration or testosterone implants upon pituitary function in hypogonadal mice bearing normal foetal preoptic area grafts. Neuroendocrinology 1987;45: 376–80.

20. Barraclough CA, Wise PM, Selmanoff MK. A role for hypothalamic catecholamines in the regulation of gonadatropin secretion. Recent Prog Horm Res 1984;40:487–529.

21. Ramirez VD, Feder HH, Sawyer CH. The role of brain catecholamines in the regulation of LH secretion: a critical inquiry. In: Martini L, Ganong WF, eds. Frontiers in neuroendocrinology, vol. 8. New York: Raven Press, 1984:27–84.

22. Ondo JG. Gamma-aminobutyric acid effects on pituitary gonadotropin secretion. Science 1974;186:738–9.

23. Adler BA, Crowley WR. Evidence for gamma-aminobutyric acid modulation of ovarian hormone effects on luteinizing hormone secretion and hypothalamic catecholamine activity in the female rat. Endocrinology 1986;118:91–7.

24. Kalra SP. Neural circuitry involved in the control of LHRH secretion: a model for preovulatory LH release. In: Martini L, Ganong WF, eds. Frontiers in neuroendocrinology, vol. 9. New York: Raven Press, 1986: 31–75.

25. Rivier C, Vale W. Effects of corticotropin-releasing factor, neurohypophyseal peptides, and catecholamines on pituitary function. Fed Proc 1985;44:189–95.

26. Kalra SP, Crowley WR. Norepinephrine-like effects of neuropeptide Y on LH release in the rat. Life Sci 1984;35:1173–6.

27. Gibson MJ, Silverman AJ. Neural tissue transplantation in neuroendocrine research. In: Greenstein B, ed. Neuroendocrine research methods. London: Harwood Academic, 1990.
28. Gibson MJ, Silverman A-J, Kokoris GJ, Zimmerman EA, Perlow MJ, Charlton HM. GnRH cell brain grafts: correction of hypogonadism in mutant mice. Ann NY Acad Sci 1987;495:296–305.
29. Sarkar DK, Chiappa SA, Fink G. Gonadotropin-releasing hormone surge in pro-estrous rats. Nature 1976;264:461–3.
30. Sarkar DK, Fink G. Luteinizing hormone releasing factor in pituitary stalk plasma from long-term ovariectomized rats: effects of steroids. J Endocrinol 1980;86:511–24.
31. Levine JE, Ramirez VD. Luteinizing hormone-releasing hormone release during the rat estrous cycle and after ovariectomy, as estimated with push-pull cannulae. Endocrinology 1982;111:1439–48.
32. Shivers BD, Harlan RE, Morrell JI, Pfaff DW. Absence of oestradiol concentration in cell nuclei of LHRH-immunoreactive neurons. Nature 1983; 304:345–7.
33. Gibson MJ, Silverman AJ, Rosenthal MF, Morrell JI. Estradiol-concentrating cells in the brains of hypogonadal female mice and in their intraventricular preoptic area implants. Exp Neurol 1989;105:127–34.
34. Silverman AJ, Kokoris GJ, Gibson MJ. Quantitative analysis of synaptic input to gonadotropin releasing hormone neurons in normal mice and hpg mice with preoptic area grafts. Brain Res 1988;443:367–72.
35. Godement P, Vanselow J, Thanos S, Bonhoeffer F. A study in developing visual systems with a new method of staining neurones and their processes in fixed tissue. Development 1987;101:697–713.
36. Silverman RC, Silverman AJ, Gibson MJ. Is outgrowth from third ventricular preoptic area (POA) grafts of the hypogonadal (hpg) mouse limited to GnRH fibers [Abstract]? Soc Neurosci Abstr 1989;15:264.
37. Olney JW, Cicero TJ, Meyer ER, DeGubareff T. Acute glutamate-induced elevations in serum testosterone and luteinizing hormone. Brain Res 1976; 112:420–4.
38. Ondo JG. Effects of the neuroexcitatory amino acids aspartate and glutamate on LH secretion. Brain Res Bull 1981;7:333–5.
39. Price MT, Olney JW, Mitchell MV, Fuller T, Cicero TJ. Luteinizing hormone releasing action of N-methyl aspartate is blocked by GABA or taurine but not by dopamine antagonists. Brain Res 1978;158:461–5.
40. Johnson MD, Whetsell JO Jr, Crowley WR. Quinolinic acid stimulates luteinizing hormone secretion in female rats: evidence for involvement of N-methyl-D-aspartate-preferring receptors. Exp Brain Res 1985;59:57–61.
41. Schainker BA, Cicero TJ. Acute central stimulation of luteinizing hormone by parenterally administered N-methyl-D, L-aspartic acid in the male rat. Brain Res 1980;184:427–37.
42. Tal J, Price MT, Olney JW. Neuroactive amino acids influence gonadotropin output by a suprapituitary mechanism in either rodents of primates. Brain Res 1983;273:179–82.
43. Gay VL, Plant TM. N-methyl-D, L-aspartate elicits hypothalamic gonadotropin-releasing hormone release in prepubertal male rhesus monkeys (*Macaca mulatta*). Endocrinology 1987;220:2289–96.

44. Wong EHF, Kemp JA, Priestly T, Knight AR, Woodruff GN, Iversen LL. The anticonvulsant MK801 is a potent N-methyl-D-aspartate antagonist. Proc Natl Acad Sci USA 1986;83:7104–8.

45. Urbanski HF, Ojeda SR. A role for N-methyl-D-aspartate (NMDA) receptors in the control of LH secretion and inactivation of female puberty. Endocrinology 1990;126:1774–6.

46. Lopez FJ, Donoso AO, Negro-Vilar A. Endogenous excitatory amino acid neurotransmission regulates the estradiol-induced LH surge in ovariectomized rats. Endocrinology 1990;126:1771–3.

47. Arslan M, Pohl CR, Plant TM. DL-2-amino-5-phosphonopentanoic acid, a specific N-methyl-D-aspartic acid receptor antagonist, suppresses pulsatile LH release in the rat. Neuroendocrinology 1988;47:465–8.

48. Saitoh Y, Silverman A-J, Gibson MJ. Effects of N-methyl D,L-aspartic acid (NMA) on LH release in normal mice and in hypogonadal mice with fetal preoptic area implants. Endocrinology 1991.

49. Bourguignon J-P, Gerard A, Franchimont P. Direct activation of gonadotropin-releasing hormone secretion through different receptors to excitatory amino acids. Neuroendocrinology 1989;49:402–8.

50. Donoso AO, Lopez FJ, Negro-Vilar A. Glutamate receptors of the non-N-methyl-D-aspartic acid type mediate the increase in luteinizing hormone-releasing hormone release by excitatory amino acids in vitro. Endocrinology 1990;126:414–20.

51. Ondo JG, Wheeler DD, Rom RM. Hypothalamic site of action for N-methyl-D-aspartate (NMDA) on LH secretion. Life Sci 1988;43:2283–6.

52. Silverman R, Silverman AJ, Gibson MJ. Identification of gonadotropin releasing hormone (GnRH) neurons projecting to the median eminence from third ventricular preoptic area grafts in hypogonadal mice. Brain Res 1989; 501:260–8.

Part III

GnRH Physiology: Animal Models

10

GnRH Subgroups: A Microarchitecture

J.C. KING AND B.S. RUBIN

Features of GnRH Cells and Fibers

GnRH cell bodies, as revealed by immunocytochemistry, are small fusiform cells with smooth or irregular profiles (Fig. 10.1). They are primarily bipolar (6 × 16 μm) or unipolar (6.5 × 10 μm) although a proportion of cells appear to be tripolar or apolar (1). Processes derived from the cells display a beaded or varicose appearance shortly after emerging from the cell body. Secondary processes originate from these primary processes (Fig. 10.1); collateralization is a common feature of these cells. The diffuse distribution of scattered GnRH cell bodies within the basal forebrain exhibits no clearly distinct organizational pattern. However, studies in our laboratory using computerized techniques, and which will be presented later in this paper, do reveal an organizational scheme of GnRH cells in the rat.

GnRH fibers directed toward the median eminence aggregate into periventricular, lateral (1), and subchiasmatic (2) pathways (Fig. 10.2), and terminate in the neurovascular zone, where they contact the basal lamina (Fig. 10.3) (3). GnRH secreted in this region enters the fenestrated capillaries and is transported to the anterior pituitary. Other sites of projection of GnRH fibers include the organum vasculosum of the lamina terminalis (OVLT), another circumventricular organ containing fenestrated capillaries. The function of GnRH fibers in the OVLT remains an enigma, given that blood of the fenestrated capillaries from the OVLT does not reach the pituitary (3, 4). One hypothesis regarding the function of these fibers is that these terminals are sensing blood factors as the circumventricular organs are outside the blood-brain barrier (3, 5).

GnRH fibers also project to multiple extrahypothalamic sites, including other circumventricular organs, such as the subfornical organ, and areas of the neuraxis intimately linked to the basal forebrain, such as the amygdala and the habenula (6, 7). These projections function to

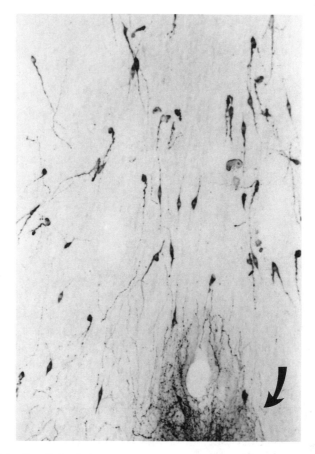

FIGURE 10.1. GnRH-immunopositive cells in the rostral preoptic area of a female proestrous rat. In this coronal section GnRH-immunopositive fibers surround the OVLT (arrow). Processes of cells closest to the midline are oriented in a dorsal-ventral direction, whereas processes of cells further from the midline are oriented in a medial-lateral direction (×100).

coordinate activity within a circuit and synchronize GnRH secretion from specific subgroups of neurons. The extrahypothalamic regions innervated by GnRH fibers also influence GnRH secretion, suggesting that GnRH neurons themselves may provide an additional level of control over this vital function. Cell bodies in extrahypothalamic regions are few in number, but those detected are located in the same regions as the fiber projections, i.e., amygdala, habenula, etc. (6).

Species Differences in GnRH Cells and Fibers

The morphology of GnRH cell bodies is strikingly similar in all vertebrate species examined, from the lamprey, a primitive vertebrate, to humans

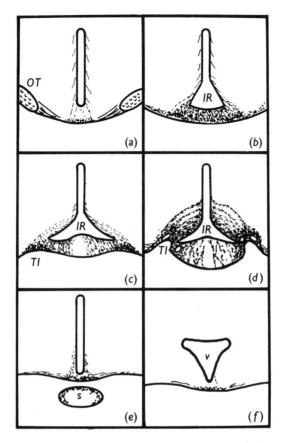

FIGURE 10.2. The rostral caudal extent of the median eminence is shown in coronal sections labeled (a) through (e). Fibers originating from GnRH cells, primarily positioned rostral to the medial basal hypothalamus, are shown entering the median eminence from the periventricular pathway and from the medial forebrain bundle. The infundibular recess (IR) is present in b–d and the tuberoinfundibular sulcus (TI) in c and d.

(6, 8). In several species, including guinea pigs, ferrets, bats, monkeys, and humans, collaterals of GnRH processes arise in close proximity to the cell body, whereas in rats collaterals arise more distally. The most fundamental variation among species is observed in the spatial distribution of cell bodies in the basal forebrain. The rostral-caudal distribution of GnRH cell bodies is most limited in the lamprey, in which GnRH perikarya are confined primarily to the preoptic area (8). The distribution is broader in rats, as GnRH cell bodies are also present in the anterior hypothalamic area and a small percentage of cells are more caudally positioned in the medial basal hypothalamus (MBH) (1, 8, 9). A greater number of cells are detected in the anterior hypothalamus and MBH of guinea pigs compared with rats. The greatest number of GnRH cell

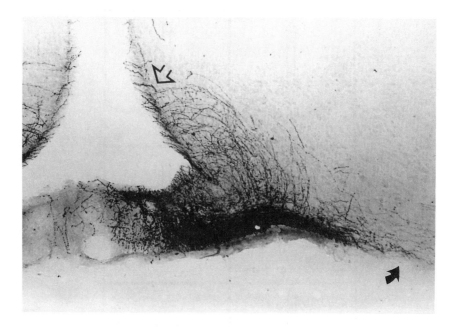

FIGURE 10.3. GnRH-immunopositive fibers enter the median eminence medially from the periventricular pathway (open arrow) and laterally from the medial forebrain bundle (closed arrow) in this coronal section. This region of the median eminence corresponds to a midregion (Fig. 10.2c) of its total rostral-caudal extent (Fig. 10.2a–e) (×86).

bodies in the MBH, however, are detected in bats, monkeys, and humans (6). GnRH cells are observed not only in the parenchyma of the hypothalamus, but also ventral to the hypothalamus in the median eminence and even within the pituitary stalk itself in ferrets, bats, monkeys, and humans (10). In some cases, the cell bodies are ventrally positioned within the stalk (Fig. 10.4), and therefore stalk-transection in these species would spare the GnRH cell bodies located within the pituitary stalk. The remaining GnRH cells in the stalk may explain the controversial data indicating that GnRH cells in the hypothalamus are not required for ovulation in primates (11). Whether there is a correlation between the number of cells spared in individual animals and the potential to ovulate has not been explored, although data from transplant studies suggest that few LHRH neurons are required to sustain ovulation (12).

Correlated with the positioning of GnRH neurons in the ventral MBH and the ME/stalk is the projection of GnRH processes into the stalk and even into the neural lobe of the pituitary (Fig. 10.4). The proportion of fibers that terminate in the external zone of the ME to those that project into the stalk or further into the neural lobe varies among species. In bats

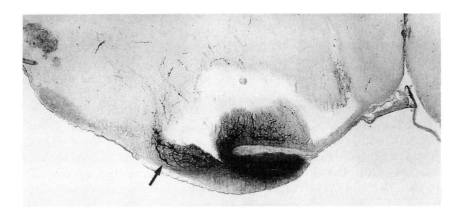

FIGURE 10.4. A parasagittal section close to the midline of the hypothalamus of a little brown bat. GnRH-immunopositive fibers are densely concentrated in the pituitary stalk and do not project to the external zone of the ME. GnRH cell bodies (arrow) are present within the pituitary stalk (×82). (Photomicrograph provided by E.L.P. Anthony.)

and ferrets the majority of fibers project into the stalk, whereas in humans and monkeys fibers terminate in both the ME and the stalk (10). The majority of GnRH fibers projecting into the stalk terminate in close association with the anterior pituitary, although others do project deeper into the neural lobe (10). It is interesting to note that the debate regarding the importance of the portal circulation was centered about the ferret, a species in which GnRH fibers project deeply into the stalk in a pattern that differs considerably from that in the commonly studied animal model, the rat (13, 14).

An important concept has emerged regarding the development of GnRH neurons and has been discussed in this symposium, namely that GnRH neurons originate in the olfactory placode and migrate into the preoptic area/hypothalamus (15, 16). If this developmental pattern can be generalized to all species, then the extent of migration may be controlled or regulated. The caudal extent of migration may be determined by a combination of factors, such as the rate of maturation or differentiation of specific regions. Some factors that might be important for migration, for example, N-CAM (17), disappear as cellular regions differentiate (18). Cellular regions often differentiate in a caudal to rostral direction, whereas migration of GnRH cells proceeds in a rostral to caudal direction. Thus, GnRH cells may migrate more caudally in species in which the factors controlling differentiation allow GnRH cell migration to continue for a longer period of time. In addition, local modulatory factors, particularly those present in circumventricular organs, may be important in guiding GnRH fibers to innervate the median eminence and the OVLT. The importance of local factors is demonstrated by transplantation studies in which GnRH cells introduced into the lateral ventricle of hypogonadal mice, a site distant to the ME, fail to innervate the ME. They do, however, contact closer extrahypothalamic sites that normally receive GnRH fibers in mice (19). Thus organizing principles operative during migration may determine the ultimate distribution of GnRH cell bodies and their projections in the basal forebrain.

Species differences are also observed in the projections of GnRH fibers to extraphypothalamic sites, such as the amygdala, habenula, and subfornical organ. For example, in bats there is a strong projection to the habenula (20), and in humans to the amygdala. In addition, projections to the OVLT are considerable in most species examined but not in the ferret (6). These variations may result from specific characteristics of the circuitry patterns unique to each species.

Variations in the Detection of GnRH Perikarya

The detection of GnRH within perikarya was problematic in early immunocytochemical studies (21). We have demonstrated that the specific binding requirements of the GnRH antibodies utilized are important factors in the detection of GnRH within cell bodies. For example, one GnRH antiserum, but not a second, was able to detect GnRH within cell bodies in equivalent sections from the same animal (22), whereas both antisera clearly detected GnRH within terminals. The antibody that detected GnRH perikarya was directed to amino acid residues in the interior of the decapeptide (23, 24). This antibody was, therefore, capable of recognizing extended forms of the decapeptide present in precursor GnRH and intermediate forms generated during processing, namely those produced upon cleavage of the signal sequence and the C-terminal peptide and amidation of the decapeptide (25). The antibody that failed to detect cell bodies required not only the entire amino acid sequence of the decapeptide, but also terminal modifications, i.e., cyclized N- and amidated C-terminal. These modifications are present only in the fully processed and physiologically active hormone (23, 24). This antibody difference in the detection of GnRH cell bodies has been confirmed in studies with more than 60 rats in various endocrine conditions—i.e., gonadectomized (26), steroid-treated (22, 27), and intact males and cycling females (28). These findings are consistent with the notion that abundance of precursor and intermediate partially processed forms of the precursor is greater than that of the fully processed decapeptide within GnRH cell bodies.

The differential ability of these antibodies to detect GnRH within cell bodies was not observed in other mammalian species, including humans, monkeys, bats, ferrets, and lampreys (6, 8, 20). One explanation of these species differences is that the fully processed hormone is more abundant in the cell bodies of these mammals. Such would be the case if vesicles that contain the precursor and proteolytic cleaving and amidating enzymes and in which the active GnRH decapeptide is generated are retained in the cell body, and not rapidly transported into the processes. The abundance of mature decapeptide would be increased as a consequence of retention of vesicles within GnRH cell bodies. Electron microscopic studies typically describe few immunopositive vesicles in GnRH cell bodies of rats (29, 30), as shown in a GnRH cell from a proestrous female rat prior to the LH surge (Fig. 10.5). In contrast, GnRH vesicles are abundant in other species, such as bats (31). Consistent with this interpretation are the results of studies in which movement of vesicles out of GnRH cell bodies is impeded in rats by the disruption of microtubules with agents such as colchicine. In these studies, the concentration of processed peptide in cell bodies would be increased. Indeed the antibody requiring the fully processed decapeptide hormone did detect GnRH within cell bodies in rats under these conditions (32). Knife-cuts provide another method of disrupting vesicle transport out of GnRH cell bodies and therefore should also result in increased con-

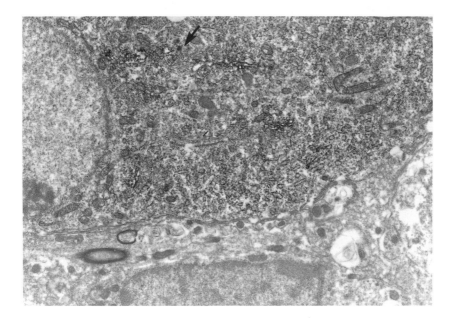

FIGURE 10.5. A GnRH-immunopositive cell from the rostral preoptic area of a proestrous female sacrificed prior to the LH surge demonstrates the paucity of vesicles (arrow) retained in the cell body, although there are several immunopositive Golgi complexes. Reaction product is also dispersed in the cytoplasm, especially in association with the rough endoplasmic reticulum (×11,266).

centrations of processed peptide. As predicted, fully processed hormone was detected within GnRH cell bodies of rats with knife-cuts that severed GnRH cell bodies from their processes (33). These two approaches suggest a variation among species regarding the time period that GnRH-generating vesicles remain in cell bodies before being transported into processes.

A second consideration in addition to the molecular forms of GnRH detected by specific primary antibodies is the immunocytochemical procedure utilized. The sensitivity of immunocytochemical procedures varies with the methodology chosen. Dilutions of a given antibody may vary by a factor of 10^3. For example, an antibody that requires a concentration of 1/1000 to yield reaction product in the peroxidase-antiperoxidase procedure (PAP) must be further diluted to a concentration of 1/10,000 in the avidin-biotin procedure (ABC) (34). In the above-mentioned example, the antibody requiring the fully processed decapeptide may be incapable of detecting GnRH cell bodies in non-colchicine-treated rats with the PAP technique but capable of detecting them when the ABC protocol is used, because of the increased level of sensitivity of the latter methodology. The abundance of the molecular forms detected by the antiserum and the sensitivity of the technique used are both important determinants in the detection of GnRH-immunopositive cells in the rat. These factors were utilized to reveal the organization of neurons within the GnRH system, discussed below.

Populations of GnRH Perikarya Detected in the Forebrain

We exploited the use of specific antibodies and the PAP technique protocol in non-colchicine-treated rats to identify GnRH cells with high concentrations of antigens. We examined the hypothesis that detectability of GnRH antigens within an individual cell varies as a function of activity, and is, in turn, related to endocrine state. The PAP technique was used, as because of its high threshold we would only detect cells in which GnRH antigens were abundant. Because of its increased sensitivity, the ABC technique would not allow discrimination between cells with high and low abundance of GnRH antigens.

We examined the distribution of cells with a high abundance of GnRH antigens in rats sacrificed at various times after gonadectomy. To do this we utilized computerized techniques to map the entire population of GnRH perikarya detected in the basal forebrain from the diagonal band of Broca to the mammillary bodies. Computerized three-dimensional reconstruction was used to define the precise position of all detectable cells within the forebrain (Fig. 10.6). This procedure required equivalent

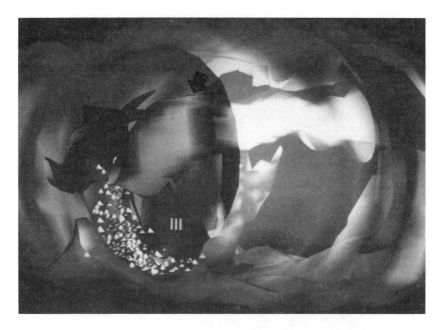

FIGURE 10.6. A computer-generated model of the rat brain rotated 45 degrees from the frontal plane, viewed from olfactory regions toward the midbrain. The cortex is made transparent to reveal the lateral and third ventricles. A three-dimensional reconstruction of the population of GnRH cell bodies from female rats 3 weeks after ovariectomy is seen as white triangles.

sampling of forebrain tissues, which was accomplished by equally dis-tributing sequential sections through the forebrain into four collection vessels (26, 28). Each vessel then contained a sample of all areas of the forebrain and was treated with one of three GnRH antisera. The fourth vessel was used as a control, i.e., GnRH antisera absorbed with GnRH before use. To standardize alignment of sections, we developed software to align individual sections with contours or profiles of sections extracted from the Koenig and Klippel atlas (35). Once sections were aligned, the position of individual cells was entered via a bitpad. Files containing the position of cells in each section were generated for each of 4 animals in a given endocrine condition. The files from the 4 animals were then concatenated to produce a single reconstruction that represented a mean population, with each animal contributing one fourth of the total number of sections through the forebrain.

Using this approach, we demonstrated alterations in populations of high-abundance GnRH perikarya that correlated with sex-specific changes in LH secretion following gonadectomy (26). The acute rise in serum LH levels detected 1 day after castration in male rats was

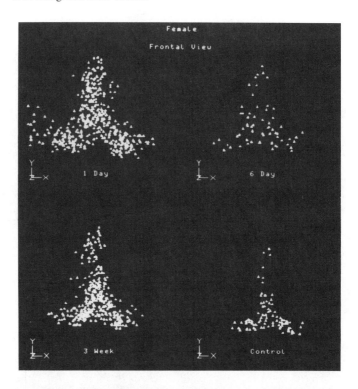

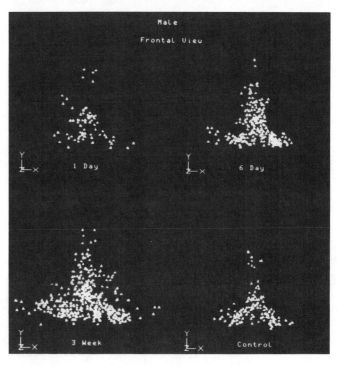

accompanied by a depletion in the population of GnRH cells, as compared with intact rats. In female rats, the acute rise in serum LH, which
is delayed until 6 days after ovariectomy, was also accompanied by a
depletion in the population of neurons with detectable levels of GnRH
(Fig. 10.7). In contrast to the acute effects, in long-term gonadectomized
animals the population of GnRH cells exceeds that of intact animals. We
propose that these differences in detectability of GnRH cells reflect
physiological differences in the functional state of these neurons. Increased
quantities of GnRH antigens generated in these GnRH cells eventually
reach the threshold for detection by the PAP technique. This is consistent
with the morphological indices of enhanced activity observed in electron
microscopic analyses of protein-synthesizing organelles within GnRH cell
bodies of long-term gonadectomized rats (30). Continuous biosynthesis
and processing in long-term gonadectomized animals results in an increased concentration of GnRH antigens.

Delineation of Subgroups of GnRH Cells

The proposed organization of GnRH cells into subgroups was examined
by utilizing computer reconstructions, as described above. Populations of
GnRH cells from animals in different endocrine conditions or in similar
endocrine conditions but treated with different antisera were compared.
Reconstructed populations were color-coded so that GnRH cells from
animals sacrificed at different times after gonadectomy could be dis-
criminated in simultaneous displays. If the populations of GnRH cells
detected by the same antibody using the same immunocytochemistry
protocol were identical, then all populations would be superimposed,
i.e., overlying each other. This was not the case; rather, this procedure
resulted in the differentiation of perikarya with threshold vs. subthreshold
quantities of GnRH moieties in animals in different endocrine states.

One subgroup of GnRH cells was consistently detected, regardless of
endocrine state. This subgroup consisted of cells in the rostral preoptic
area surrounding the OVLT. Surrounding this subgroup were cells in
which GnRH was variably detected as a function of sex and time after
gonadectomy. For example, in females there was a subgroup of cells in
which GnRH was detected 1 day and 3 weeks after ovariectomy, but not
detected 6 days after ovariectomy. This subgroup circumscribed the

◄────────────────────────────────

FIGURE 10.7. Frontal views of the reconstructed forebrain populations of GnRH-
immunopositive cell bodies from female and male rats sacrificed 1 or 6 days, and 3
weeks after gonadectomy are shown independently. The X plane represents the
medial lateral dimension, the Y plane the dorsal ventral dimension, and the Z
plane the rostral caudal dimension. Note that the most widely dispersed population of females is observed 1 day after ovariectomy. In males the most widely
dispersed population is observed 3 weeks after castration.

central subgroup. Finally, a subgroup of cells in which GnRH reached detectable levels on only one of the three time periods after gonadectomy surrounded the other two subgroups and was most superficial. This third subgroup, consisting of cells in which detection of GnRH was the most variable, was particularly large in males (Fig. 10.5).

Subgroups of neurons containing detectable levels of GnRH were arranged in a laminar onion-skin-like organization, with the focus being the central subgroup of GnRH cells in the midline rostral preoptic area. The other subgroups emanated from this central subgroup, consisting of GnRH cells that surrounded and enveloped the central group, extending more laterally in the diagonal band of Broca, preoptic area, and anterior hypothalamic area, ventrally dorsally, and caudally. These findings are consistent with the hypothesis that the apparently diffuse forebrain distribution of GnRH cells is actually composed of defined subgroups of GnRH cells with a precise organization. The configuration of these subgroups differs considerably from that of prototypic subgroups within a nucleus, such as the subdivisions of the ventromedial nucleus or the paraventricular nucleus (36).

A similar laminar organizational pattern was revealed in studies of intact rats sacrificed on different days of the estrous cycle (28). A more widespread distribution of GnRH cells was observed on proestrus than on estrus (Fig. 10.8). Independent analyses of GnRH populations detected with antisera with differing binding requirements also revealed this

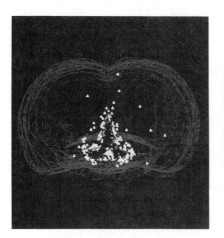
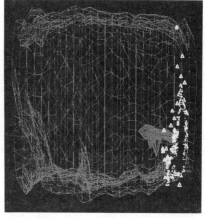

FIGURE 10.8. GnRH-immunopositive cells detected in proestrous, but not estrous rats are shown from (a) a frontal and (b) a lateral view. The cortex and the anterior commissure of the rat brain are shown as light gray wire-frame structures. GnRH cells, shown as white pyramids, are detected on proestrus but not on estrus, using our protocol. This subgroup constitutes one of the lamina in the microarchitecture.

laminar pattern of organization. In this case, although both antisera required interior amino acids for binding, the length of the required sequence differed. Whereas the central subgroup was detected by both antisera, the more superficial subgroups were only detected by the antiserum requiring the shorter sequence. Thus it appears that the basic organization of GnRH cell bodies can be characterized by a laminar pattern. We refer to this onion-skin-like laminar pattern of GnRH subgroups as the microarchitecture of the GnRH system.

Functional Significance of the Laminar Organization

This analytical approach provides a unique insight into the organization of GnRH cell bodies and raises several issues. For example, is the laminar organization of subgroups of GnRH neurons related to differences in functional activity? This is consistent with the data that threshold levels of GnRH are consistently detected in the midline central GnRH cells under all conditions. In contrast, GnRH is variably detected in GnRH cells positioned more widely, i.e., successively expanding from the central group, as a function of endocrine condition or antiserum binding requirements. If this is indeed the case, the pattern of innervation to successive lamina may differ, resulting in a microenvironment that is unique to each of the GnRH subgroups.

For example, there are two major routes of inputs to the hypothalamus, a periventricular midline route and a lateral route via the medial forebrain bundle. Consider that afferents projecting via the periventricular route innervate the preoptic/hypothalamus. The density of innervation may form a gradient with the heaviest innervation closest to the midline and the sparsest innervation most lateral (Fig. 10.9). Conversely, afferents projecting via the medial forebrain bundle may densely innervate lateral regions and only sparsely innervate regions closest to the midline. A pattern of innervation imposed by these two gradients would result in different microenvironments that vary as a function of distance from the midline (Fig. 10.9c). The precise pattern of innervation may be further modified by additional innervation originating from local interneurons resident in the preoptic/hypothalamus.

Furthermore, a hierarchy of function within the population of GnRH cells may exist such that the central focal group has a unique function. For example, GnRH cells in this region may influence the activity of GnRH neurons in other subgroups, i.e., the central group could innervate the more superficial subgroups (31). Although their spatial distribution has not been examined, there are several reports of GnRH-GnRH contacts (31, 37–39). If indeed this is the case, is GnRH itself the neurotransmitter, or do other peptides colocalized in these cells, such as galanin or delta-sleep-inducing-peptide, serve as neurotransmitters (40, 41)?

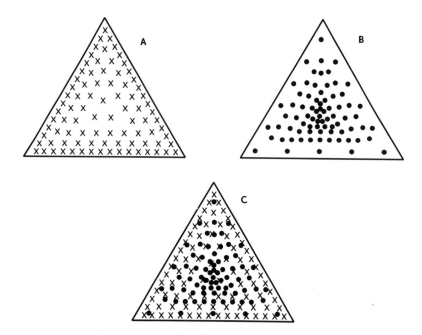

FIGURE 10.9. This diagram represents afferents projecting to the three-dimensional population of GnRH cells. In panel A the projections are heaviest in the superifical zones of the population and probably originate from fibers entering from a lateral pathway. Panel B represents afferents that project most heavily to the center of the population, which is in the midline. These fibers probably represent a periventricular pathway. The bottom panel (C) represents the superimposition of these two afferent projections and demonstrates the microenvironments in the proposed lamina of the population.

In addition to the pattern of afferents, is the pattern of efferent projections distinct for GnRH cells in specific subgroups? For example, do GnRH processes originating from cells in each subgroup terminate in restricted, defined regions of the median eminence, OVLT, or other regions of the neuraxis? Regarding the ME, is there a point-to-point relationship of position of GnRH cells to position of termination in the ME, as has been suggested in birds (42)? Currently, we are analyzing GnRH terminals and processes in coronal sections throughout the ME, as described in Figure 10.2. Image analysis is being used to identify regions of the ME in which the quantity of GnRH reaction product changes as a function of the LH surge. A similar approach is being used in electron microscopic studies to quantitate GnRH reaction product in individual neurovascular terminals and to determine their distance from the basal lamina in gonadectomized rats. Ongoing analyses of recent data suggest that sites of GnRH release within the ME of proestrous (43, 44) and gonadectomized animals are restricted.

If GnRH neurons do project to select, restricted regions of the ME, is there an organizational pattern such that terminals contacting specific capillaries superfuse restricted, defined regions of the anterior pituitary? Are specific gonadotropes, for example, more important in the periovulatory release of LH? Recent evidence suggests that gonadotropes in the rostral area contribute more to the periovulatory surge than do those located in other regions of the anterior lobe (45). These gonadotropes may receive a greater GnRH stimulus on proestrus due in part to the enlarged neurovascular zone of the portal capillaries present in female rats (46). If these speculations regarding an organizational pattern are true, they may reflect a hierarchical and sex-specific function of specific GnRH subgroups.

To date there have been many attempts to define the specific GnRH cells that project to the ME by using a number of retrograde tracers, i.e., horseradish peroxidase and wheat germ agglutinin. The estimates have varied from a low of 50% (47) to a high of 70% (48). In some cases, uptake of the tracer necessarily reflects the activity of the GnRH terminals, as the tracer must be incorporated by endocytosis. Therefore, 50% may represent an underestimate of the percentage of GnRH cells projecting to the ME. It is possible that only 50% of the terminals were actively secreting GnRH during the time period sampled. The conclusion that the remaining 50% of GnRH neurons do not project to the ME but project to other sites in the neuraxis is based on the assumption that individual GnRH cells project to a single site. The possibility that GnRH cells project to multiple sites via branching collaterals, which have been frequently observed, must also be considered. For example, individual GnRH cells projecting to the ME may also project to other parts of the neuraxis. This yoking of secretion of GnRH at the level of the ME with simultaneous release at other sites may be important to ensure the complex synchrony of GnRH secretion related to ovulation and other physiological and behavioral processes required for reproduction.

In summary, we propose that the apparently diffuse distribution of GnRH cells possesses a distinct microarchitecture. It is composed of subgroups of GnRH cells arranged to optimize integration of signals from the internal and external environment and to trigger a sequence of events that maximize to potential for reproductive success.

Acknowledgments. The authors thank Akira A. Arimura, U.S.-Japan Biomedical Research Laboratories, New Orleans, LA, and Robert P. Millar, University of Cape Town Medical School, Capetown, South Africa, for generously providing antisera to LHRH. The authors also thank Stu Tobet for reading the manuscript and providing useful suggestions and Stan Vernon for photographic assistance. This work was supported by Grants NIH HD19803 and NSF DCB 9004498 (JCK) and NIH HD 19174 (BSR).

References

1. King JC, Tobet SA, Snavely FL, Arimura AA. LHRH immunopositive cells and their projections to the median eminence and organum vasculosum of the lamina terminalis. J Comp Neurol 1982;209:287–300.
2. Hoffman GE, Gibbs FP. LHRH pathways in rat brain: "deafferentation" spares a sub-chiasmatic LHRH projection to the median eminence. Neuroscience 1982;7:1979–1993.
3. Ambach G, Kivovics P, Palkovits M. The arterial and venous blood supply of the preoptic region in the rat. Acta Morphol Acad Sci Hung 1978;26:21–41.
4. Weindl A, Sofroniew MV. Neurohormones and circumventricular organs. In: Scott DE, Kozlowski GP, Weindl A, eds. Brain-endocrine interaction, III: neural hormones and reproduction. Basel: Karger, 1978:117–137.
5. Katsuura G, Arimura A, Koves K, Gottschall PE. Involvement of organum vasculosum of lamina terminalis and preoptic area in interleukin 1 beta-induced ACTH release. Am J Physiol 1990;258:E163–E171.
6. King JC, Anthony EL. LHRH neurons and their projections in humans and other mammals: species comparisons. Peptides 1984;5:195–207.
7. Stopa EG, Koh-Tongju E, Svendsen CN, Rogers W, Schwaber J, King JC. 3-D mapping of gonadotropin-releasing hormone (GnRH) in human basal forebrain and amgydala. Soc Neurosci 1988.
8. King JC, Sower SA, Anthony EL. Neuronal systems immunoreactive with antiserum to lamprey gonadotropin-releasing hormone in the brain of *Petromyzon marinus*. Cell Tissue Res 1988;253:1–8.
9. King JC, Tobet SA, Snavely FL, Arimura AA. The LHRH system in normal and neonatally androgenized female rats. Peptides 1980;1 (suppl 1):85–100.
10. Anthony EL, King JC, Stopa EG. Immunocytochemical localization of LHRH in the median eminence, infundibular stalk, and neurohypophysis: evidence for multiple sites of releasing hormone secretion in humans and other mammals. Cell Tissue Res 1984:236:5–14.
11. Wildt L, Hausler A, Hutchison JS, Marshall G, Knobil E. Estradiol as a gonadotropin releasing hormone in the rhesus monkey. Endocrinology 1981;108:2011–2013.
12. Gibson MJ, Silverman AJ, Kokoris GJ, Zimmerman EA, Perlow MJ, Charlton HM. GnRH cells brain grafts: correction of hypogonadism in mutant mice. Ann NY Acad Sci 1987;495:296–305.
13. Donovan BT, Harris GW. Effect of pituitary stalk section on light-induced oestrus in the ferret. Nature 1954;174:503–504.
14. Thomson APD, Zuckerman S. Functional relations of the adenohypophysis and hypothalamus. Nature 1953;171:970.
15. Wray S, Nieburgs A, Elkabes S. Spatiotemporal cell expression of luteinizing hormone-releasing hormone in the prenatal mouse: evidence for an embryonic origin in the olfactory placode. Dev Brain Res 1989;46:309–318.
16. Schwanzel-Fukuda M, Pfaff DW. Origin of luteinizing hormone-releasing hormone neurons. Nature 1989;338:161–164.
17. Schwanzel-Fukuda M, Abraham S, Crossin KL, Edelman GM, Pfaff DW. Immunocytochemical demonstration of neural cell adhesion molecule along the migration route of luteinizing hormone-releasing hormone neurons in mice [Abstract]. Soc Neurosci Abstr 1990;16.

18. Chuong CM, Edelman GM. Alterations in neural cell adhesion molecules during development of different regions of the nervous system. J Neurosci 1984;4:2354–2368.

19. Kokoris GJ, Silverman AJ, Zimmerman EA, Perlow MJ, Gibson MJ. Implantation of fetal preoptic area into the lateral ventricle of adult hypogonadal mutant mice: the pattern of gonadotropin-releasing hormone axonal outgrowth into the host brain. Neuroscience 1987;22:159–167.

20. King JC, Anthony EL, Gustafson AW, Damassa DA. Luteinizing hormone-releasing hormone (LH-RH) cells and their projections in the forebrain of the bat *Myotis lucifugus lucifugus*. Brain Res 1984;298:289–301.

21. King JC, Parsons JA, Erlandsen SL, Williams TH. Luteinizing hormone-releasing hormone (LH-RH) pathway of the rat hypothalamus revealed by the unlabeled antibody peroxidase-antiperoxidase method. Cell Tissue Res 1974;153:211–217.

22. King JC, Anthony EL. Biosynthesis of LHRH: inferences from immunocyto-chemical studies. Peptides 1983;4:963–970.

23. Arimura A. Recent developments in the study of hypothalamic hormones with special reference to LHRH and somatostatin. Folia Endocrinol Jpn 1976;52:1159–1183.

24. Millar RP, Denniss P, Tobler C, et al. Presumptive prohormonal forms of hypothalamic peptide hormones. In: Vincent JD, Kordon C, eds. Cell biology of hypothalamic neurosecretion. Bordeaux: Coll. Int. du Centre National de la Recherche Scientifique, 1977:487–510.

25. Adelman JP, Mason AJ, Hayflick JS, Seeburg PH. Isolation of the gene and hypothalamic cDNA for the common precursor of gonadotropin-releasing hormone and prolactin release-inhibiting factor in human and rat. Proc Natl Acad Sci USA 1986;83:179–183.

26. King JC, Kugel G, Zahniser D, Wooledge K, Damassa DA, Alexsavich B. Changes in populations of LHRH-immunopositive cell bodies following gonadectomy. Peptides 1987;8:721–735.

27. King JC, Anthony EL, Damassa DA, Elkind Hirsch KE. Morphological evidence that luteinizing hormone-releasing hormone neurons participate in the suppression by estradiol of pituitary luteinizing hormone secretion in ovariectomized rats. Neuroendocrinology 1987;45:1–13.

28. Hiatt ES, Seiler GR, Brunetta PG, King JC. Cyclic changes in numbers of LHRH neurons in female rats [Abstract]. Soc Neurosci 1988;18th annual meeting:#161.10–80.

29. Seiler GR, Brunetta PG, King JC. Subcellular features of LHRH neurons in cycling female rats [Abstract]. Soc Neurosci 1988;18th annual meeting: #161.9–80.

30. King JC, Seiler GR. Ultrastructural evidence suggests variations in bio-synthesis and processing within LH-RH neurons as a function of ovariectomy in rats. Brain Res 1988;452:127–140.

31. Anthony ELP, Weston PJ, Montvilo JA, Bruhn TO, Neel K, King JC. Dynamic aspects of the LHRH system associated with ovulation in the little brown bat (*Myotis lucifugus*). J Reprod Fertil 1989;87:671–686.

32. Setalo G, Vigh S, Schally AV, Arimura A, Flerko B. LH-RH-containing neural elements in the rat hypothalamus. Endocrinology 1975;96:135–142.

33. Setalo G, Vigh S, Schally AV, Arimura A, Flerko B. Immunohistological study of the origin of LH-RH-containing nerve fibers of the rat hypothalamus. Brain Res 1976;103:597–602.
34. Sternberger LA. Immunocytochemistry. 3rd ed. New York: John Wiley & Sons, 1986:168–171.
35. Koenig JFR, Klippel RA. The rat brain: a stereotaxic atlas of the forebrain and lower parts of the brain stem. Huntington, NY: RK Krieger Publ. Co., 1970.
36. Bleier R, Byne W. Septum and hypothalamus. In: Paxinos G, ed. The rat nervous system, vol. 1: Forebrain and midbrain. New York: Academic Press, 1985:87–118.
37. Leranth C, Segura LM, Palkovits M, MacLusky NJ, Shanabrough M, Naftolin F. The LH-RH-containing neuronal network in the preoptic area of the rat: demonstration of LH-RH-containing nerve terminals in synaptic contact with LH-RH neurons. Brain Res 1985;345:332–336.
38. Pelletier G. Demonstration of contacts between neurons staining for LHRH in the preoptic area of the rat brain. Neuroendocrinology 1989;46:457–459.
39. Chen WP, Witkin JW, Silverman AJ. Sexual dimorphism in the synaptic input to gonadotropin releasing hormone neurons. Endocrinology 1990; 126:695–702.
40. Coen CW, Montagnese C, Opacka-Juffry J. Coexistence of gonadotrophin-releasing hormone and galanin: immunohistochemical and functional studies. J Neuroendocrinol 1990;2:107–111.
41. Merchenthaler I, Lopez FJ, Negro-Vilar A. Colocalization of galanin and luteinizing hormone-releasing hormone in a subset of preoptic hypothalamic neurons: anatomical and functional correlates. Proc Natl Acad Sci USA 1990;87:6326–6330.
42. Oksche A. Evolution, differentiation and organization of hypothalamic systems controlling reproduction. In: Scott DE, Kozlowski GP, Weindl A, eds. Brain-endocrine interaction, III: Neural hormones and reproduction. Basel: Karger, 1978:2–15.
43. King JC, Rubin BS, Yao P. Changes in LHRH neuronal populations associated with the LH surge in young and middle-aged female rats [Abstract]. Soc Neurosci Abstr 1990;16.
44. King JC, Letourneau RJ, Brenner JF. LHRH within individual neurovascular terminals is increased in proestrous compared to estrous rats. Endocrine Society Meeting, 1990.
45. Goldman JM, Cooper RL, Rehnberg GL, Booth KC, McElroy WK, Hein JF. Regional patterning of hormones in the female rat anterior pituitary: disproportionate changes over the estrous cycle. Endocr Res 1988;14:263–282.
46. Rethelyi M. Regional and sexual differences in the size of the neuro-vascular contact surface of the rat median eminence and pituitary stalk. Neuroendocrinology 1979;28:82–91.
47. Silverman AJ, Jhamandas J, Renaud LP. Localization of luteinizing hormone-releasing hormone (LHRH) neurons that project to the median eminence. J Neurosci 1987;7:2312–2319.
48. Merchenthaler I, Setalo G, Petrusz P, Negro-Vilar A, Flerko B. Identification of hypophysiotropic luteinizing hormone-releasing hormone (LHRH) neurons by combined retrograde labeling and immunocytochemistry. Exp Clin Endocrinol 1989;94:133–140.

11

Exactitude in the Relationship Between GnRH and LH Secretion

I.J. Clarke

In the past decade a number of new techniques have been made available for the collection of hypophyseal portal blood and the measurement of the secretion of gonadotropin releasing hormone. With the consequent accumulation of data on real-life secretion of GnRH and the way in which this relates to the secretion of luteinizing hormone, it seems appropriate to review our understanding of the exact relationship between the secretions of the two. It is well established that the pulsatile secretion of LH from the pituitary is a direct reflection of the pulsatile secretion of GnRH from the hypothalamus (1–4), but the exact relationship between the amplitude of GnRH pulses and the amplitude of LH pulses can vary, depending on various factors such as pulse frequency, the influence of steroids, and the inclusion of small GnRH pulses between major events. This chapter will analyze these aspects in detail. In addition, it has been postulated that the shape of the GnRH pulse is an important determinant of the LH response (5), and this issue will be examined also. In particular, we have focused on the question by taking portal blood samples at intervals of 2.5 min to characterize GnRH pulse shape and pulse duration in ovariectomized ewes.

GnRH Pulse Shape and Duration

An in vitro study of perfused ovine pituitary cells indicated that the LH response to a given amount of GnRH increased as the pulse width was shortened (5). To examine the same question, we conducted studies in OVX ewes that had been subjected to surgical hypothalamo-pituitary disconnection (HPD) to remove all central neuroendocrine inputs to the pituitary gland (6). We used a dose of 250 ng GnRH administered as a bolus IV injection or as a "pulse" of 6-, 12-, or 18-min duration, and found that the peak of the LH response and the total amount of LH released declined as the "pulse" width increased (7). When one-third of the dose was given as a bolus followed by two-thirds as an infusion, the LH response was also lower than that obtained with a bolus injection of the total dose. Thus, GnRH pulses of short duration and high amplitude will give a larger LH response than broader GnRH pulses of lower amplitude.

The question remained as to the shape of GnRH pulses in real life. To address this issue, we took hypophyseal portal blood samples from 4 OVX sheep at intervals of 2.5 min over 4–5-W periods, whereas previous

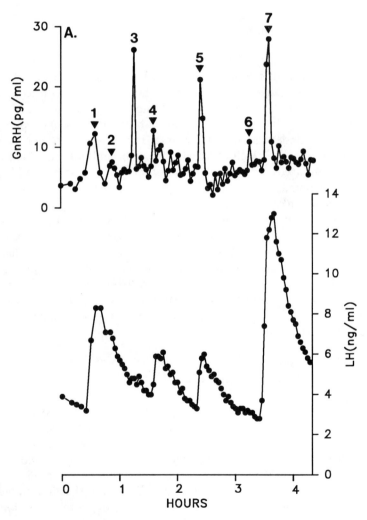

FIGURE 11.1. Portal GnRH and jugular LH levels, in two OVX ewes sampled at 2.5-min intervals.

sampling intervals had been 5–10 min. In this series we did not take account of any plasma effect in the GnRH assay, which is usually correct baseline values. This was done to maximize the chances of detecting small GnRH pulses. The data for 2 sheep are shown in Figure 11.1. We detected 24 pulses, 17 of which (71%) caused LH pulses. GnRH pulses that occurred independently of LH pulses were generally smaller than those occurring with LH pulses, although this was not always the case (compare pulses 3 and 4 in Fig. 11.1A). LH pulses were always associated with GnRH pulses. In 33% of cases the GnRH pulses had a width of at least 3 sampling intervals (7.5 min), whereas 83% of all pulses had a width of at least 2 intervals (5 min). In 14 of 24 cases (58%) the peak of the GnRH pulse was achieved in the first sample—e.g., pulse 1, Fig. 11.1B. In other cases GnRH pulses appeared to have a slow onset and then a "spike" component (pulse 2, Fig. 11.1B). Some more complex situations (pulse 4, Fig. 11.1A) were also seen, in which low-amplitude wide pulses were seen. There was clear evidence that the GnRH pulses that occurred in the absence of LH pulses (pulse 2, in Fig. 11.1A; pulse 6, in Fig. 11.1B) were not isolated, aberrant samples, since the shape of

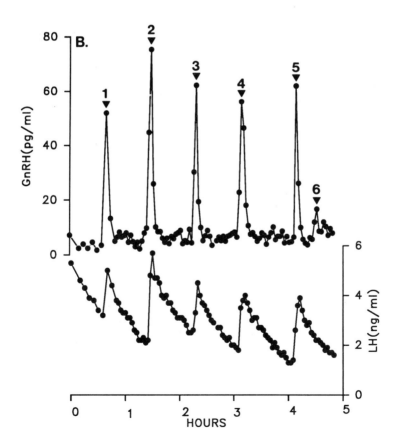

these pulses was that which one would expect following a secretory episode—i.e., peak followed by a decay phase. These data indicate the following:

1. The majority of GnRH pulses last more than 5 min.
2. More than half of GnRH pulses have a leading edge of approximately 2.5 min.
3. "Silent" pulses occur.
4. There is considerable variation in pulse shape.

Changing Pulse Frequency

The amplitude of a pulse of LH in peripheral plasma is inversely proportional to the frequency of pulses at a given time. This has been demonstrated in various models. In OVX monkeys with lesions in the region of the arcuate nucleus that eliminate gonadotropin secretion, pulsatile GnRH replacement was given in various frequency/amplitude modes (8). When 6-μg pulses were given at hourly intervals, the plasma LH and FSH levels were in the normal range for OVX animals; but when the frequency was increased to 2–5 pulses/h, a decline in mean LH and FSH levels was seen. When the GnRH pulse frequency was decreased to 1 pulse/3 h, then mean LH levels fell and mean FSH levels rose. Comparing data between experiments, but not in the same animals, it appeared that reduced GnRH pulse frequencies led to increased LH pulse amplitudes. Whereas the response to very rapid pulses of GnRH can be attributed to a desensitization phenomenon, the reason that plasma LH levels went down but plasma FSH levels went up when the frequency of pulses was reduced is less clear.

In another laboratory, the testosterone-replaced castrated male rat has been employed as a model in which GnRH secretion is suppressed. Using this, Katt et al. (9) showed that LH responses to 25-ng IV pulses of GnRH could be obtained when the frequency of administration was every 30 min; responses were much less at higher or lower pulse frequencies. The concentration of pituitary membrane GnRH receptors was found to be maximal with replacement or the 30-min frequency, suggesting a direct relationship between GnRH pulse frequency, GnRH receptor level, and LH pulse amplitude. A later paper (10) showed that the 30-min frequency was also optimal for the expression of the LHβ subunit gene.

Our studies on this issue in sheep have relied on the use of our hypophyseal portal blood collection model and HPD sheep (6). Replacement with 250-ng IV pulses of GnRH to OVX-HPD ewes gave plasma gonadotropin levels in the castrate range (11). Changes in the frequency of GnRH pulses led to immediate changes in LH pulse amplitude; a reduction in frequency led to an increased LH pulse amplitude, and vice versa (11). When amounts were maintained on hourly or 3-h pulses of GnRH (250 ng/pulse) for 1 week, there was no difference between the two groups in pituitary GnRH receptor affinity or number or total pituitary LH content (12). We did find, however, that the mean ($\pm$SD) pool of LH that was able to be released by a high-dose infusion of GnRH (area under curve) was much larger (P < 0.01) in the ewes given 3-h pulses (7562 $\pm$ 871 mm^2) than in those given hourly pulses (2940 $\pm$ 1354 mm^2) (13). The infusions were commenced at the time these ewes would otherwise have received their next GnRH pulse, and thus indicated the amount of LH available for release at that time. These data are in general accord with those of Wildt et al. (8). The greater the time interval between GnRH pulses, the greater is the accumulation of releasable LH, leading to increased LH pulse amplitudes.

Plasma FSH concentrations were not found to change in the short term when GnRH pulse frequencies were altered in OVX-HPD ewes (11). We have not measured long-term changes in plasma FSH levels in our OVX-HPD across changes in GnRH pulse frequencies. In another study in which gonad-intact rams were subjected to HPD and then given IV GnRH pulses at hourly, 2-h, or 4-h pulse frequencies at weekly intervals, the plasma FSH levels remained stable, suggesting little influence of GnRH pulse frequency on FSH secretion. This contrasts with the data of Wildt et al. (8), which could be explained by a species difference.

From the above, it can be concluded that the LH response to a given amplitude pulse of GnRH depends on the frequency with which pulses reach the pituitary gland. Our data from the HPD sheep strongly support the view that the inverse relationship is due to the time available between pulses to accumulate releasable LH, whereas the data from the more complicated T-replaced castrated rat model suggests that changes in GnRH-R and posttranslational steps in gonadotropin assembly may be important (10). Our simplistic interpretation is easily applied to the estrous/menstrual cycle, where LH pulses occur at a greater frequency and have a lower amplitude during the follicular phase than during the luteal phase (14–16). This is not, however, the only mechanism operative during the cycle. Hypophyseal portal GnRH concentrations have been monitored across the estrous cycle of the ewe, and the increase in GnRH pulse frequency in the follicular phase is accompanied by a decrease in GnRH pulse amplitude, compared with that of the luteal phase (17). This point will be expanded upon below.

The Follicular Phase of the Estrous/Menstrual Cycle

The follicular phase of the estrous/menstrual cycle is a unique situation in which responsiveness to GnRH is altered by the influence of estrogen. Various studies have shown that responsiveness is increased in the late follicular phase of the estrous cycle of the sheep (18) and other species. A most dramatic demonstration of this is the enhancement of the so-called "self-priming effect." This was discovered when two pulses of GnRH were given to proestrous rats 30–240 min apart and the response to the second injection was found to be greater than the response to the first (19). The ratio of the response to the second pulse over the response to the first pulse can be referred to as the "priming effect index," and this is markedly increased in the rat during proestrus (19) and also in the late follicular phase of the sheep estrous cycle (20). This provides potential for an increase in GnRH pulse frequency to cause a markedly increased output of LH. Thus the signal-to-response relationship between GnRH and LH could increase in the lead-up to the LH surge. It seems likely that such an increase in GnRH pulse frequency is a predominant factor in the generation of the LH surge.

Although there is a markedly enhanced responsiveness to GnRH around the onset of estrus in the sheep (21), which is the time of the LH surge (22), there is a less complete picture of the events leading up to the LH surge. We have reexamined the patterns of GnRH secretion and responsiveness to GnRH in the late luteal phase and in the mid-late follicular phase of the ewe. Hypophyseal portal blood samples were taken for at least 6 h at 5- or 10-min intervals from 5 sheep during the late luteal phase of the estrous cycle (day 10) or 24 h (n = 5) or 48 h (n = 6) after an IM injection of 125 µg prostaglandin analog (cloprostenol) on day 10 of the cycle to cause regression of the corpus luteum and the progression of a follicular phase. Table 11.1 shows the frequency and amplitude of GnRH pulses in the 3 groups, essentially confirming our earlier work (17). During the follicular phase, GnRH pulses were more rapid and of lower amplitude than during the luteal phase. Sheep that were sampled after 24-h or 48-h cloprostenol injections had more frequent GnRH pulses than sheep sampled during the luteal phase of the estrous cycle.

TABLE 11.1. GnRH pulse amplitudes and interpulse intervals.

Group	GnRH pulse amplitude (ng/ml)	GnRH interpulse interval (min)	LH response to GnRH (ng/ml)
Luteal phase	13.3 ± 1.9 (11)[b]	152 ± 37 (8)	8.2 ± 1.5 (4)
Follicular phase (+24 h)[a]	8.2 ± 1.5 (34)	55 ± 6 (29)***	13.6 ± 1.4 (4)
Follicular phase (+48 h)	5.5 ± 0.4 (44)*	53 ± 3 (40)***	22.1 ± 5.4 (3)*

Note: Mean (±SEM) amplitudes of GnRH pulses and frequencies of GnRH pulses in hypophyseal portal plasma of ewes during the late luteal phase and during the follicular phase of the estrous cycle, and responses (plasma LH pulse amplitudes) in response to 1 µg IV injections of GnRH at similar times. Luteal phase ewes were given 125 µg prostaglandin analog (cloprostenol) IM to generate the follicular phase series. Responses to GnRH were tested in ewes under halothane anesthesia.
[a] Sampling commenced 24 or 48 h after cloprostenol.
[b] Number of ewes in parentheses.
* P < 0.05, *** P < 0.001 compared with luteal phase by ANOVA.

GnRH pulse amplitudes were lower (P < 0.07) in the early follicular phase than in the luteal phase, but a significant (P < 0.05) difference in pulse amplitude was observed only between luteal phase and late follicular phase.

To test pituitary responsiveness, we injected 1 μg GnRH (IV) into ewes on day 10 or 24 or 48 h after giving cloprostenol to luteal-phase animals. The injections were made 1 h after anesthetic induction and the sheep were maintained on halothane/oxygen in stage 2–3 anesthesia to block endogenous GnRH secretion (23). Blood samples were taken at 10-min intervals for 1 h before injection and for 1.5 h afterwards for plasma LH assays.

Responsiveness to GnRH injection increased between the luteal and the early follicular phase and there was a more substantial rise in the late follicular phase (Table 11.1). Thus, a progressive decrease in amplitude of GnRH pulses occurred across a time when responsivity to GnRH increased between the luteal phase and early follicular phase, and a further increase was seen in the late follicular phase. This clearly represents a gradual divergence in the relationship between GnRH pulse amplitude and LH response, but in real life plasma LH pulse amplitude is reduced during the follicular phase and LH levels either are maintained (24, 25) or fall (26, 27) across the follicular phase. This conforms with the predicted relationship between GnRH pulse frequency and LH pulse amplitude mentioned above. The increase in responsivity is in accord with an observed increase in GnRH receptor number across the follicular phase (28), which is most likely due to a direct pituitary action of estrogen (29). These dynamic relationships are summarized in Figure 11.2.

If responsivity to GnRH is enhanced during the follicular phase but LH pulse amplitude does not rise, this could be due, in part, to the observed reduction in GnRH pulse amplitude (Table 11.1). An additional factor could be that rising levels of estrogen exert a "clamp" on the pituitary response to LH, which is supported by the data from the studies of Scaramuzzi and Radford (26) and Thomas et al. (27), showing that LH pulse amplitudes decline between the early and late follicular phase in sheep. This negative feedback "clamp" is seen in OVX ewes immediately after an IM injection of 50 μg estradiol benzoate is given, and is a direct effect on the pituitary gland (30). The more profound negative feedback effect that follows IV injection of estrogen also involves a reduction in GnRH secretion (31), but this is probably an unphysiological response, due to a sudden large increase in circulating estrogen levels.

The LH Surge

There is now unequivocal evidence from a variety of species showing that the preovulatory LH surge is dependent upon a rise in GnRH secretion, but an issue that requires further elucidation is the *pattern* of the GnRH

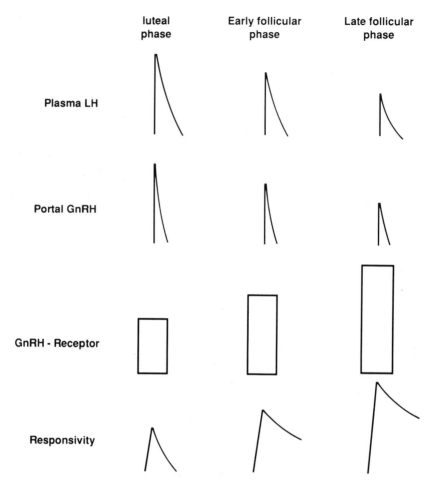

FIGURE 11.2. Changes in GnRH pulse amplitude, GnRH receptor number (from Ref. 28), responsivity to GnRH, and LH pulse amplitude across the late luteal phase and follicular phase of the ewe.

rise. In our earlier work we found variable patterns of GnRH at the time of the cyclic LH surge (17), and in OVX ewes treated with estrogen (32). The latter result was explicable in terms of procedural artifact, since we sampled from the median eminence rather than the portal vessels, but the former result was more puzzling. Recently Karsch and Moenter have obtained evidence of more consistent rises in GnRH secretion at the time of the LH surge (see Chapter 15 of this volume).

In the context of this chapter, I shall limit discussion to the extent to which the formal relationship between GnRH and LH diverges at the time of the LH surge. Is the LH surge simply a result of markedly increased GnRH pulse frequency, or is the form of GnRH secretion during the LH surge due to an "outpouring" of GnRH?

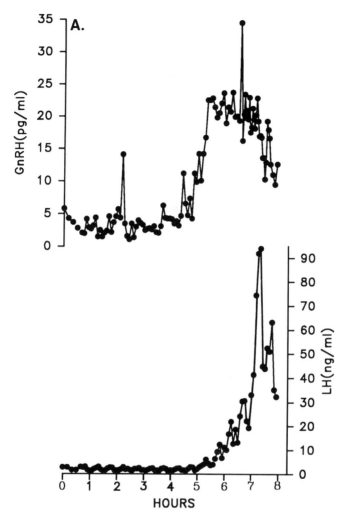

FIGURE 11.3. Concentrations of GnRH in the hypophyseal portal plasma and LH levels in jugular venous plasma of three OVX ewes given 50 μg estradiol benzoate IM. (continues)

Based on studies in OVX-HPD ewes given exogenous GnRH (33) and other sheep models (34), it was clear that a full LH surge could not be obtained in response to estrogen by gradually or abruptly increasing the GnRH pulse frequency, at least to a frequency of one pulse/30 min. An abrupt increase in frequency to 4 pulses/h (34) or a volley of four 10-min pulses (35) could produce an LH surge in estrogen-primed animals. This suggests that the signal for the onset of the LH surge is an abrupt and sustained increased in GnRH secretion. If this is due to an increase in pulse frequency, then rapid (2.5–5 min) sampling may be required to

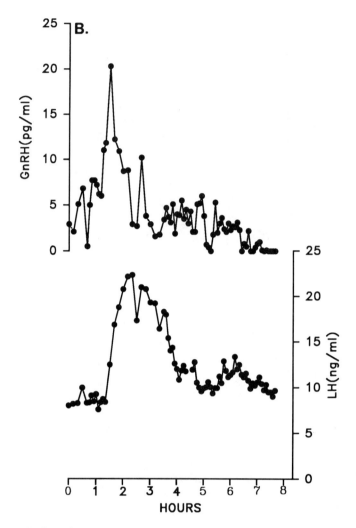

FIGURE 11.3. (cont.)

discern pulses occurring with a frequency of less than 10 min. We have examined GnRH secretory profiles in OVX ewes given 50 μg estradiol benzoate (IM) to induce an LH surge and sampled at 5- or 10-min intervals. Figure 11.3 shows examples of the type of GnRH secretion that occurred during the LH surge and emphasizes the variability in the *patterns* of secretion between animals. In some sheep there was a brief but sustained increase in GnRH secretion at the onset of the LH surge, whereas in other sheep the GnRH rise was more prolonged. Figure 11.3A shows data from an animal sampled at 5-min intervals, with pulses of GnRH clearly evident. Note the burst of rapid pulses that occurred after 1540 h and coincided with a marked increase in LH secretion. In Figure

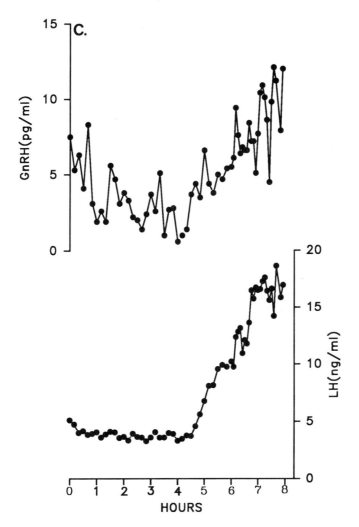

FIGURE 11.3. (cont.)

11.3B there was a sustained rise of GnRH secretion at the onset of the surge, but this did not appear to be composed of GnRH pulses. In Figure 11.3C is an example in which a large GnRH pulse occurred at the onset of the LH surge followed by a rise in GnRH secretion; in this case GnRH pulses did not relate to LH pulses during the surge. A common feature of the data from all sheep was the sustained elevation of GnRH secretion, suggesting that a rise in basal secretion rather than an increase in GnRH pulse frequency is a most important factor in the positive feedback mechanism. This divergence from the one-to-one GnRH-to-LH pulse relationship is quite possibly the mechanism for the generation of the LH surge. These data also suggest that the GnRH input required for an estrogen-induced LH surge can vary in form. In some animals a sustained but transient rise in GnRH secretion (Fig. 11.3B) is observed at the onset of the surge, whereas in others (Fig. 11.3A) high-frequency GnRH pulses are seen across the surge. Another reason why the explicit pulse-for-pulse GnRH/LH relationship is lost during the LH surge is that the LH responses to GnRH pulses are prolonged at this time (30, 36). Because of this, LH pulsatility would not be apparent with rapid GnRH pulses.

Conclusions

It is clear that LH pulses are generated by GnRH pulses, but there are a number of overriding factors that influence the exactitude of this relationship. The shape of GnRH pulses can vary, and the existence of "silent" GnRH pulses can alter the shape of LH pulses. The amplitude of LH pulses probably reflects the amplitude of GnRH pulses, although this has not been formally studied. It is quite clear, however, that the amplitude of LH pulses is dependent upon the frequency of GnRH pulses. It is clear that steroidal feedback has a marked effect on the relationship between GnRH and LH secretion, leading to a divergence in the relationship in the follicular phase of the estrous cycle. At the time of the LH surge the explicit pulse-for-pulse relationship can disappear.

References

1. Clarke IJ, Cummins JT. The temporal relationship between gonadotropin releasing hormone (GnRH) and luteinizing hormone (LH) secretion in ovariectomized ewes. Endocrinology 1982;111:1737–1739.
2. Levine JE, Pau K-YF, Ramirez VD, Jackson GL. Simultaneous measurement of luteinizing hormone-releasing hormone and luteinizing hormone release in unanesthetized, ovariectomized sheep. Endocrinology 1982;111: 1449–1455.
3. Caraty A, Locatelli A, Schanbacher B. Augmentation by naloxone of the frequency and the amplitude of LH-RH pulses in hypothalamo-hypohyseal portal blood in castrated ram. C R Acad Sci (Paris) 1987;305:369–374.
4. Levine JE, Norman RL, Gliessman PM, Oyama TT, Bangsberg DR, Spies HG. In vivo gonadotropin-releasing hormone release and serum luteinizing hormone measurements in ovariectomized, estrogen-treated rhesus monkeys. Endocrinology 1985;117:711–721.
5. McIntosh RP, McIntosh JEA. Influence of the characteristics of pulses of gonadotrophin releasing hormone on the dynamics of luteinizing hormone release from perfused sheep pituitary cells. J Endocrinol 1983;98:411–421.
6. Clarke IJ, Cummins JT, DeKretser DM. Pituitary gland function after disconnection from direct hypothalamic influences in the sheep. Neuroendocrinology 1983;36:376–384.
7. Handelsman DJ, Cummins JT, Clarke IJ. Pharmacodynamics of gonadotropin-releasing hormone: I. Effects of gonadotropin releasing hormone pulse

contour on pituitary luteinizing hormone secretion in vivo in sheep. Neuro-endocrinology 48:432–438.

8. Wildt L, Hausler A, Marshall G, et al. Frequency and amplitude of gonadotropin-releasing hormone stimulation and gonadotropin secretion in the rhesus monkey. Endocrinology 1981;109:376–385.

9. Katt JA, Duncan JA, Herbon L, Barkan A, Marshall JC. The frequency of gonadotropin-releasing hormone stimulation determines the number of pituitary gonadotropin-releasing hormone receptors. Endocrinology 1985; 116:2113–2115.

10. Haisenleder DJ, Katt JA, Ortolano GA, et al. Influence of gonadotropin-releasing hormone pulse amplitude, frequency and treatment duration on the regulation of luteinizing hormone (LH) subunit messenger ribonucleic acids and LH secretion. Mol Endocrinol 1988;2:338–343.

11. Clarke IJ, Cummins JT, Findlay JK, Burman KJ, Doughton BW. Effects on plasma luteinizing hormone and follicle stimulating hormone of varying the frequency and amplitude of gonadotropin-releasing hormone pulses in ovariectomized ewes with hypothalamo-pituitary disconnection. Neuro-endocrinology 1984;39:214–221.

12. Clarke IJ, Cummins JT, Crowder ME, Nett TM. Pituitary receptors for GnRH in relation to changes in pituitary and plasma LH in hypothalamo-pituitary disconnected ewes: I. Effects of changing GnRH pulse frequency. Biol Reprod 1987;37:749–754.

13. Clarke IJ, Cummins JT. GnRH pulse frequency determines LH pulse amplitude by altering the amount of releasable LH in the pituitary gland. J Reprod Fertil 1985;73:425–431.

14. Baird DT. Pulsatile secretion of LH and ovarian estradiol during the follicular phase of the sheep estrous cycle. Biol Reprod 1978;18:359–364.

15. Reame N, Saunder SE, Kelch RP, Marshall JC. Pulsatile gonadotropin secretion during the human menstrual cycle: evidence for altered frequency of gonadotropin-releasing hormone secretion. J Clin Endocrinol Metab 1984; 59:328–337.

16. Filicori M, Santoro N, Merriam GR, Crowley WR. Characterization of the physiological pattern of episodic gonadotropin secretion throughout the human menstrual cycle. J Clin Endocrinol Metab 1986;62:1136–1144.

17. Clarke IJ, Thomas GB, Yao B, Cummins JT. GnRH secretion throughout the ovine estrous cycle. Neuroendocrinology 1987;46:82–88.

18. Hooley RD, Baxter RN, Chamley WA, Cumming IA, Jonas HA, Findlay JK. FSH and LH response to gonadotropin-releasing hormone during the ovine estrous cycle and following progesterone administration. Endocrinology 1974;95:937–942.

19. Aiyer MS, Fink G, Grieg F. Changes in the sensitivity of the pituitary gland to luteinizing hormone releasing factor during the oestrous cycle of the rat. J Endocrinol 1974;60:47–64.

20. Stelmasiak T, Cumming IA. Two pools of pituitary LH: an hypothesis explaining the control of the preovulatory surge of LH in the ewe [Abstract]. Theriogenology 1977;8:131.

21. Reeves JJ, Arimura A, Schally AV. Pituitary responsiveness to purified luteinizing hormone-releasing hormone (LH-RH) at various stages of the estrous cycle in sheep. J Anim Sci 1971;32:123–126.

22. Cumming IJ, Buckmaster JM, Blockey MA, Goding JR, Winfield CG, Baxter RW. Constancy of interval between luteinizing hormone release and ovulation in the ewe. Biol Reprod 1973;9:24–29.
23. Clarke IJ, Doughton BW. Effects of various anaesthetics on resting plasma concentrations of luteinizing hormone follicle stimulating hormone and prolactin in ovariectomized ewes. J Endocrinol 1977;98:79–89.
24. Baird DT, Swanston IA, McNeilly AS. Relationship between LH FSH and prolactin concentration and the secretion of androgens and estrogens by the preovulatory follicle in the ewe. Biol Reprod 1981;24:1013–1025.
25. Karsch FJ, Foster DL, Legan SJ, Ryan KD, Peter GK. Control of the pre-ovulatory endocrine events in the ewe: interrelationship between estradiol, progesterone and luteinizing hormone. Endocrinology 1979;105:42–46.
26. Scaramuzzi RJ, Radford HM. Factors regulating ovulation rate in the ewe. J Reprod Fertil 1983;69:353–367.
27. Thomas GB, Martin GB, Ford JR, Moore PM, Campbell BK, Lindsay DR. Secretion of LH, FSH and oestradiol-17β during the follicular phase of the oestrous cycle in the ewe. Aust J Biol Sci 1988;41:303–308.
28. Crowder ME, Nett TM. Pituitary content of gonadotropins and receptors for gonadotropin-releasing hormone (GnRH) and hypothalamic content of GnRH during the periovulatory period of the ewe. Endocrinology 114: 234–239.
29. Clarke IJ, Cummins JT, Crowder ME, Nett TM. Pituitary receptors for GnRH in relation to changes in pituitary and plasma gonadotrophins in ovariectomized hypothalamo-pituitary disconnected ewes: II. A marked rise in receptor number during acute feedback effects of estradiol. Biol Reprod 1988;39:349–354.
30. Clarke IJ, Cummins JT. Direct pituitary effects of estrogen and progesterone on gonadotropin secretion in the ovariectomized ewe. Neuroendocrinology 1984;39:267–274.
31. Caraty A, Locatelli A, Martin GB. Biphasic response in the secretion of gonadotrophin-releasing hormone (GnRH) in ovariectomized ewes injected with estradiol. J Endocrinol 1989;123:375–382.
32. Clarke IJ, Cummins JT. Increased GnRH pulse frequency associated with estrogen-induced LH surges in ovariectomized ewes. Endocrinology 1985; 116:2376–2383.
33. Clarke IJ, Cummins JT, Jekins M, Phillips DJ. The oestrogen-induced surge of LH requires a "signal" pattern of gonadotrophin-releasing hormone input to the pituitary gland in the ewe. J Endocrinol 1989;122:127–134.
34. Kaynard AH, Malpaux B, Robinson JE, Wayne NL, Karsch FJ. Importance of pituitary and neural actions of estradiol in induction of the luteinizing hormone surge in the ewe. Neuroendocrinology 1988;48:296–303.
35. Phillips DJ, Cummins JT, Clarke IJ. Effects of modifying gonadotrophin-releasing hormone input prior to and following the estrogen-induced luteinizing hormone surge in ovariectomized hypothalamo-pituitary disconnected ewes. J Endocrinol 1990;127:223–233.
36. Crighton D, Foster JP. Luteinizing hormone release alter two injections of synthetic luteinizing hormone releasing hormone in the ewe. J Endocrinol 1977;72:59–67.

12

Studies of LHRH Secretion into the Hypophyseal Portal Blood of the Ram: Gonadal Regulation of LH Secretion Is Exerted Mainly at the Hypothalamic Level

Alain Caraty, Philippe Bouchard, and Michel R. Blanc

LHRH is the most important peptide involved in the regulation of reproduction, and the pattern of LHRH secretion is the major control that governs, directly or indirectly, every reproductive process (1). During almost all stages of reproductive life, LHRH is secreted as a pulse from the median eminence into the hypophyseal portal vasculature and reaches gonadotropes in the antehypophysis, where it evokes an LH pulse (2–4). The secretion of FSH from the pituitary gland is also stimulated by LHRH, but under many circumstances this secretion does not appear closely linked to LHRH secretion (5), but appears to be regulated largely by gonadal steroids, as well as by inhibin-like peptides (6). The control of the reproductive system depends mainly on the frequency of LHRH pulses, but only to a minor extent on their amplitude (7). In fact, many reproductive processes, like the timing of puberty, the ovulatory cycle, the induction of ovulation, seasonal changes of sexual activity, and recovery from postpartum anestrus, are governed by changes in LHRH pulse frequency. The "LHRH pulse generator," a hypothetical control center controlling the pulsatility of LHRH, is under the influence of various physiological stimuli (i.e., photoperiod, olfaction, social cues, and feedback by gonadal products) (8). As a consequence, knowledge of the activity of the LHRH pulse generator is essential to understanding and modulating reproductive endocrine functions, and has been a major subject for debate for many years.

In the ram, as in all large domestic animal species, measurement of LH in peripheral blood is relatively simple, whereas it is more difficult to sample hypophyseal portal blood. Thus, most of our knowledge of the

LHRH pulse generator has been deduced from LH levels in peripheral blood, and is based on the largely untested axiom that every LH pulse in peripheral blood is preceded by a corresponding LHRH pulse in the hypophyseal portal blood. However, due to a paucity of direct LHRH measurements, some questions still remain to be clarified. For example, it is well known that negative feedback of gonadal steroid is one of the components of the hypothalamo-pituitary axis, which modulates the release of gonadotropins by the anterior pituitary gland, but the principal site at which testosterone in the ram exters negative feedback has been conjectural for a long time. Therefore, experiments reported here were designed to determine the respective roles of gonadal hormones either on the physiological regulation of the LHRH pulse generator or at the pituitary level in transducing the LHRH hypothalamic signal. Particular attention was focused on (1) the role of steroids in the regulation of LHRH pulse frequency, (2) the timing of action of this steroid on LHRH pulse generator activity, and (3) the capacity of testosterone to modulate the transduction of the LHRH signal by gonadotropes. Finally, the interaction between the opioid pathway and gonadal hormones on the regulation of LHRH secretion was also examined.

Effects of Gonadectomy in the Ram: LHRH and LH Secretion

In the ram, blood concentrations of LH are characterized by pulses of low amplitude and low frequency (9–12), and there is general agreement that the frequency of these pulses increases from the nonbreeding to the breeding season (13–15). Negative feedback by gonadal steroids is well documented in this species. Administration of testosterone can suppress LH in prepubertal (16), pubertal (17), and mature (18–22) animals. Castration induces a rapid increase in mean LH concentration (23) through an increase in both frequency and amplitude (24, 25). In addition, this increase in pulse frequency and amplitude is more rapid when daylengths are stimulatory than when they are inhibitory (26). Furthermore, within 1 month after castration basal plasma levels of LH reach high values that partially hide the pulsatile nature of this secretion. Testosterone replacement from the time of castration induces a dose-suppressive effect on both LH pulse frequency and pituitary responsiveness 6 weeks later (27). This supports a dual action with effects of testosterone at both the hypothalamic and the pituitary levels. But the question of how LHRH secretion is involved in the phenomena induced by castration remains to be answered.

Increased LHRH Pulse Frequency After Castration?

Using our technique of hypophyseal portal blood collection (3, 4) we have obtained the first direct information on LHRH secretion in the ram.

Portal and peripheral blood samples were simultaneously obtained from conscious, unrestrained intact rams, or rams castrated 2–15 days before (short-term castration) or 1–6 months before (long-term castration). In all three models, LHRH secretion is clearly pulsatile, and analysis of coincidence between LHRH concentrations in hypophyseal portal blood and those of LH in peripheral blood in the same ram provide evidence of a simple, direct cause-and-effect relationship in almost all cases (Fig. 12.1). Only for some long-term castrated animals was the temporal relationship between LHRH pulses and LH pulses not so clear, as the LH pulses in peripheral blood were not well defined because of high basal levels and small pulse amplitudes (24). Following gonadectomy, the major effect was a clear and progressive increase in LHRH pulse frequency. LHRH pulses occurred at intervals of 180, 70, and 36 min in intact, short-term castrated and long-term castrated rams, respectively. In consequence, the good temporal relationship between LHRH and LH pulses indicates that the increase in LH pulse frequency results from the increase of LHRH pulse generator activity. In addition, the great increase in the secretion of the decapeptide may be the reason for the decrease in LHRH hypothalamic tissue content observed after castration (28).

Delay After Castration Necessary to Increase LHRH Pulse Generator Activity

The first experiment having clearly established that removal of gonadal hormones by gonadectomy is followed by an increase of the LHRH pulse frequency in hypophyseal portal blood, the next step was to try to determine how long a period after the removal of negative feedback was necessary to observe an increase in the LHRH pulse generator activity. Because of the large quantities of heparin administered during portal blood collection, surgical castration of animals being sampled cannot be used to answer this question. Recently, LHRH analogs have been synthesized that bind to the LHRH receptors of the gonadotropes but do not elicit a release of LH (29). These antagonists, by blocking the pituitary LHRH receptors, suppress pituitary LH secretion and reduce serum concentration of gonadals steroids (30), providing a method of fast and reversible "chemical castration."

The first indirect evidence that injection of a potent LHRH antagonist leads to a compensatory increase of LHRH secretion was obtained in the sexually active ram (31). This was deduced from the occurrence of a higher LH pulse frequency when the antagonist was cleared from the system and the pituitary regained its ability to respond to the hypothalamic signal. By contrast, we have recently demonstrated that extended blockade of LH secretion by LHRH antagonist administration in castrated rams is not associated with a change in the pattern of LHRH secretion in portal blood (32). Taken together, these two experiments give a good indication that the compensatory increase of the LHRH pulse generator

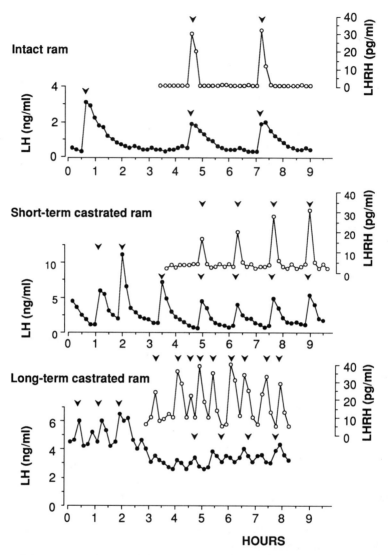

FIGURE 12.1. Time course of LHRH concentrations in hypophyseal portal blood (open circles) and LH concentrations in the peripheral circulation (closed circles) of one representative intact ram (top panel), one short-term castrated ram (middle panel), and one long-term castrated ram (lower panel) sampled every 10 min for 8–9 h. Black arrows indicate algorithm-identified pulses. Reprinted with permission from Ref. 3.

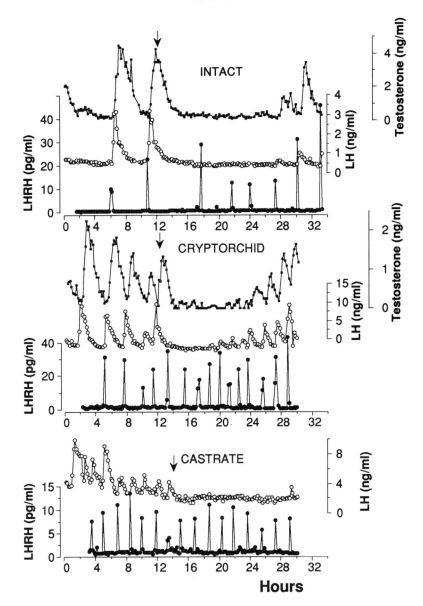

FIGURE 12.2. Time course of LHRH concentrations in hypophyseal portal blood (closed circles) and LH (open circles) and testosterone concentrations in the systemic circulation (closed squares) of a representative intact (top panel), cryptorchid (middle panel), and castrated ram (lower panel). For this experiment, animals were left intact or castrated or rendered cryptorchid by surgery, respectively, 7 and 45 days before blood collection. Portal and peripheral blood were collected every 10 min for 30 to 34 h, and about 10 h after the beginning of blood collection 1 mg of a potent LHRH antagonist (Nal-Glu: Ac-D2-Nal1, D4-Cl-Phe2, D3-Pal3, Arg5, D4-p-methoxybenzoyl-2-aminobutyric acid6, D-Ala10 GnRH) was given intravenously (arrows).

activity observed in the sexually active ram after LHRH antagonist treatment was the result of a decrease in the circulating concentration of gonadal hormones, and not a consequence of a decline of circulating LH levels (short loop feedback) or a result of a blockade of the hypothalamic LHRH receptors putatively involved in the autoregulation of LHRH (ultrashort loop feedback).

To further analyze this point, we have recently carried out an experiment to study the effect of a transitory decrease of gonadal hormones on the LHRH pulse generator activity. We compared the effects of administration of a potent LHRH antagonist (Nal-Glu) on endogenous LHRH secretion in hypophyseal portal blood of intact, cryptorchid, and castrated rams. LHRH antagonist administration was able to suppress LH pulses fully for 14–20 h in the three groups of animals, and suppression took place within 10 min (Fig. 12.2). Testosterone secretion was also suppressed for the same duration in intact and cryptorchid animals. In castrated rams LHRH secretion did not change following Nal-Glu administration, as previously reported (32). By contrast, in intact and cryptorchid animals a clear increase in LHRH pulse frequency following LHRH antagonist administration was observed (Fig. 12.3). The LHRH pulse frequency was increased more than twofold between 10 and 20 h after Nal-Glu administration in intact animals, whereas the increase was only about 50% in cryptorchid animals during the same period. There were no changes in LHRH pulse amplitude at any time in any of the three groups. These results strongly suggest that the increase in frequency evident in the cryptorchid and intact rams reflects the rapid escape of the

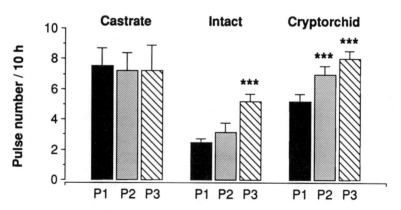

FIGURE 12.3. LHRH pulse frequency in castrated, cryptorchid, and intact rams during the 10 h before (P1, black bars) and during 0–10 h (P2, dotted bars) and 10–20 h (P3, hatched bars) after IV administration of 1 mg of the LHRH antagonist Nal-Glu (mean ± SEM, n = 6). ***$P < 0.001$, compared with P1 (paired t-test). For details see Figure 12.2.

LHRH pulse generator from the negative feedback of gonadal hormones. Indirect evidence indicates that testosterone (or its metabolites) seems to be the major gonadal hormone implicated in this mechanism. In testosterone-implanted castrated rams, administration of LHRH antagonist did not induce a compensatory increase in the frequency of LH pulses when the pituitary regained its responsiveness to LHRH as compared with castrated rams (33). In addition, because naloxone administration is able to increase LHRH frequency in castrated rams under treatment by the LHRH antagonist (32), it cannot be assumed that LHRH pulse frequency was maximum in this model and cannot be increased by Nal-Glu administration.

From these results it can be concluded that a decrease in the negative feedback of gonadal hormones (probably mainly testosterone or its metabolites) induces an acceleration of LHRH pulse generator activity within a few hours.

Role of Testosterone in Transduction of the LHRH Hypothalamic Signal by the Pituitary

Testosterone is the major gonadal steroid in the male, and many experiments have been conducted to determine its role in the hypothalamo-pituitary axis. In the ram, it has been suggested that testosterone can modulate gonadotropin secretion by acting at both the pituitary and the hypothalamic level (34, 35). In addition, androgen and estrogen receptors have been demonstrated to be present in both the hypothalamus and the pituitary (36, 37), although the cells containing these receptors within the pituitary are still unidentified in the ram. However, pharmacological doses of steroid and decapeptide were used in the first studies showing an effect of testosterone on the pituitary responsivenes to the LHRH in this species (38). More recently, experiments with lower amounts of testosterone in castrated animals have led to contradictory results. Testosterone implants administered at the time of castration for 6 weeks, which maintained constant levels of steroid in plasma of around 4 ng/ml, induced a decrease of pituitary responsiveness to LHRH (27), whereas perfusion of the same steroid for 10 h, leading to a plasma level of about 10 ng/ml in castrated animals, did not (39). However, as testosterone secretion is pulsatile in the ram, constant administration is probably not the best way to reproduce the moment-to-moment regulation of pituitary responsiveness by this steroid. To test this aspect of gonadal regulation of the hypothalamo-pituitary axis, we used a model developed in our laboratory (40).

This model was designed to determine pituitary responsiveness to LHRH. It combines suppression of the endogenous secretion of LHRH

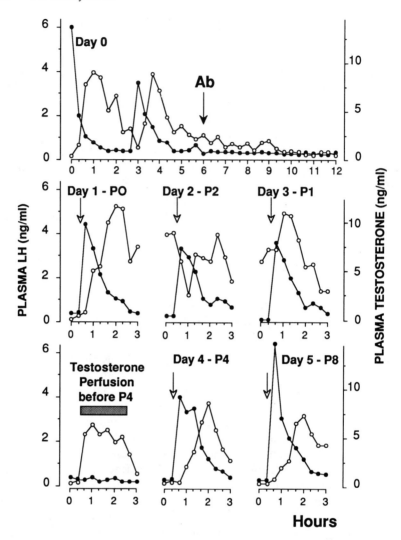

FIGURE 12.4. Changes in LH (closed circles) and testosterone (open circles) plasma level of one representative ram before and after IV injection of LHRH antiserum (Ab) on day 0, during 3-h windows for the 5 following days, and during the testosterone perfusion given on day 4. For this experiment 100 ml of a potent LHRH antiserum was given IV to five intact Prealpes du Sud rams (day 0). This treatment has previously been shown to be able to block LH secretion for at least 3 weeks by immunoneutralization of the decapeptide (40). On the 5 following days (days 1–5), pituitary LHRH responsiveness was tested by IV administration of doses of 400 ng of the LHRH agonist (LHRH Des-Gly10-ethylamide) given at the same time (2 pm) (white arrows). A testosterone perfusion (4 mg/2 h) that mimics an endogenous pulse pattern of testosterone was given 1, 2, 4, or 8 h (P1, P2, P4, and P8, respectively) or not given (P0) before the administration of the LHRH analog. The order of these perfusions was random. Blood samples were

through passive immunization against the decapeptide with administration of an LHRH agonist (LHRH Des-Gly10-ethylamide) that is not recognized by the injected antibodies. For this experiment a potent LHRH antiserum was given IV to intact rams. For 5 days afterwards pituitary LHRH responsiveness was tested by IV administration of the LHRH agonist. A testosterone perfusion that mimics an endogenous pulsatile pattern of testosterone was given or not given 1, 2, 4, or 8 h before the administration of the LHRH analog. The pattern of LH and testosterone plasma levels for one representative ram during this experiments is shown in Figure 12.4. Clear endogenous LH and testosterone pulses were obsered in peripheral blood before LHRH antiserum administration, whereas neutralization of endogenous LHRH induced a rapid and deep suppression of both LH and testosterone secretion. The administration of the agonist induced a qualitative (Fig. 12.4) and quantitative LH response (Fig. 12.5) that resembled an endogenous LH pulse, as previously described (40). Furthermore, the perfusion of testosterone mimicked an endogenous pulse of testosterone (Fig. 12.4). In relation to the beginning of the testosterone perfusion, testosterone levels were quite different at the time of injection of the analog (high at 1 and 2 h, low at 4 and 8 h or when none was given). However, LHRH agonist was always able to induce a clear LH pulse. In fact, there were no changes either in LH pulse amplitude or in the amount of LH secreted in relation to the time of the testosterone perfusion—i.e., to the steroid plasma levels at the time of injection of the analog (Fig. 12.5). These results indicate that individual testosterone pulses play no role at the pituitary level in the moment-to-moment pituitary responsiveness to the hypothalamic signal. Recent similar findings have been obtained by another group (A. Tilbrook and I. Clarke, personal communication). These authors first observed that treatments by subcutaneous administration of testosterone propionate or dihydrotestosterone benzoate or estradiol benzoate for 1 week was able to decrease both mean LH plasma concentrations and LH pulse frequency in wethers to levels normal in intact rams. Furthermore, using "hypothalamo-pituitary-disconnected" wethers maintained under continuous administration of exogenous LHRH (125 ng every 2 h), they found that the same treatments did not affect the amplitude of LH pulses.

In conclusion, taken together these data indicate that negative feedback action of steroids at the level of the adenohypophysis plays no major role in the moment-to-moment regulation of LH secretion in this species.

---

taken every 20 min for 6 h before and after administration of the antiserum on day 0, for 3 h on each following day starting 30 min before the injection of the analog, and for 3 h starting 30 min before the perfusion of testosterone (P4).

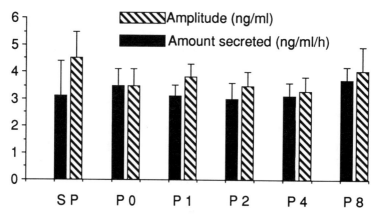

FIGURE 12.5. Parameters (mean + SEM) of spontaneous LH pulses (SP, n = 6) or LH pulses induced by IV administration of 400 ng of the LHRH analog (n = 5) given 1, 2, 4, or 8 h after the beginning of the testosterone perfusion (P1, P2, P4, and P8, respectively) or given without testosterone perfusion (P0). For details see Figure 12.4.

Role of Endogenous Opiates in the Regulation of LHRH Secretion

In species that breed continuously, much evidence indicates that endogenous opioid peptides play a role in the inhibitory control of LH secretion. In the rat, for example, administration of β-endorphin, morphine, or met-enkephalin inhibits LH secretion (41, 42), while β-endorphin antiserum or an antagonist of opiate receptors such as naloxone increases LH secretion (43, 44). The action of endogenous opiates on LH secretion takes place at the hypothalamic level because (1) β-endorphins (45) or morphine (46) did not reduce the LH response induced by injection of LHRH, (2) the increase of LH secretion induced by naloxone was inhibited by an LHRH antagonist (47), and (3) morphine (48) or met-enkephalin (49) inhibits in vitro LHRH secretion, whereas LHRH release is increased by naloxone (50). Furthermore, castration induces an important decrease in the LH response to naloxone (51), as well as decreasing brain opioid reeptors (52) and pituitary portal blood concentrations of β-endorphins (53). All these effects are reversed by sex steroid replacement in castrated animals. These data indicate that neurones synthesizing endogenous opiates or bearing opiate receptors are involved in the steroid feedback inhibition of LHRH secretion.

In the ram, which breeds seasonally, there is also indirect experimental evidence that opioid peptides are involved in the homeostatic regulation of LH secretion. Morphine infusion abruptly suppresses LH secretion in castrates without any effects on pituitary responsiveness to exogenous

LHRH (54), indicating a decrease in LHRH secretion. Naloxone infusion induces an immediate release of LH secretion in intact rams and wethers implanted with testosterone or estradiol, whereas, in contrast, the same treatment of wethers altered the pattern of LH secretion without affecting mean serum LH concentrations (54). These results indicate that steroids are involved in the mechanism whereby endogenous opiates affect the hypothalamo-pituitary axis in the ram. However, in view of the inhibition of LH secretion induced by morphine infusion in whethers, it must be hypothesized that opiate receptors persist after castration. In addition, while changes from stimulatory to inhibitory photoperiods result in an increase in the sensitivity of the hypothalamo-pituitary axis to the negative effects of gonadal steroids (55), the response to naloxone suggests that there is a decrease in opioid activity under inhibitory photoperiods (56). In fact, a clear dose-response increase in mean LH concentration was observed following naloxone administration in the intact and testosterone-treated castrated rams under stimulatory photoperiods, whereas even the highest dose failed to elicit LH release in the intact animal, and produced only a very small effect in testosterone-treated castrated rams during inhibitory photoperiods. Thus, inhibition of LHRH secretion in photo-inhibited rams does not appear to be due to opioid-dependent mechanisms but must involve other inhibitory mechanisms.

Using direct measurements of LHRH secretion, we have reinvestigated the interplay between the steroid and opioid pathways on the control of LHRH release during breeding season. In a first study, we found that naloxone administration was able to induce an increase of LHRH release in the hypophyseal portal blood of short-term castrated rams (57). In addition, the response of the hypothalamus was dependent on the dose of naloxone administered. With one IV injection (about 2 mg/kg) only an increase in LHRH pulse amplitude was observed, whereas multiple injections increased both the frequency and the amplitude of the LHRH pulses. More recently, we examined the time course effect of gonadectomy of the release of LHRH induced by the same dose of naloxone. Multiple injections of naloxone were given to intact, short-term castrated or long-term castrated rams. As previously observed (3; Figs. 12.1 and 12.2), before naloxone administration both LHRH and LH pulse frequency increased from the intact group to the long-term castrated group. In all groups administration of naloxone was able to induce a clear increase in both LHRH and LH secretion. However, the magnitude of the response (expressed as percentage of increase) was quite different (Figs. 12.6 and 12.7; LHRH: 1710, 243, and 66%; LH 534, 93, and 12%, for intact and short-term and long-term castrated rams, respectively). Thus, opioid inhibitory tone as estimated by the percentage of increase in LHRH release following naloxone is strongly diminished during the escape from gonadal hormones in the ram. These data are in agreement with previous reports showing that naloxone can induce a large release of LH secretion

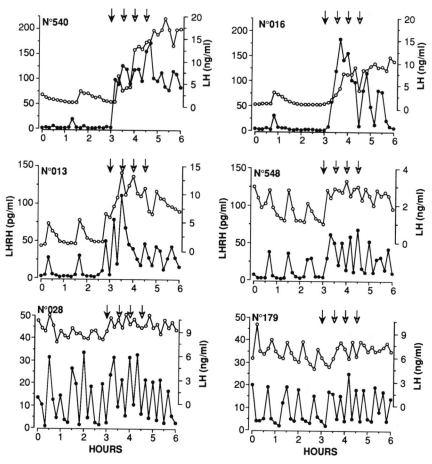

FIGURE 12.6. Time course of LHRH concentrations in hypophyseal portal blood (closed circles) and LH concentration in the peripheral circulation (open circles) of two representative intact rams (top panel), short-term castrated rams (middle panel), and long-term castrated rams (lower panel) before and after IV administration of naloxone. For this experiment, intact, short-term castrated (6–8 days after castration), or long-term castrated Romanov rams (1 month after castration) were used during the breeding season. Portal and peripheral blood were obtained simultaneously every 10 min for 6 h. After 3 h of blood sampling, one intravenous injection of naloxone (100 mg, black arrows) was given followed by three additional injections (50 mg each) given 30, 60, and 90 min after the first one (white arrows).

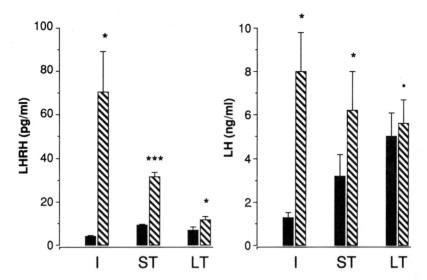

FIGURE 12.7. Mean LHRH (left panel) and LH concentrations (right panel) circulating during a 3-h period (mean ± SEM) before (black bars) and after (striped bars) naloxone administration in intact rams (I, n = 4), long-term castrated rams (ST, n = 4), and long-term castrated rams (LT, n = 4). For details see Figure 12.6.

in intact, testosterone-implanted or estradiol-implanted wethers but not in untreated wethers (54). However, we also report a small increase in both LHRH and LH secretion in long-term castrated rams following naloxone administration, suggesting that both endogenous opiates and opiate receptors persist in castrated male sheep.

In conclusion, in view of the difference of LHRH response to the administration of naloxone in the presence or in the absence of sex steroids, our results, together with previously published data (54), suggest that endogenous opiates can regulate the LHRH pulse generator by coupling to a steroid-sensitive neuronal system within the hypothalamus of male sheep during the breeding season. During the nonbreeding season this coupling may be disconnected.

Summary and Conclusions

Our results demonstrate that in the ram the LHRH pulse generator is physiologically under the control of gonadal hormones, probably mainly sex steroids. In addition, we have shown that the suppression of gonadal hormone secretions for only a few hours is sufficient to free the LHRH pulse generator from their inhibitory effects, resulting in an increase in the frequency of LHRH pulses. We thus can assume that testosterone (or its metabolites) is one of the major factors regulating from moment to moment the frequency of the LHRH pulse generator. However, as it has been shown that an increase in LH pulse amplitude occurs within 1 day after gonadectomy (58), and there is an inverse relationship between the frequency and the amplitude of the LH pulses in LHRH-pulsed hypothalamo-pituitary-disconnected ewes (59), an increase in LHRH pulse amplitude also takes place a few days following gonadectomy.

By contrast, the abrupt rise of testosterone concentration in the peripheral circulation following the occurrence of each LH pulse does not appear to be able to change the parameters of the next LH pulse by a direct action at the pituitary level. By means of a different approach others (A. Tilbrook and I.J. Clarke, personal comunication) have reached similar conclusions. We thus propose that the feedback mechanism by gonadal steroids expressed at the level of the pituitary is not important in the short-term regulation of LH secretion in the ram and is involved in the long-term effects of castration. Therefore, gonadal regulation of LH secretion in male sheep appears similar to that previously proposed for male rhesus monkeys (60).

Finally, our findings, showing a change in sensitivity of LHRH secretion following gonadectomy to the antagonistic effect of naloxone, suggest a functional role for endogenous opiates for the tonic regulation of LHRH secretion during the breeding season and provide insight into the hormonal mechanisms regulating reproductive functions in the male sheep.

References

1. Lincoln DW. LHRH: pulse generation. In: Leng G, ed. Pulsatility in neuro-endocrine systems. Boca Raton, FL: CRC Press, 1988:35–60.
2. Clarke IJ, Cummins JT. The temporal relationship between gonadotropin releasing hormone (GnRH) and luteinizing hormone (LH) secretion in ovariectomized ewes. Endocrinology 1982;11:1737–39.
3. Caraty A, Locatelli A. Effect of castration on the secretion of LHRH and LH in the ram. J Reprod Fertil 1988;82:263–9.
4. Caraty A, Moenter SM, Locatelli A, Martin GB, Karsch FJ. Gonadotropin releasing hormone (GnRH) secretion during the preovulatory luteinizing hormone (LH) surge in the ewe. In: Bouchard P, Haour F, Franchimont P, Schatz B, eds. Recent progress on GnRH and gonadal peptides. Paris: Elsevier, 1989:59–70.
5. Culler MD, Negro-Vilar A. Evidence that pulsatile follicle-stimulating hormone secretion is independent of endogenous luteinizing hormone-releasing hormone. Endocrinology 1986;118:609–12.
6. Ling N, Ying SY, Ueno N, et al. Pituitary FSH is released by a heterodimer of the β-subunits from the two forms of inhibin. Nature 1986;321:779–82.

7. Knobil E. The neuroendocrine control of the menstrual cycle. Recent Prog Horm Res 1980;36:53–88.
8. Lincoln DW, Fraser HM, Lincoln GA, Martin GB, McNeilly AS. Hypothalamic pulse generators. Recent Prog Horm Res 1985;41:369–85.
9. Bolt DJ. Changes in the concentration of LH in plasma of rams following administration of oestradiol, progesterone, or testosterone. J Reprod Fertil 1971;24:435–48.
10. Katongole CP, Naftolin F, Short RV. Seasonal variations in blood LH and testosterone in rams. J Endocrinol 1974;60:101–6.
11. Sanford LM, Winter JSD, Palmer WM, Howland BE. The profile of LH and testosterone secretion in the ram. Endocrinology 1974;95:627–31.
12. D'Occhio MJ, Schanbacher BD, Kinder JE. Relationship between serum testosterone concentration and patterns of luteinizing hormone secretion in male sheep. Endocrinology 1982;110:1547–54.
13. Lincoln GA. Seasonal variation in the episodic secretion of luteinizing hormone and testosterone in the ram. J Endocrinol 1976;69:213–26.
14. Schanbacher BD, Ford JJ. Seasonal profiles of plasma luteinizing hormone, testosterone and estradiol in the ram. Endocrinology 1976;99:752–7.
15. D'Occhio MJ, Schanbacher BD, Kinder JE. Profiles of luteinizing hormone, follicle-stimulating hormone, testosterone and prolactin in rams of diverse breeds: effect of contrasting short (8L:16D) and long (16D:8L) photoperiods. Biol Reprod 1984;30:1039–54.
16. Crim LW, Geschwind II. Patterns of FSH and LH secretion in the developing ram: the influence of castration and replacement therapy with testosterone propionate. Biol Reprod 1972;7:47–54.
17. Schanbacher BD. Testosterone regulation of luteinizing hormone and follicle stimulating hormone secretion in young male lambs. J Anim Sci 1980;51: 679–84.
18. Pelletier J. Mode of action of testosterone propionate on the secretion and release of luteinizing hormone releasing hormone (LHRH) in the castrated ram. Acta Endocrinol 1970;63:290–8.
19. Bolt DJ. Changes in the concentration of luteinizing hormone in plasma of rams following administration of oestradiol, progesterone, or testosterone. J Reprod Fertil 1971;24:435–8.
20. Garnier DH, Terqui M, Pelletier J. Plasma concentrations of LH and testosterone in castrated rams treated with testosterone and testosterone propionate. J Reprod Fertil 1977;49:359–61.
21. Schanbacher BD, Ford JJ. Gonadotropin secretion in cryptorchid and castrated rams and acute effects of exogenous steroids treatment. Endocrinology 1977; 100:387–93.
22. Bremner WJ, Findlay JK, Lee VWK, DeKretser DM, Cumming IA. Feedback effects of the testis on pituitary responsiveness to luteinizing hormone-releasing hormone infusions in the ram. Endocrinology 1980;106:329–36.
23. Pelletier J. Elévation du taux de LH dans le plasma sanguin du bélier aprés castration. Ann Biol Anim Biochem Biophys 1968;8:313–5.
24. Riggs BL, Malven PV. Spontaneous patterns of LH release in castrate male sheep and the effects of exogenous estradiol. J Anim Sci 1974;21:1239–45.
25. Schanbacher BD, D'Occhio MJ. Hypothalamic control of the post castration rise in serum LH concentration in rams. J Reprod Fertil 1984;72:537–42.

26. Lincoln GA, Short RV. Seasonal breeding: nature's contraceptive. Recent Prog Horm Res 1980;36:1–52.

27. D'Occhio MJ, Schanbacher BD, Kinder JE. Relationship between serum testosterone concentration and patterns of luteinizing hormone secretion in male sheep. Endocrinology 1982;110:1547–53.

28. Caraty A. Ram hypothalamic-pituitary-gonadal interactions: effects of castration and cryptorchidism. Acta Endocrinol 1983;102:292–8.

29. Karten MJ, Rivier JE. Gonadotropin-releasing hormone analogue design: structure-function studies toward the development of agonists and antagonists: rationale and perspective. Endocr Rev 1986;7:44–64.

30. Pavlou SN, Wakefield G, Schlechter NL, et al. Mode of suppression of pituitary and gonadal function after acute or prolonged administration of a luteinizing hormone-releasing hormone antagonist in normal men. J Clin Endocrinol Metab 1989;68:446–54.

31. Lincoln GA, Fraser HM. Compensatory response of the luteinizing-hormone (LH)-releasing hormone (LHRH)/LH pulse generator after administration of a potent LHRH antagonist in the ram. Endocrinology 1987;120:2245–50.

32. Caraty A, Locatelli A, Delaleu B, Spitz M, Schatz B, Bouchard P. Gonadotropin-releasing hormone (GnRH) agonists and GnRH antagonists do not alter endogenous GnRH secretion in short-term castrated rams. Endocrinology 1990;127:2523–9.

33. Lincoln GA, Fraser HM. Negative feedback regulation of pulsatile LH secretion during treatment with an LHRH antagonist in rams. J Androl 1990; 11:287–92.

34. Galloway DB, Pelletier J. Luteinizing hormone release in entire and castrated rams following injection of synthetic luteinizing hormone releasing hormone and effect of testosterone propionate pre-treatment. J Endocrinol 1975;64: 7–16.

35. Garnier DH, Terqui M, Pelletier J. Plasma concentration of LH and testosterone in castrated rams treated with testosterone or testosterone propionate. J Endocrinol 1977;49:359–61.

36. Thieulant ML, Pelletier J. Evidence for androgen and estrogen receptors in castrated ram pituitary cytosol: influence of time after castration. J Steroid Biochem 1979;10:677–87.

37. Pelletier J, Caraty A. Characterisation of cytosolic 5a-DHT and 17β-oestradiol receptors in the ram hypothalamus. J Steroid Biochem 1981;14: 603–11.

38. Pelletier J. Decrease in the pituitary response to synthetic LH-RH in castrated rams following testosterone propionate treatment. J Reprod Fertil 1974; 41:397–402.

39. D'Occhio M, Kinder JE, Schanbacher BD. Pattern of LH secretion in castrated bulls (steers) during intravenous infusion of androgenic and estrogenic steroids: pituitary response to exogenous luteinizing hormone-releasing hormone. Biol Reprod 1982;26:249–57.

40. Caraty A, Martin GB, Montgomery G. A new method for studying pituitary responsiveness in vivo using pulses of LH-RH analogue in ewes passively immunized against native LH-RH. Reprod Nutr Dev 1984;24:439–48.

41. Bruni JF, Van Vugt D, Marshall S, Meites J. Effects of naloxone, morphine and met-enkephalin on serum prolactin, LH, FSH, TSH and GH. Life Sci 1977;21:461–6.

42. Kinoshita F, Nakai Y, Katakami H, Kato Y, Yajima H, Imura H. Effect of β-endorphin on pulsatile LH release in conscious castrated rats. Life Sci 1980;27:843–6.
43. Schulz R, Wilhelm A, Pirke KM, Gramsch G, Herz A. β-endorphin and dynorphin control of serum luteinizing hormone level in immature female rats. Nature 1981;294:757–9.
44. Sylvester PW, Van Vught DA, Aylswort CA, Hanson EA, Meites J. Effect of morphine and naloxone on inhibition by ovarian hormones of pulsatile release of LH in ovariectomized rats. Neuroendocrinology 1982;34:269–73.
45. Weisner JB, Koening JI, Krulich L, Moss RL. Site of action for β-endorphin-induced changes in plasma luteinizing hormone and prolactin in ovariectomized rats. Life Sci 1984;34:1463–73.
46. Ferin M, Wehremberg WB, Lam NY, Alston EJ, Van de Wiele RL. Effects and site of action of morphine on gonadotropin secretion in the female rhesus monkey. Endocrinology 1982;111:1652–6.
47. Blank MS, Robert DL. Antagonist of gonadotropin-releasing hormone blocks naloxone-induced elevations in serum luteinizing hormone. Neuro-endocrinology 1982;35:309–12.
48. Drouva SV, Epelbaum J, Heri M, Tapia Arancibia L, Laplante E, Kordon C. Neuroendocrinology 1981;32:163–7.
49. Rasmussen DD, Liu JD, Wolf PL, Yen SS. Endogenous opioid regulation of gonadotropin-releasing hormone release from the human fetal hypothalamus in vitro. J Clin Endocrinol Metab 1983;57:881–6.
50. Wilkes MM, Yen SS. Augmentation by naloxone of efflux of LRF from superfused medial basal hypothalamus. Lifes Sci 1981;28:2355–9.
51. Cicero TJ, Schainker BA, Meyer ER. Endogenous opioids participate in the regulation of hypothalamic-pituitary-luteinizing hormone axis and testosterone's negative feedback control of luteinizing hormone. Endocrinology 1979;104:1286–91.
52. Hahn F, Fishman J. Castration affects male rat brain opiate receptor content. Neuroendocrinology 1985;41:60–3.
53. Sarkar DJ, Yen SSC. Changes in β-endorphin-like immunoreactivity in pituitary portal blood during estrous cycle and after ovariectomy in rats. Endocrinology 1985;116:2075–9.
54. Schanbacher BD. Endogenous opiates and the hypothalamic-pituitary-gonadal axis in male sheep. Domestic Animal Endocrinology 1985;2:67–75.
55. Lincoln GA. Central effect of photoperiod on reproduction in the ram revealed by the use of a testosterone clamp. J Endocrinol 1984;103:233–41.
56. Ebling FJP, Lincoln GA. Endogenous opioids and control of seasonal LH secretion in Soay rams. J Endocrinol 1985;107:341–53.
57. Caraty A, Locatelli A, Schanbacher BD. Augmentation par la naloxone de la fréquence et de l'amplitude des pulses de LH-RH chez le bélier castré. C R Acad Sci 1987;305:369–74.
58. Blanc M. Etude du rétro-contrôle testiculaire de la sécrétion des hormones gonadotropes chez le mouton (ovis aries): composantes protéiques et stéroidiennes. Thèse de Doctorat en Sciences Naturelles, Université Pierre et Marie Curie, Paris VI, 1987.
59. Clarke IJ, Cummins JT, Crowder ME, Nett TM. Pituitary receptors for gonadotropin-releasing hormone in relation to changes in pituitary and plasma luteinizing hormone in ovariectomized-hypothalamo pituitary dis-

connected ewes: effect of changing frequency of gonadotropin-releasing hormone pulses. Biol Reprod 1987;37:749–54.
60. Plant TM. Gonadal regulation of hypothalamic gonadotropin-releasing hormone release in primates. Endocr Rev 1986;7:75–88.

13

Gonadal Feedback Regulation of LHRH Release and Actions in the Rat

JANICE H. URBAN, JOHN M. MEREDITH,
ANGELA C. BAUER-DANTOIN, FRANK J. STROBL,
AND JON E. LEVINE

It is now well established that the intermittent discharge of luteinizing hormone releasing hormone into the hypophyseal portal vasculature serves as the primary neural determinant of pulsatile LH secretion (1–7). The endocrine (nonneural) regulation of pulsatile LH secretion, by contrast, is dominated by the actions of gonadal steroid hormones operating in both negative (males and females) and positive (females) feedback modes. Both forms of gonadal feedback regulation appear to be mediated by alterations in the amount or pattern of pulsatile LHRH release, as well as by modulation of pituitary responsiveness to the decapeptide. Given the central importance of these feedback loops in the maintenance of reproductive viability, it is not surprising that much attention has been focused on the nature of the neural and endocrine mechanisms that mediate both types of hormonal feedback. In the work summarized below, we have used a variety of approaches to measure, manipulate, and mimic LHRH and LH release patterns, so that we might analyze and compare the mechanisms by which positive and negative feedback actions may be manifest. The concept is advanced that negative and positive feedback regulations at the hypothalamic level differ not only in sign, but also in the fundamental mechanisms by which LHRH neurons may ultimately mediate these processes. Specifically, a case is made for frequency and amplitude modulation as the primary bases for negative and positive feedback regulation, respectively. In addition, it is also proposed that there exist qualitative differences in the manner by which negative and positive feedback actions are exerted at the level of the pituitary gland.

Negative Feedback Regulation of LHRH/LH Secretion in Male Rats

Modulation at the Hypothalamic Level

Romoval of circulating testicular hormones by castration produces robust and continued increases in LH and FSH levels, and in LH pulse amplitude and frequency (8). In the male rat these parameters are significantly elevated even by 24 h postcastration (8). Treatment with physiologic levels of testosterone returns LH pulse amplitude and frequency to levels characteristic of the testes-intact animal (9). The site(s) and mechanism(s) by which testosterone may exert these negative feedback actions have remained unclear, given the previous unexpected findings that LHRH levels in stalk-transected, anesthetized rats are not changed following castration (10). One hypothesis, proposed on the basis of studies with monkeys bearing lesions of the arcuate nucleus (11), has held that testosterone may retard the activity of the LHRH pulse generator, and through this mechanism exert its negative feedback suppression of LH secretion. According to this view, castration of male animals would be expected to result in an acceleration of the activity of the LHRH pulse generator—i.e., in an increase in the frequency of pulsatile LHRH release.

To test this hypothesis in intact and short-term (24–30 h) castrated rats, push-pull perfusion of the mediobasal hypothalamic (MBH)/median eminence region and peripheral blood sampling were used to monitor LHRH//LH in both intact and castrated rats (7). In the castrate group, both LHRH and LH pulses occurred at a higher frequency than in the sham-operated (testes-intact) animals (Table 13.1); no significant changes in either LHRH pulse amplitude or LHRH mean levels were observed. In more recent experiments, pituitary microdialysis was similarly used to examine LHRH release patterns following castration; in these experiments, levels of LHRH were monitored at the "receiving end" of the portal vessels, in the extracellular fluid of the anterior pituitary gland. Similarly, as in the push-pull perfusion experiments, removal of gonadal

TABLE 13.1. Effect of gonadectomy on GnRH pulse parameters as determined by push-pull perfusion.

	Intact	Castrate
Pulse frequency (pulses/h)	0.83 ± 0.13	1.30 ± 0.16
Pulse amplitude (pg, trough to peak)	0.83 ± 0.24	0.58 ± 0.06
Hormone level (pg/10 min)	0.46 ± 0.11	0.47 ± 0.04

Note: Mean $\pm$ SEM; n = 7 per group.
Source: Data from Ref. 7.

steroids were found to produce an increase in LHRH pulse frequency (0.87 ± 0.06 [intact] vs. 1.30 ± 0.26 pulses/h [castrate]), with no significant change in either LHRH pulse amplitude (0.42 ± 0.06 [intact] vs. 0.24 ± 0.03 ng/ml [castrate]) or mean levels (0.48 ± 0.06 [intact] vs. 0.37 ± 0.04 ng/ml [castrate]). The results of both studies suggest that the postcastration rise in LH secretion is at least partially due to a postcastration acceleration of LHRH pulse frequency. Both findings are also entirely consistent with the idea that testicular feedback at the level of the hypothalamus is mediated by deceleration of the LHRH pulse generator (7).

In the earlier push-pull perfusion studies, examination of the LHRH and LH pulse profiles from individual castrated animals showed that almost every LHRH pulse was associated with an LH pulse. However, in the testes-intact animals, LHRH pulses were less frequent, and "silent" LHRH pulses (those pulses that do not produce an LH pulse) were more common. These results suggest that in addition to inhibiting the LHRH pulse generator at the hypothalamic level, gonadal steroids may also alter the responsiveness of the pituitary to the decapeptide. From these findings and previous observations on LH/testosterone relationships (12) we have proposed a model for the reproductive axis of the male rat. The model holds that a continual cycling of the following events occurs in the adult male rat: LHRH pulses initiate LH pulses, one or more LH pulses evoke(s) a testosterone secretory episode, and testosterone suppression at the level of the pituitary gland is momentarily augmented. The pituitary effects of testosterone are self-limiting, as they temporarily eliminate LH support for secretion of the steroid. The model holds that there is little, if any, acute endocrine regulation of LHRH release, providing that testosterone remains within physiological limits. According to our model, the homeostasis within the axis is maintained by the ebb and flow of feedback and feedforward between pituitary and gonad. Longer-term shifts in the activity of the axis, or compensatory responses to unusual perturbations such as castration, are mediated via changes in the frequency of LHRH pulse generation (7).

Modulation at the Pituitary Level

We have recently conducted experiments in which the pituitary component of the foregoing model was directly assessed. Based on our working model, we reasoned that castration should result in not only an acceleration of LHRH pulsatility, but also an enhancement of LH secretion resulting from disinhibition of pituitary responsiveness to LHRH. To test this hypothesis, an in vivo isolated pituitary paradigm was developed so that controlled GnRH pulses could be delivered to a functioning pituitary that is devoid of hypothalamic input (13, 14). Hypophysectomized rats receive anterior pituitary transplants under the kidney capsule. The animals are then fitted with concentric atrial catheters to allow for both infusion of GnRH and blood sampling through a side port. The animal can move freely and receive GnRH infusions for an unlimited amount of time. Male rats were prepared in this manner and maintained on pulsatile GnRH infusions (50 ng/min, 5-min duration, hourly) for 5 days prior to and throughout the experimental sessions. After 5 days of pulsatile infusions, the rats were either castrated or sham-operated. Plasma samples were collected 2 h before surgery and every 2 h for the next 24 h after castration or sham surgeries. As depicted in Figure 13.1, support was indeed gained from these experiments for direct feedback suppression of LHRH-induced LH secretion (13). In hypophysectomized, pituitary-grafted rats that received sham surgeries, LH levels remained constant throughout the postsurgery period. By contrast, plasma LH levels in the hypophysectomized, pituitary-grafted rats increased steadily until they reached a plateau at 18 h after surgery. Since pulsatile LHRH stimulation was not changed during the course of the experiments, one can only conclude that the rise resulted from the removal of direct pituitary feedback suppression by the testes. That this reflects the response of the normal pituitary is suggested by the fact that the absolute amounts of immunoreactive LH and the trajectory of the LH rise in the hypophysectomized, pituitary-grafted castrates closely mimicked those in normal castrates during the initial 20 h following

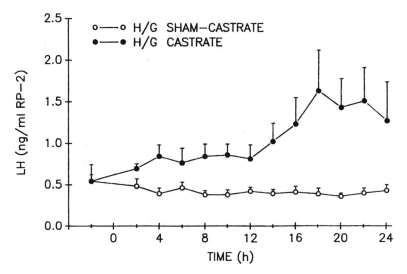

FIGURE 13.1. Plasma LH levels in hypophysectomized rats bearing anterior pituitary transplants and receiving hourly GnRH infusions, at successive time-points after castration or sham-surgery. Data represented as mean ± SEM. Reprinted with permission from Ref. 13, © by The Endocrine Society, 1989.

removal of the testes (13). Interestingly, these similarities were absent at longer times following castration, suggesting that additional hypothalamic input figures more importantly in elevating LH levels at longer post-castration intervals.

Positive Feedback Regulation of the LH Surge by Gonadal Steroids

Pulsatile LH secretion during the ovulatory cycle of the rat is maintained at low levels on estrus, metestrus, diestrus, and the morning of proestrus through the negative feedback actions of gonadal steroids (15). The hypothalamo-hypophyseal unit abruptly discharges the preovulatory LH surge on the afternoon of proestrus, an event that has long been known to be dependent upon the preovulatory release of estrogen and a daily signal generated by a 24-h neuronal clock (16). Progesterone released just prior to or during the surge appears to amplify the event and prevent its reoccurrence on the following afternoon (17, 18). These positive feed-back actions of ovarian steroids can be reproduced in ovariectomized animals, in which LH surges of physiological amplitude and timing can be reproduced by proper sequential administration of estrogen and progesterone (19). Prolonged administration of estrogen alone via silastic capsule implants has also been shown to produce daily LH surges (20), although they are diminished in amplitude and more variable in timing than those in normal proestrous rats (20) or ovariectomized animals treated with estrogen and progesterone.

The intra- and intercellular routes by which steroids exert these effects have received much attention, and several hypotheses have been pro-posed to explain the succession of events that intervene between steroid binding and the generation of the LH surge. There exists much evidence, for example, that noradrenergic neurons may, in part, mediate the positive feedback actions of estrogen and progesterone (21). In the succeeding discussion, however, we consider only how these feedback actions may ultimately be exerted on the LHRH secretory process, and how they may also be complemented by steroid-dependent effects on pituitary respon-siveness to the decapeptide.

Modulation at the Hypothalamic Level

Sarkar et al. (22) first demonstrated that the culmination of the neural events leading to the LH surge is an acute increase in LHRH neuro-secretion on the afternoon of proestrus. Since this landmark finding, several approaches have been taken in various species to characterize the form of this preovulatory rise in LHRH—i.e., to determine if LHRH amplitude and/or pulse frequency is increased during the initiation of the surge. Analysis of LH pulses during the ascending limb of the LH surge in the female rat has yielded one important clue (23): LH pulse frequency is not significantly increased during the dramatic rise in LH levels that constitutes the initiation of the preovulatory surge.

Push-pull perfusion studies have provided data that are consistent with these results (3, 24). In original push-pull perfusion studies by Levine and Ramirez (3), it was determined that the underlying LHRH release patterns in proestrous rats (2), or in ovariectomized rats receiving estrogen and progesterone (2), also give no indication that there is an abrupt increase in LHRH pulse frequency during the ascending limb of the LH surge. Rather, the increase in LHRH release appears to be composed of pulses of LHRH that are increased in amplitude. A recent analysis of LHRH patterns in the pituitary gland itself (24) has borne out this view. The effects of higher, sustained doses of estrogen in the absence of progesterone treatment have been more difficult to document, probably as a result of the diminished magnitude and variable timing of surges evoked by this steroid regimen. For example, implantation of estrogen capsules has been shown to stimulate high-amplitude LHRH release in one study (25), but injections of the steroid did not augment overall release in another (26). Nevertheless, based on the data from estrogen/progesterone-treated rats (2), and from rats sampled on the afternoon of proestrus (3), it appears likely that the rapid ascent of LH levels during the onset of the LH surge is driven, in part, by a punctuated increase in the amplitude of LHRH release. The increase in LHRH release may, in turn, result from an augmentation of LHRH production (27) or the delivery of an acute, stereotyped set of synaptic signals that superimposes a surge-generating stimulus upon the pulsatile electrophysiological rhythm. This issue will not be thoroughly addressed until higher resolution of LHRH pulse analyses is possible in rats, as has become possible in the ewe (28).

Modulation at the Pituitary Level

The timing of the preovulatory LH surge appears to be determined largely by the timing of the antecedent increase in LHRH amplitude. The magnitude of the surge, however, depends upon a combination of factors that likely include the size and form of the LHRH trigger and the degree to which the responsiveness of the pituitary gland is augmented (29–31). It is well documented that the rising tide of estrogen secreted by the developing follicle not only activates the circuitry that delivers the afternoon LHRH neurosecretory trigger, but also serves to sensitize the pituitary gland to the actions of the decapeptide. The sensitivity of the pituitary gland is gradually increased from late diestrus through early proestrus, in parallel with circulating estrogen levels (29, 30). The sensitivity of the pituitary is then acutely augmented on the afternoon of proestrus, yielding a total increase in sensitivity that is 50-fold greater than previous levels. The gradual increase in pituitary sensitivity has been attributed to the direct priming actions of estrogen (30), while the acute increase in responsiveness on the afternoon of proestrus has been thought to occur as a result of the direct pituitary actions of progesterone (30) and/or the self-priming actions of LHRH (31). There is little direct evidence, however, that these mechanisms can fully account for the massive, 50-fold increase in pituitary sensitivity.

We recently used the in vivo isolated pituitary paradigm to estimate the degree to which physiologic levels of estrogen and progesterone can modify the LHRH-induced LH secretion by the ectopic pituitary gland (32). Hypophysectomized, pituitary-grafted rats with pituitary transplants were maintained on pulsatile LHRH infusions for 4 days and then treated with estrogen, or estrogen and progesterone, in regimens that produce LH surges in normal animals. Treatment with estrogen, or sequential treatment with estrogen and progesterone, initially suppressed LH secretion to a degree comparable with that produced in pituitary-intact animals. The response was followed by a rise in LH secretion in response to the unvarying LHRH pulsatile infusions, giving levels that were approximately 3-fold greater than suppressed values. Although these results are consistent with the hypothesis that circulating estrogen is responsible for the initial phase of pituitary priming, they fail to confirm a role for either steroid in the acute priming phase.

It therefore remains a viable possibility that some other circulating hormone, or some additional neurosecretory factor, may participate in the priming of the pituitary gland and thereby operate as an important component of the LH surge-generating process. It was recently suggested that neuropeptide Y (NPY) may operate in this manner, inasmuch as passive immunoneutralization of the peptide attenuates steroid-induced LH surges (33). We have recently tested this concept by examining the in vivo actions of NPY in pentobarbital-blocked, proestrous rats. Animals were fitted with atrial catheters and at 1300 h received either saline vehicle or pentobarbital (40 mg/kg ip) to block endogenous LHRH secretion. In the animals treated with anesthetic, pulsatile LHRH infusions (15, 150, or 1500 ng/pulse) were administered at 30-min intervals from 1400 h to 1800 h, and were found to produce subphysiological, physiological, and supraphysiological LH surges, respectively. Superimposition of NPY on the LHRH infusions caused a clear-cut, dose-dependent enhancement of the LHRH-induced LH surges (Fig. 13.2). Infusions of NPY alone were without effect, confirming that these actions are modulatory in nature. These findings are consistent with the idea that NPY operates as a neuroendocrine modulator during generation of the preovulatory LH surge. In addition to modifying LHRH secretion directly (34, 35), NPY appears to be secreted into the hypophyseal portal vessels on the afternoon of proestrus to prime the pituitary gland to the actions of LHRH.

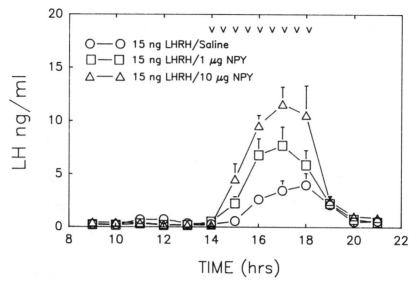

FIGURE 13.2. Potentiation of LH response to LHRH pulses by NPY (1 or 10 μg) in pentobarbital-blocked proestrous rats. Reprinted with permission from Ref. 36, © by The Endocrine Society, 1991.

This contention has derived further support from our recent finding that the priming actions of exogenous NPY are specifically demonstrable in animals undergoing LH surges, and not in ovariectomized rats that have not received steroid priming (36, 37).

To further test the involvement of NPY neurons in the generation of preovulatory LH surges, we recently conducted a set of in situ hybridization experiments in which we analyzed NPY gene expression in proestrous rats (38). Neuropeptide Y mRNA levels were measured by quantitative autoradiography, throughout the arcuate nucleus of proestrous rats at 0900, and every 2 h from 1400 to 2200 h. Comparisons of data obtained at these time points revealed a clear, step-wise increase in NPY gene expression throughout the day of proestrus. At 1600 h, when LH values were significantly greater than 0900 values, NPY mRNA levels were significantly greater than 0900 intensities ($P < 0.01$). By 1800 h, the time at which the LH surge peaked, NPY mRNA levels also peaked (Fig. 13.3), and were 3-fold greater than levels observed at 0900 h ($P < 0.01$). NPY mRNA levels remained elevated above 0900 values, but by 2200 h had decreased significantly from 1800 levels ($P < 0.05$). No significant changes in NPY mRNA levels were observed in cerebral cortex during the same time periods. Thus, NPY gene expression in the arcuate nucleus is augmented in parallel with LH levels throughout the generation of the preovulatory LH surge. The increase in NPY gene expression may occur

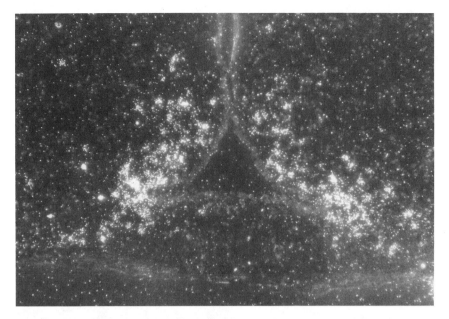

FIGURE 13.3. Darkfield photomicrograph showing labeling of NPY mRNA in cells of the arcuate nucleus (atlas level −2.60 mm caudal to bregma) from a proestrous rat at 1800 h. Probe was an ^{35}S-labeled oligonucleotide complementary for NPY mRNA.

in preparation for the increased release of NPY during the surge, or as a rebound replenishment of NPY stores following the acute release of the peptide. In either case, the changes in NPY mRNA that we have observed during the elaboration of the LH surge are consistent with the hypothesis that NPY-producing neurons participate in the generation of preovulatory LH surges, through the release of NPY and subsequent potentiation of the release (35) and/or actions of LHRH (34, 36).

Summary and Conclusions

There is now abundant evidence that both the negative and the positive feedback influences of gonadal hormones are conveyed through complementary mechanisms at hypothalamic and pituitary levels. We have attempted to summarize evidence that suggests that negative feedback actions, at least in male rats, and positive feedback actions in female rats, may differ not only in sign but also in the fundamental mechanisms by which they are expressed. At least two qualitative differences in the two feedback modes appear to exist. First, negative feedback at the hypothalamic level appears to involve regulation of the LHRH pulse generator, inasmuch as LHRH pulse frequency in both the median eminence (7) and the anterior pituitary (39) is increased in short-term castrates. By contrast, positive hypothalamic feedback actions appear to be mediated by punctuated changes in the amplitude of LHRH release (2, 3, 25). Second, while both types of gonadal feedback involve direct steroid actions on the adenohypophysis, the actions of neurohormonal "comodulators," such as NPY, may be enlisted as additional components of positive feedback effects at the pituitary level.

Acknowledgments. We thank NIADDK, Dr. Gordon Niswender, and Dr. Leo Reichert, Jr. for supplying gonadotropin RIA materials, and Drs. William Ellinwood and Martin J. Kelly for supplying the EL-15 LHRH antiserum. This work was supported by NIH RO1 HD-20677 (J.E.L.), NIH T32 HD-07068 (J.E.L./N.B. Schwartz), NIH PO1 HD-21921 (J.E.L./N.B. Schwartz), and KO4 00879 (RCDA to J.E.L.).

References

1. Carmel PW, Araki S, Ferin M. Pituitary stalk blood collection in rhesus monkeys: evidence for pulsatile release of gonadotropin releasing hormone (GnRH). Endocrinology 1976;99:243–8.
2. Levine JE, Ramirez VD. In vivo release of luteinizing hormone-releasing hormone estimated with push-pull cannulae from the mediobasal hypothalami of ovariectomized, steroid-primed rats. Endocrinology 1980;107:1782–91.
3. Levine JE, Ramirez VD. Luteinizing hormone releasing hormone during the rat estrous cycle and after ovariectomy, as estimated with push-pull cannulae. Endocrinology 1982;111:1439–48.
4. Levine JE, Pau-K-YP, Ramirez VD, Jackson GL. Simultaneous measurement of luteinizing hormone-releasing hormone and luteinizing hormone release in unanesthetized, ovariectomized sheep. Endocrinology 1982;111:1449–55.
5. Clark IJ, Cummins JT. The temporal relationship between gonadotropin releasing hormone (GnRH) and luteinizing hormone secretion in ovariectomized ewes. Endocrinology 1982;111:1737–9.
6. Levine JE, Norman RL, Gleissman PM, Oyama TT, Bangsberg DR, Spies HG. In vivo gonadotropin-releasing hormone release and serum luteinizing hormone measurement in ovariectomized, estrogen treated rhesus macaques. Endocrinology 1985;117:711–21.
7. Levine JE, Duffy MT. Simultaneous measurement of luteinizing hormone-releasing hormone, LH and follicle-stimulating hormone release in intact and short-term castrate rats. Endocrinology 1988;122:2211–21.
8. Ellis GB, Desjardins C. Orchidectomy unleashes pulsatile luteinizing hormone secretion in the rat. Biol Reprod 1984;30:619–27.
9. Steiner RA, Bremner WJ, Clifton DK. Regulation of luteinizing hormone pulse frequency and amplitude in the adult male rat. Endocrinology 1982;111:2055–61.

10. Brar AK, McNeilly AS, Fink G. Effects of hyperprolactinemia and testosterone in the release of luteinizing hormone releasing hormone and the gonadotropins in intact and castrated rats. J Endocrinol 1985;104:35–42.
11. Plant TM, Dubey AK. Evidence from the rhesus monkey (*Macaca mulatta*) for the view that negative feedback control of luteinizing hormone secretion by the testes is mediated by a deceleration of the hypothalamic gonadotropin-releasing hormone pulse frequency. Endocrinology 1984;115:2145–53.
12. Ellis GB, Desjardins C. Male rats secrete luteinizing hormone and testosterone episodically. Endocrinology 1982;110:1618–24.
13. Strobl FJ, Gilmore CA, Levine JE. Castration induces luteinizing hormone (LH) secretion in hypophysectomized pituitary-grafted rats receiving pulsatile LH-releasing hormone infusions. Endocrinology 1989;124:1140–4.
14. Strobl FJ, Levine JE. Estrogen inhibits luteinizing hormone but not follicle stimulating hormone in hypophysectomized, pituitary grafted rats receiving pulsatile luteinizing hormone-releasing hormone infusions. Endocrinology 1988;123:622–30.
15. Leipheimer R, Bona-Gallo A, Gallo W. The influence of progesterone and estradiol in the acute changes in pulsatile luteinizing hormone release induced by ovariectomy on diestrous day 1 in the rat. Endocrinology 1984;114:1605–12.
16. Everett JW, Sawyer CH. A 24-hour periodicity in the "LH-release apparatus" of female rats, disclosed by barbiturate sedation. Endocrinology 1950;47:198–218.
17. Kalra SP, Kalra PS. Neural regulation of leteinizing hormone secretion in the rat. Endocrinol Rev 1983;4:311–51.
18. Freeman ME, Dupke KC, Croteau CM. Extinction of the estrogen-induced daily signal for LH release in the rat: a role for the proestrous surge of progesterone. Endocrinology 1976;99:223–9.
19. Caligaris L, Astrada JJ, Taleisnik S. Biphasic effect of progesterone on the release of gonadotropin in rats. Endocrinology 1977;89:331–7.
20. Legan SL, Karsch FJ. A daily signal for the LH surge in the rat. Endocrinology 1975;96:57–62.
21. Barraclough CA, Wise PM. The role of catecholamines in the regulation of pituitary LH and FSH secretion. Endocrinol Rev 1982;3:91–119.
22. Sarkar DK, Chiappa SA, Fink G. Gonadotropin releasing hormone surge in proestrous rats. Nature 1976;264:461–3.
23. Fox SR, Smith MS. Changes in the pulsatile pattern of luteinizing hormone secretion during the rat estrous cycle. Endocrinology 1985;116:1485–92.
24. Park O-K, Ramirez VD. Spontaneous changes in LHRH release during the rat estrous cycle, as measured with repetitive push-pull perfusions of the pituitary gland in the same female rats. Neuroendocrinology 1989;50:66–72.
25. Levine JE. Hypothalamic neuropeptide release in conscious rats. Ann NY Acad Sci 1986;473:503–6.
26. Dluzen DE, Ramirez VD. In vivo LHRH output of ovariectomized rats following estrogen treatment. Neuroendocrinology 1986;43:459–65.
27. Wise PM, Rance N, Selmanoff MK, Barraclough CA. Changes in radio-immunoassayable luteinizing hormone releasing hormone in discrete brain regions of the rat at various times on proestrus, diestrous day 1 and after phenobarbital administration. Endocrinology 1981;108:2179–85.

28. Karsch FJ, Moenter SM, Caraty A. The preovulatory surge of GnRH: characterization and regulation. In: Conn PM, Crowley WF, eds. Modes of action of GnRH and GnRH analogs, 1991. (*See* Chapter 15, this volume.)
29. Aiyer MS, Fink G, Grieg F. Changes in the sensitivity of the pituitary gland to luteinizing hormone releasing factor during the oestrous cycle of the rat. J Endocrinol 1974;60:47–64.
30. Aiyer MS, Fink G. The role of sex steroid hormones in modulating the responsiveness of the anterior pituitary gland to luteinizing hormone releasing factor in the female rat. J Endocrinol 1974;553–72.
31. Pickering AJ, Fink G. Priming effect of luteinizing hormone releasing factor in vitro: role of protein synthesis, contractile elements, calcium and cyclic AMP. J Endocrinol 1979;81:223–34.
32. Strobl FJ, Levine JE. In vivo tissue culture: use of the ectopic anterior pituitary gland to study steroid and neuropeptide actions on adenohypophysial tissue. In: Conn PM, ed. Methods in neuroscience, vol 2: Cell culture. San Diego: Academic Press, 1990:316–29.
33. Sutton SW, Toyama TT, Otto S, Plotsky PM. Evidence that neuropeptide Y (NPY) released into the hypophysial portal circulation participates in priming gonadotropes to the effects of gonadotropin releasing hormone (GnRH). Endocrinology 19888;123:1208–10.
34. Crowley WR, Kalra SP. Neuropeptide Y stimulates the release of luteinizing hormone releasing hormone in vitro: modulation by ovarian hormones. Neuroendocrinology 1987;46:97–103.
35. Sabatino FD, Collins P, McDonald JK. Neuropeptide-Y stimulation of luteinizing hormone-releasing hormone secretion from the median eminence in vitro by estrogen-dependent and extracellular Ca^{++}-independent mechanisms. Endocrinology 1989;124:2089–98.
36. Bauer-Dantoin AC, McDonald JK, Levine JE. Neuropeptide Y potentiates luteinizing hormone (LH)-releasing hormone stimulated LH surges in pentobarbital-blocked, proestrous rats. Endocrinology 1991.
37. Bauer-Dantoin AC, Levine JE. Neuropeptide Y (NPY) potentiation of LHRH-induced LH secretion is steroid-dependent. Soc Neurosci 1991.
38. Bauer-Dantoin AC, Urban JH, Levine JE. Neuropeptide Y (NPY) gene expression in the arcuate nucleus is increased during preovulatory LH surges. Soc Neurosci 1991.
39. Levine JE, Meredith JM. Effects of short-term castration on LHRH patterns in intra-hypophysial microdialysates. Soc Neurosci 1990:168.4.

14

Gonadotropin Releasing Hormone Gene Expression During the Rat Reproductive Cycle

Ok-Kyong Park, Sajiv Gugneja, and Kelly E. Mayo

The synthesis and secretion of the anterior pituitary gonadotropins luteinizing hormone and follicle stimulating hormone are regulated by both neural and peripheral hormones (1–4). The 10-amino-acid hypothalamic neuropeptide gonadotropin releasing hormone plays a predominant role in controlling the tonic release of the gonadotropins and in initiating the preovulatory gonadotropin surge (5). GnRH-producing cells originate from the olfactory placode during embryonic development and migrate predominantly into brain regions including the diagonal band of Broca (DBB), the organum vasculosum of the lamina terminalis (OVLT), and the preoptic area (POA) (6). These neurosecretory cells send terminals to the median eminence and secrete GnRH into the hypophyseal portal vessels (7, 8) by which it reaches the anterior pituitary and activates GnRH receptors (9).

The secretory profile of GnRH is pulsatile (10), and GnRH neuronal activity is thought to be regulated by diverse stimuli both during tonic release of GnRH and during the preovulatory surge (5). The anatomical proximity of GnRH neurons to catecholaminergic (11), opioidergic (12), and GABA-ergic (13) neurons supports the idea that these neurotransmitters play a role in modulating the activity of GnRH neurons, perhaps mediating informational input from the environment, such as photoperiodic (14, 15) and chemicosensory signals (16, 17). In addition, ovarian steroids exert at least some of their effects on gonadotropin secretion by directly regulating the release of GnRH (18, 19). Clearly, the GnRH neuronal system is complex and is regulated in a multifactorial fashion.

Following the isolation of GnRH cDNA clones and the elucidation of the structure of the GnRH precursor protein (20, 21), it became possible to study the biosynthesis of GnRH at the molecular level. GnRH RNA

223

expression in the hypothalamus has been analyzed by using dot blot or solution hybridization assays (22, 23) as well as in situ hybridization (24–28). We have previously isolated a rat hypothalamic GnRH cDNA clone and have utilized in situ hybridization to localize GnRH mRNA-expressing neurons in the female rat hypothalamus (29). In this chapter, we use this in situ hybridization assay to examine the relationship between changes in GnRH gene expression and changes in GnRH secretion, as monitored by serum LH levels. Several animal models, including cycling, steroid-treated, and lactating rats have been investigated.

Materials and Methods

Animals

Control or pregnant female Sprague-Dawley rats (200–240 g) were purchased from Charles River (Wilmington, MA) or Harlan (Indianapolis, IN) breeding laboratories, respectively. Animals were kept in a 14L:10D photoperiod with lights on at 0500 h. Food and water were freely available. Three experimental groups were included in this study: intact cycling rats, ovariectomized animals, and lactating animals. Estrous cycle experiment: Cycle stages were determined by monitoring vaginal cytology, and only those rats demonstrating at least 2 consecutive 4-day cycles were used. Animals were sacrificed at 1100 h of each day of the cycle and at 1400, 1600, 1800, 2000, and 2200 h on proestrus. A group of proestrous rats were injected ip with either sodium pentobarbital (100 mg/kb BW) or saline at 1100 h and sacrificed at 1800 h. Trunk blood was collected for serum LH determination, and the brain was rapidly removed and stored at $-80°C$. Steroid-replacement experiment: Animals were bilaterally ovariectomized under metofane anesthesia. After 7–9 days, animals were implanted with either a crystalline E_2 silastic capsule (Dow-Corning, Medfield, MA; 5 mm; id = 0.062 in; od = 0.095 in) or an empty capsule. At 0900 h 2 days later, animals were injected sc with either progesterone (1.5 mg in mineral oil) or vehicle only. Rats were sacrificed at either 1100 or 1800 h of the same day, and brains and trunk blood were collected as described above. Lactation experiment: The day of delivery was designated day 0. On day 2, bilateral ovariectomy was performed and litter size was adjusted to 8–10 pups. On day 8 after delivery, pups were removed from appropriate groups. At 1000–1100 h on day 10 after delivery, rats were sacrificed, and brains and trunk blood were collected as described above.

Immunocytochemistry

Coronal brain sections (20 µm) were cut on a Reichert 820 cryostat (Buffalo, NY) at $-20°C$ and mounted onto gelatin and poly-L-lysine-coated glass slides. Sections were post-fixed in 5% paraformaldehyde for

10 min, and washed in PBS-T buffer (cold PBS containing 0.04% Triton X-100). Sections were incubated in 1% hydrogen peroxide in PBS-T buffer for 30 min, washed in PBS-T buffer for 30 min, and incubated in 3.3% normal goat serum for 30 min. Sections were then incubated overnight with the primary rabbit anti-GnRH sera (1:4000 dil in PBS containing 0.4% Triton X-100) generously provided by Dr. Robert Benoit (Children's Hospital, Montreal). After extensive washing in PBS-T buffer, sections were treated for staining using immunoperoxidase by the avidin-biotin complex method (Vectastain Inc., Burlingame, CA). Cells were counter-stained with eosin.

In Situ Hybridization

Coronal brain sections (20 µm) were cut throughout the entire area encompassing the DBB, OVLT, and POA. Sections were fixed in 5% paraformaldehyde (pH 7.5) for 5 min, washed in 2X SSC for 5 min, rinsed in distilled deionized water and in 0.1 M triethanolamine, and incubated in 0.25% acetic anhydride in 0.1 M triethanolamine for 10 min. Sections were dehydrated through an ethanol serres and vacuum-dried until hybridization. Antisense and sense [^{35}S]UTP-labeled RNA probes were synthesized using SP6 polymerase from a rat hypothalamic GnRH cDNA clone. Probe (10^7 cpm/ml) was applied to the slides in standard hybridization buffer, a coverslip was applied, and the slides were incubated at 47°C for 15 h. After hybridization, coverslips were removed in 4X SSC and the sections were treated with RNAse A (20 µg/ml) at 37°C for 30 min, washed in 0.1X SSC at 55°C, and dehydrated through an ethanol series. Sections were exposed to Kodak XAR-5 film overnight, then coated with Kodak NTB-2 liquid emulsion for autoradiography. After development, sections were stained with cresyl violet and observed by microscopy, and GnRH mRNA-expressing cells were manually counted. For quantification of specific hybridization in GnRH cells located in the OVLT-POA region, an Image-1/AT program from Universal Imaging Corporation was used (30). Using 100X dark-field optics, an area of $75 \times 75 \, \mu m^2$ was examined to determine grain density. Nearby negative cells were measured as a control to determine background density. Manual grain counts were shown to be linearly related to the values obtained using the image-analysis system.

Radioimmunoassay

LH concentrations were determined using an ovine:rat RIA system with NIH LH S-25 as the standard and anti-rat antibody S-10 from the NIDDK kit. The intra- and inter-assay coefficients of variation for the LH RIA were 5.0% and 6.0%, respectively. FSH concentrations were determined using the rat:rat NIDDK kit with NIH FSH RP-2 as the standard. The intra- and inter-assay coefficients of variation were 3.0% and 2.5%, respectively.

Results

Use of In Situ Hybridization to Study GnRH Gene Expression

Figure 14.1 briefly outlines the in situ hybridization procedure that was used to examine GnRH gene expression. Frozen tissue sections were cut on a cryostat, fixed, and processed for hybridization to a labeled GnRH antisense RNA probe. Hybridization was detected by subsequent autoradiography, and GnRH mRNA-expressing cells were counted and/or examined using computer-enhanced image analysis. In each experiment, all tissue sections were processed simultaneously and a single preparation of probe was used.

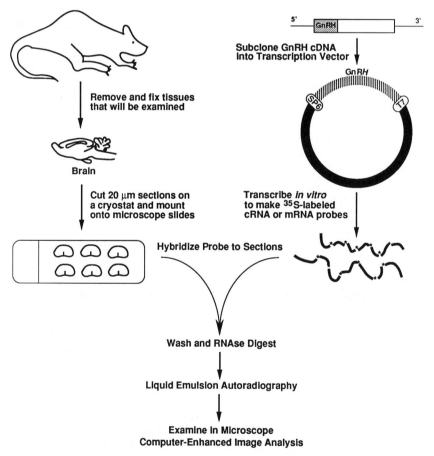

FIGURE 14.1. Schematic diagram of the procedures used to detect GnRH mRNA by in situ hybridization. Details are described in Materials and Methods.

One reason that in situ hybridization is particularly applicable to study-ing GnRH gene expression is that the GnRH neurons are broadly dis-tributed throughout the hypothalamus. As shown in Figure 14.2, growth hormone releasing hormone (GHRH), corticotropin releasing hormone (CRH), and somatostatin-expressing neurons are localized to discrete hypothalamic nuclei (the arcuate, paraventricular, and periventricular nuclei, respectively), while the GnRH-expressing neurons are at best clustered in a few predominant locations, such as the preoptic area. Thus while it is possible to microdissect defined regions expressing mRNAs such as GHRH, CRH, or somatostatin for blot or solution hybridization assays, this is more difficult for detection of GnRH mRNA.

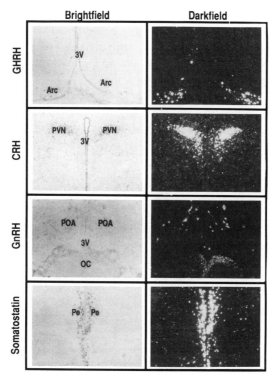

FIGURE 14.2. Localization of neuropeptide mRNAs in the rat brain. Sections from the hypothalamus were hybridized to probes for growth hormone releasing hor-mone (GHRH), corticotropin releasing hormone (CRH), GnRH, or somatostatin as indicated. The left panels are brightfield photomicrographs of the brain region, the right panels are darkfield photomicrographs that show the hybridization. GHRH, CRH, and somatostatin-expressing cells are highly localized, whereas GnRH-expressing neurons are much more dispersed. (Arc = arcuate nucleus, PVN = paraventricular nucleus, Pe = periventricular nucleus, 3V = third ventricle.)

228   O.-K. Park et al.

An example of the type of hybridization detected with the GnRH probe is shown in Figure 14.3. This shows a field of GnRH mRNA-expressing cells in the OVLT/preoptic area. The hybridization is readily distinguished from background, and individual GnRH mRNA-expressing cells can easily be counted. At higher magnification, silver grains are heavily clustered over single cell bodies; this magnification was used for all image analysis procedures to determine grain densities over single cells. When similar sections were hybridized to a sense-strand GnRH RNA probe, or when the antisense GnRH RNA probe was hybridized to other tissues such as liver, no specific hybridization was observed (not shown). In addition, this same GnRH cDNA probe detects a single transcript of approximately 500 nucleotides when it is used to probe hypothalamic polyadenylated RNA by Northern RNA blot analysis (not shown).

The location, morphology, and number of GnRH mRNA-expressing cells are all similar to what is observed in using GnRH immunocyto-chemistry. An example of this is shown in Figure 14.4, which compares

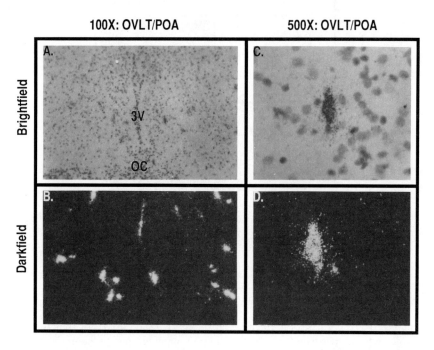

FIGURE 14.3. Detection of GnRH mRNA expressing cells in the rat brain. The upper panels (A, C) are brightfield photomicrographs of the OVLT/preoptic area at the indicated magnifications. The lower panels (B, D) are corresponding darkfield photomicrographs. (3V = third ventricle, OC = optic chiasm.) Reprinted with permission from Ref. 29, © by The Endocrine Society, 1990.

the two assays on brain sections in close proximity. One difference appears to be sensitivity, in that more GnRH mRNA-expressing cells are seen than GnRH-immunoreactive cells. We are currently attempting to colocalize the mRNA and peptide in individual cells.

GnRH Gene Expression During the Estrous Cycle

In order to examine the relationship between the release and synthesis of GnRH, we measured serum LH levels (as an index of GnRH secretion) and GnRH mRNA expression (by in situ hybridization) during the 4-day estrous cycle. We focused on the proestrous-to-estrous transition, since increased GnRH secretion at this time is thought to drive the pre-ovulatory LH surge (31). For these experiments, we counted the number of GnRH mRNA-expressing cells in a brain region including the DBB, OVLT, and POA, and normalized the data to the value observed at 1800 h metestrus. As shown in Figure 14.5 (panel B), serum LH levels in these animals increase by 1600 h proestrus, peak at 1800 h proestrus, then

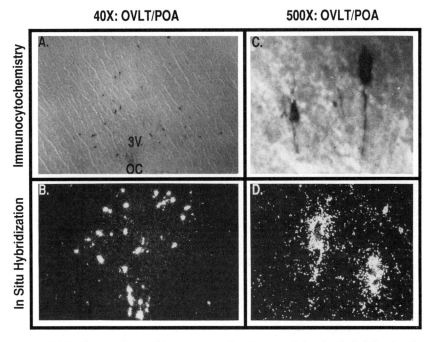

FIGURE 14.4. Comparison of immunocytochemistry and in situ hybridization for detection of GnRH-expressing neurons. Sections from the same brain region (OVLT/POA) were processed for immunocytochemistry (A, C) or in situ hybridization (B, D) as indicated. Two magnifications are shown. (3V = third ventricle, OC = optic chiasm.)

slowly decline to basal levels by estrous morning. During the early part of
the estrous cycle, no significant changes in the number of GnRH mRNA-
expressing cells were observed; however, after the onset of the preovulatory LH surge the number of GnRH mRNA-expressing cells nearly
doubled. Significant increases were observed at 1800 and 2000 h on
proestrus (Fig. 14.5, panel A).

We also quantified GnRH mRNA expression by individual neurons,
using computer-based image analysis. Cells were scored for their relative
expression of GnRH mRNA, as determined by grain density measurements. Figure 14.6 shows data from about 300–370 cells located in
the OVLT-POA region of proestrous rats. In early proestrus (P1100 to

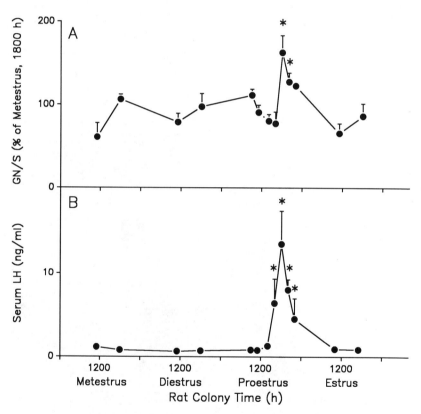

FIGURE 14.5. Changes in the number of GnRH mRNA-expressing cells and in
serum LH levels during the rat estrous cycle. Panel A shows the average number
of GnRH mRNA-expressing cells per brain section (GN/S); values are expressed
as a percentage of GN/S at 1800 h on metestrus. Panel B shows serum LH levels
in the corresponding animals. *P < 0.05 as compared with other groups, n = 4–5
for each. Reprinted with permission from Ref. 29, © by The Endocrine Society,
1990.

P1600), the majority of cells express mRNA at relatively low levels. After the onset of the LH surge (P1800 and P2000), the distribution is shifted such that more cells express higher levels of GnRH mRNA. As the LH surge is terminated (P2200), the distribution begins to return toward that observed prior to the surge.

Because of the temporal correlation between the increase in GnRH mRNA-expressing cells and the preovulatory LH surge, we attempted to explore further the role of the LH surge in GnRH mRNA expression in proestrous animals treated with pentobarbital. Barbituate treatment

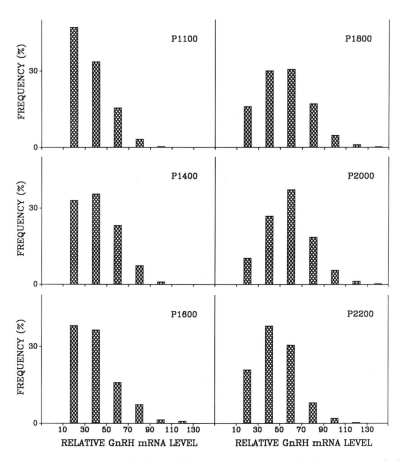

FIGURE 14.6. Changes in GnRH mRNA expression by individual neurons during the afternoon and evening of proestrus. The relative expression of GnRH mRNA by individual cells was determined by using a computer-based image analysis system. Results are plotted as the frequency at which cells with a particular grain density are represented (n = 300–370). The time of sacrifice on proestrus is indicated at the upper right corner of each individual plot.

before the critical period is known to block the LH surge, probably through an effect on GnRH release (14). Animals were treated with pentobarbital at 1100 h proestrus and sacrificed at 1800 h proestrus, a time when we observed an increased number of GnRH mRNA-expressing cells in control animals. The results are shown in Figure 14.7. Pentobarbital completely blocked the LH surge and eliminated the increase in the number of GnRH mRNA-expressing cells normally observed on proestrous evening.

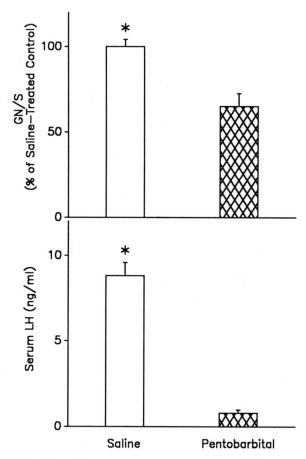

FIGURE 14.7. The effect of pentobarbital treatment on GnRH gene expression at the time of the preovulatory LH surge. The upper panel shows the relative number of GnRH mRNA-expressing cells, while the lower panel shows serum LH levels. Proestrous rats were treated with either pentobarbital or saline at 1100 h and sacrificed at 1800 h. *P < 0.05, n = 4 for each group. Reprinted with permission from Ref. 29, © by The Endocrine Society, 1990.

Effects of Ovarian Steroids on GnRH mRNA Expression

Ovarian steroids are thought to modulate gonadotropin secretion by acting both at the pituitary and the hypothalamic level. Because steroid hormones act on target tissues to control the expression of specific genes, we wanted to determine whether they might directly modulate GnRH gene expression. We utilized ovariectomized rats that received estrogen implants to generate a constant level of hormone. Some animals

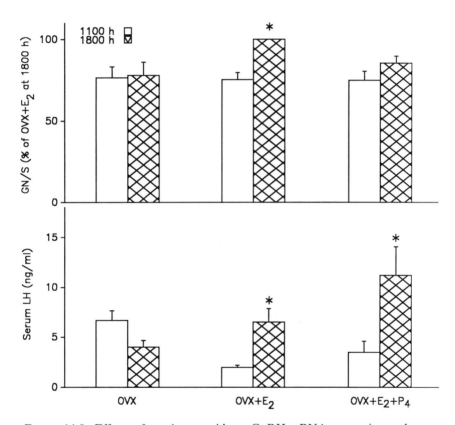

FIGURE 14.8. Effects of ovarian steroids on GnRH mRNA expression and serum LH levels in ovariectomized rats. The top panel shows the numbers of GnRH mRNA-expressing cells, normalized to the value at 1800 h in estrogen-replaced rats. The bottom panel shows serum LH levels. Two times, 1100 h (open bars) and 1800 h (hatched bars), were analyzed as indicated. Groups were ovariectomized (OVX), estrogen-replaced (OVX + E$_2$), or estrogen and progesterone-replaced (OVX + E$_2$ + P$_4$). *P < 0.05, n = 4 for each group. Reprinted with permission from Ref. 29, © by The Endocrine Society, 1990.

also received a single injection of progesterone shortly before sacrifice. The results of these experiments are shown in Figure 14.8. When ovariectomized or steroid-replaced animals were examined for GnRH mRNA expression at 1100 h, no significant differences between the groups were observed. Interestingly, when these same groups were examined at 1800 h, estrogen replacement resulted in a significant increase in the number of GnRH mRNA-expressing cells. In these estrogen-replaced animals, daily LH surges occur between 1500 and 1800 h. Curiously, estrogen plus progesterone-replaced animals showed no significant increase in GnRH mRNA expression. This might be due to a progesterone-induced advance in the time of the daily LH surge (1, 5).

Changes in GnRH Gene Expression Induced by Lactation

One well-characterized animal model in which the tonic release of LH is altered, presumably through changes in GnRH secretion, is the lactating rat (32, 33). We used this animal model to determine whether the established suppression of serum LH during lactation was correlated with reduced expression of the GnRH gene. Groups of animals with identically sized litters (8–10) were maintained for 8 days following delivery, and then pups were removed from appropriate groups for 2 days prior to assay. To determine whether ovarian steroids might mediate any of the effects of suckling on GnRH secretion, we also examined similar groups of animals that had been ovariectomized 2 days after delivery. These results are shown in Figure 14.9.

As expected, groups with pups had lower serum LH levels than those without (Fig. 14.9, panel C), both in intact and in ovariectomized animals. Ovariectomy resulted in a large increase in serum LH levels. The presence of pups had no effect on serum FSH levels, which were also increased by ovariectomy (Fig. 14.9, panel D). In examining the number of GnRH mRNA-expressing cells in these animals, we noticed that changes in GnRH gene expression appeared to be confined to GnRH neurons in the preoptic/OVLT area. In animal groups with pups, the number of GnRH mRNA-expressing cells in the POA/OVLT was decreased to $68.6 \pm 6.7\%$ of control in intact animals and to $69.6 \pm 5.3\%$ of control in ovariectomized animals (Fig. 14.9, panel A). No significant changes in the number of GnRH mRNA-expressing cells were observed between any of the groups when cells in the septal area/DBB were scored separately (Fig. 14.9, panel B). This suggests that a suckling stimulus might differentially regulate GnRH gene expression in anatomically discrete neuronal populations. Ovariectomy had no effect on the suckling-induced suppression of GnRH gene expression.

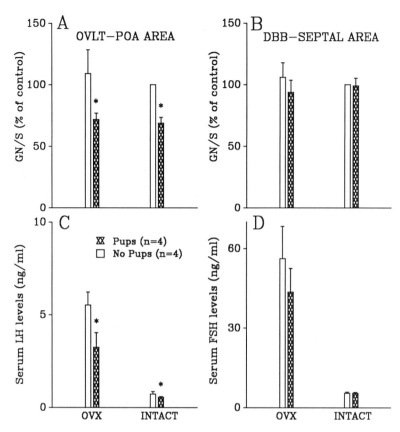

FIGURE 14.9. Effect of lactation on GnRH gene expression and serum gonadotropin levels. Panels A and B show the number of GnRH mRNA-expressing neurons in the OVLT-POA and DBB-septal areas, respectively. Values are normalized to those of intact rats without pups. Panels C and D show serum LH and FSH levels, respectively. Open bars indicate animals with pups and hatched bars indicate animals without pups. Ovariectomized (OVX) and intact groups are indicated. *P < 0.05, n = 4 for each group.

Discussion

Despite considerable evidence supporting the notion that GnRH secretion from the hypothalamus is highly regulated (1, 5, 10, 31), the specific details of how the biosynthetic activity of the GnRH neuron is modulated have remained elusive. With the molecular cloning of the GnRH precursor (20, 21, 29, 34) it has become possible to directly measure changes in GnRH mRNA production and to try to correlate these to changes in GnRH secretion. We have employed an in situ hybridization assay for the measurement of GnRH mRNA expression. This is a particularly appropriate technique for examining GnRH gene expression because of the scattered location of GnRH mRNA-expressing neurons in the rat brain. We have shown that in situ hybridization detects neurons that have a distribution and morphology similar to those observed using immuno-cytochemistry. Others have recently demonstrated colocalization of the peptide and mRNA in single neurons by using combined in situ hybridiza-tion and immunocytochemical approaches (35). While both assays detect the same population of GnRH neurons, in situ hybridization appears to be more sensitive and detects cells not readily observed using immuno-cytochemistry (35, and our unpublished results).

As an index of GnRH gene expression, we have counted the number of GnRH mRNA-expressing cells within a brain region including the DBB, OVLT, and POA. In adult cycling female rats, we found that both the number of GnRH mRNA-expressing cells and the average level of mRNA expression per cell were significantly increased at the time of the preovulatory LH surge. The timing of this increase suggests that GnRH gene expression might be changing in response to the increased GnRH secretory activity occurring late on proestrous afternoon. Consistent with this, blockade of the preovulatory LH surge, and presumably of GnRH secretion, with pentobarbital eliminates the increase in GnRH mRNA expression normally seen between 1800 and 2000 h proestrus.

It is likely that a subpopulation of the GnRH cells actively participate in the generation of the preovulatory LH surge. Not all GnRH neurons in the OVLT-POA region send terminals into the median eminence (7, 8), and only some GnRH cells in the POA express the activation marker c-*fos* during the critical period preceding the LH surge (36, 37). It is therefore interesting that both by in situ hybridization (our results) and by immunocytochemistry (38) there appears to be a recruitment of additional GnRH-expressing cells following the preovulatory LH surge. The signal for this recruitment remains unclear, but secretion-synthesis coupling seems to be one important component for activation of the GnRH system.

Steroid hormones clearly play important roles in the generation of the preovulatory LH surge and in the feedback regulation of gonadotropin secretion. Although GnRH-expressing cells are reported to lack estrogen receptors (39), estrogen appears to be able to modulate GnRH gene expression (23, 25, 26, 27, 40). In our experiments, we observed a significant increase in the number of GnRH mRNA-expressing cells in ovariectomized, estrogen-replaced animals at 1800 h, but not at 1100 h. Since these animals have a daily LH surge at about 1500–1800 h, our data are consistent with a model in which increased LH secretion serves as the specific signal for enhanced GnRH gene expression, and the role of estrogen is more indirect.

Last, we examined lactating rats with differing suckling stimuli (pups or no pups) to determine whether the suppression of LH secretion by a suckling stimulus is coupled to decreases in GnRH gene expression. Surprisingly, we found an anatomical segregation of GnRH mRNA-expressing cells responsive to the suckling stimulus. There was a significant decrease in GnRH mRNA expression in animals with pups in the OVLT/POA, but not in the DBB/septal area. These results are consistent with the suggestion that GnRH secretion in lactating animals is decreased (32, 33) and again suggests a close coupling of GnRH secretion and GnRH gene expression in this animal model.

Our results in these diverse animal models are all suggestive of secretion-synthesis coupling as one component important for the appropriate regulation of the GnRH neuron. Clearly, more direct effects of neurotransmitters or hormones on expression of the GnRH gene are in no way precluded by these results. It should also be noted that we, and most others, have to date measured only changes in GnRH mRNA abundance, and not in GnRH gene transcription. Based upon these types of in vivo experiments, it should now be possible to study directly the transcriptional regulation of the GnRH gene in in vitro systems, such as the recently described GnRH-expressing neuronal cell line (41).

Acknowledgments. We thank Dr. A.F. Parlow and the NIDDK for the LH and FSH RIA kits. We acknowledge Robert Valadka for radioimmunoassays and Elena Burtea for experimental assistance. This work was supported by grants from the Searle Scholars Program (87-G-113), the NSF PYI Program (DCB-8552977), the McKnight Foundation, and the NIH (HD-21921).

References

1. Fink G. Gonadotropin secretion and its control. In: Knobil E, Neill JD, eds. Physiology of reproduction, vol. 1. New York: Raven Press, 1988:1349–77.
2. Freeman ME. The ovarian cycle of the rat. In: Knobil E, Neill JD, eds. Physiology of reproduction, vol. 2. New York: Raven Press, 1988:1893–928.
3. Andrews WV, Maurer R, Conn PM. Stimulation of rat luteinizing hormone β-messenger RNA levels by gonadotropin-releasing hormone. J Biol Chem 1988;263:13755–61.
4. Wierman ME, Rivier JE, Wang C. Gonadotropin-releasing hormone-dependent regulation of gonadotropin subunit messenger ribonucleic acid levels in the rat. Endocrinology 1989;124:272–8.
5. Kalra SP. Neural circuitry involved in the control of LHRH secretion: a model for the preovulatory LH release. In: Ganong WF, Martini L, eds. Frontiers in neuroendocrinology, vol. 9. New York: Raven Press, 1986: 311–51.

6. Swanzel-Fukuda M, Pfaff DW. Origin of luteinizing hormone-releasing hormone neurons. Nature 1989;338:161–4.

7. Merchenthaler I, Setalo G, Csontos C, Petrusz P, Flerko B, Negro-Vilar A. Combined retrograde tracing and immunocytochemical identification of luteinizing hormone-releasing hormone and somatostatin-containing neurons projecting to the median eminence of the rat. Endocrinology 1988;125:2812–21.

8. Silverman AJ, Jhamandas J, Renand L. Localization of luteinizing hormone-releasing hormone (LHRH) neurons that project to the median eminence. J Neurosci 1987;7:2312–9.

9. Clayton RN. Gonadotropin-releasing hormone: its actions and receptor. J Endocrinol 1989;120:11–9.

10. Levine JE, Ramirez VD. Luteinizing hormone-releasing hormone release during the rat estrous cycle and after ovariectomy as estimated with push-pull cannulae. Endocrinology 1982;111:1439–48.

11. Watanabe T, Nakai Y. Electron microscopic cytochemistry of catecholaminergic innervation of LHRH neurons in the medial preoptic area of the rat. Arch Histol Jpn 1987;50:103–12.

12. Rotsztejun WH, Drouva SV, Pollard H, Sokoloff P, Pattou E, Kordon C. Further evidence for the existence of opiate binding sites on neurosecretory LHRH mediobasal hypothalamic nerve terminals. Eur J Pharmacol 1982;80:139–41.

13. Leranth C, Maclusky N, Salamoto H, Shanabrongh M, Naftolin F. Glutamic acid decarboxylase-containing axons synapsing on LHRH neurons in the rat medial preoptic area. Neuroendocrinology 1985;40:536–9.

14. Everett JW, Sawyer CH. A 24-hour periodicity in the "LH-releasing apparatus" of female rats, disclosed by barbituate sedation. Endocrinology 1950;47:198–218.

15. Hoffman JC. Light and reproduction in the rat: effect of lighting schedule on ovulation blockade. Biol Reprod 1969;1:185–8.

16. Dluzen DE, Ramirez VD, Carter CS, Getz LL. Male vole urine changes luteinizing hormone-releasing hormone and norepinephrine in female olfactory bulb. Science 1981;212:573–5.

17. Vandenbergh JG. Pheromones and mammalian reproduction. In: Knobil E, Neill JD, eds. The physiology of reproduction, vol. 2. New York: Raven Press, 1988:1679–96.

18. Dluzen DE, Ramirez VD. In vivo LHRH output of ovariectomized rats following estrogen treatment. Neuroendocrinology 1986;43:459–65.

19. Ramirez VD, Dluzen DE, Lin D. Progesterone administration in vivo stimulates release of luteinizing hormone-releasing hormone in vitro. Science 1980;208:1037–9.

20. Adelman JP, Mason AJ, Hayflick JS, Seeburg PH. Isolation of the gene and hypothalamic cDNA for the common precursor of gonadotropin-releasing hormone and prolactin release-inhibiting factor in human and rat. Proc Natl Acad Sci USA 1986;83:179–83.

21. Bond CT, Hayflick JS, Seeburg PH, Adelman JP. The rat gonaodtropin-releasing hormone: SH locus structure and hypothalamic expression. Mol Endocrinol 1989;3:1257–62.

22. Kim K, Lee BJ, Park Y, Cho WK. Progesterone increases messenger ribonucleic acid (mRNA) encoding luteinizing hormone-releasing hormone (LHRH) level in the hypothalamus of ovariectomized estradiol-primed prepubertal rats. Mol Brain Res 1989;6:151–8.
23. Roberts JL, Dutlow CM, Jakubowski M, Blum M, Millar RP. Estradiol stimulates preoptic area-anterior hypothalamic proGnRH-GAP gene expression in ovariectomized rats. Mol Brain Res 1989;6:127–33.
24. Pfaff DW. Gene expression in hypothalamic neurons: luteinizing hormone-releasing hormone. J Neurosci Res 1986;16:109–15.
25. Rothfeld J, Heytmancik JF, Conn PM, Pfaff DW. In situ hybridization for LHRH mRNA following estrogen treatment. Mol Brain Res 1989;6:121–6.
26. Wray S, Zoeller RT, Gainer H. Differential effects of estrogen on luteinizing hormone-releasing hormone gene expression in slice explant cultures prepared from specific rat forebrain regions. Mol Endocrinol 1989;3:1197–206.
27. Zoeller RT, Seeburg PH, Young WS III. In situ hybridization histochemistry for messenger ribonucleic acid (mRNA) encoding gonadotropin-releasing hormone (GnRH): effect of estrogen on cellular levels of GnRH mRNA in female rat brain. Endocrinology 1988;122:2570–7.
28. Kelly MJ, Garrett J, Bosch MA, et al. Effects of ovariectomy on GnRH mRNA, proGnRH, and GnRH levels in the preoptic hypothalamus of the female rat. Neuroendocrinology, 1989;49:88–97.
29. Park OK, Gugneja S, Mayo K. Gonadotropin-releasing hormone gene expression during the rat estrous cycle: effects of pentobarbital and ovarian steroids. Endocrinology 1990;127:365–72.
30. Kornhauser JM, Nelson DE, Mayo KE, Takahashi JS. Photic and circadian regulation of c-fos gene expression in the hamster suprachiasmatic nucleus. Neuron 1990;5:127–34.
31. Sarkar DK, Chiappa SA, Fink G, Sherwood NM. Gonadotropin-releasing hormone surge in pro-oestrous rats. Nature 1976;264:461–3.
32. Smith MS, Lee LR. Modulation of pituitary gonadotropin-releasing hormone receptors during lactation in the rat. Endocrinology 1989;124:1456–61.
33. McNeilly AS. Suckling and the control of gonadotropin secretion. In: Knobil E, Neill JD, eds. The physiology of reproduction, vol. 2. New York: Raven Press, 1988:2323–49.
34. Radovick S, Wondisford FE, Nakayama Y, Yamada M, Cutler GB, Weintraub BD. Isolation and characterization of the human gonadotropin-releasing hormone gene in the hypothalamus and placenta. Mol Endocrinol 1990;4:476–80.
35. Ronnekleiv OK, Naylor BR, Bond CT, Adelman JP. Combined immunohistochemistry for gonadotropin-releasing hormone (GnRH) and pro-GnRH and in situ hybridization for GnRH mRNA in the rat brain. Mol Endocrinol 1989;3:363–71.
36. Lee WS, Smith MS, Hoffman GE. Progesterone enhances the surge of luteinizing hormone by increasing the activation of luteinizing hormone-releasing hormone neurons. Endocrinology 1990;127:2604–6.
37. Lee WS, Smith MS, Hoffman GE. Luteinizing hormone-releasing hormone (LHRH) neurons express c-fos during the proestrous surge. Proc Natl Acad Sci USA 1990;87:5163–7.

38. King JC, Rubin BS, Yao P. Changes in LHRH neuronal populations associated with the LH surge in young and middle-aged female rats [Abstract]. 20th annu mtg Neurosci Soc, 1990;abstract 168.11.
39. Shivers BD, Harlan RE, Morrel JI, Pfaff DW. Absence of oestradiol concentration in cell nuclei of LHRH immunoreactive neurons. Nature 1983; 304:345-7.
40. Sierman ME, Wang C, Sun W, Raynolds MV, Gordon DF, Wood WM. Negative regulation of the rat gonadotropin releasing hormone (GnRH) gene by estrogen [Abstract]. 72nd annu mtg Endocrine Soc, 1990;abstract 1054.
41. Mellon PL, Windle JJ, Goldsmith PC, Padula CA, Roberts JL, Weiner RI. Immortalization of hypothalamic GnRH neurons by genetically targeted tumorigenesis. Neuron 1990;5:1-10.

15

The Preovulatory Surge of Gonadotropin Releasing Hormone

Fred J. Karsch, Suzanne M. Moenter, and Alain Caraty

The regulation of gonadotropin releasing hormone secretion during the preovulatory surge of luteinizing hormone has been a focus of neuroendocrinological investigation for decades. Although it is clear that an increase in estradiol secretion from the developing follicle is an essential ovarian signal for the LH discharge, a fundamental question remains: Does estradiol elicit the LH surge by stimulating the secretion of GnRH? Despite the importance of this question, it is only in the laboratory rat that there has been general agreement and ample direct evidence for heightened secretion of GnRH (1–6). In the rat, however, an increased secretion of GnRH at the time of the LH surge would seem a virtual certainty, for the surge in this species is precisely timed by a circadian clock located in the brain (5–7). The circadian signal emanating from the clock would be expected to be relayed to the pituitary via a hypophyseotropic stimulus discharged into pituitary portal blood. In species in which the preovulatory LH surge is not tightly coupled to a circadian clock, for example in primates (8) and sheep (9), enhanced secretion of GnRH at the time of the LH surge is not necessarily expected, nor is there consistent evidence that such an increase actually exists. Further, a stimulatory action of estradiol upon the anterior pituitary gland is documented to be one mode by which this steroid elicits the preovulatory LH discharge (10–16), and in at least one species, the rhesus monkey, this pituitary action of estradiol may itself be sufficient for LH-surge induction (16). Therefore, the fundamental question remains: Does estradiol induce the preovulatory LH surge by enhancing the secretion of GnRH?

A major hurdle to answering this question has been methodological, namely the lack of a technique that allows direct monitoring of the time course of GnRH secretion throughout the LH surge of conscious animals. In recent years, several procedures have been developed for measurement of GnRH secretion in nonanesthetized sheep (17–19), making this species ideal for approaching the question of GnRH secretory dynamics during the LH surge. Of these techniques, the method of Caraty and Locatelli (19) allows sequential sampling of hypophyseal portal blood over a period sufficient to span the entire LH surge in the same animal. Initial studies employing this technique to monitor GnRH identified an unambiguous increase in secretion at the time of the LH surge induced in ovariectomized ewes treated with bolus injections of estradiol (20). We have now used this method to assess the secretory pattern of GnRH both during the preovulatory LH surge of the estrous cycle of the ewe and in a physiological endocrine model for the follicular phase. This chapter constitutes a progress report of our studies, which are being performed as a collaborative effort at the Institut National de la Recherche Agronomique (France) and the University of Michigan. Since the technique for obtaining samples for monitoring GnRH secretion is so critically important, we begin this report with a brief description of methodology.

Method for Sampling Hypophyseal Portal Blood

Our procedure for obtaining portal blood is a modification of the method described by Caraty and Locatelli (19). It consists of surgical implantation of a sampling apparatus and subsequent automated blood collection at a site remote to the sheep. The first step is construction of the sampling apparatus. This is done by cementing two 75-mm blunt-tip hypodermic needles and a polypropylene cup together with dental acrylic such that the rim of the cup extends 2–3 mm beyond the blunted needle tips (see Fig. 15.1). The top needle serves initially as a guide tube for a stylet used to cut portal vessels and subsequently as an air vent during removal of portal blood. The bottom needle is used to aspirate portal blood.

The second step is implantation of the apparatus into the head of the ewe. A medial triangular incision is made between the eyes; a bone flap is cut; and the turbinates in the caudal nasal cavity are removed to expose the cribriform plate. With the aid of an operating microscope, a midline tunnel is drilled through the bone under the optic chiasm until the dura mater covering the anterior face of the pituitary gland is exposed (Fig. 15.1). After measuring of the distance to the pituitary to the nearest millimeter, the dura mater is cut and removed to create a "window" through which portal vessels can be seen. The collection apparatus is next positioned such that the rim of the cup fits snugly against the bone surrounding the dural window, creating a water-tight seal. The collection apparatus is then cemented in place with dental acrylic, filled with saline, and capped, and the incision is closed. After recovery, the ewe is maintained by usual husbandry procedures until sampling, which is usually performed at least 1 week after surgery to allow healing and thus minimize bleeding from the surgical field.

The third step is the sampling of portal blood. Two ewes, each fitted

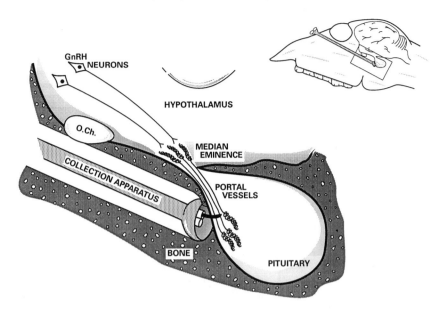

FIGURE 15.1. Surgical approach for placement of apparatus for portal blood collection. The inset in the upper right shows the position of the apparatus in the skull; the area within the rectangle is enlarged below. The curved heavy line extending from the collection apparatus depicts a stylet used to cut a portion of the portal vasculature. Reprinted with permission from Ref. 21. © by The Endocrine Society, 1990.

with a collection apparatus, are penned in adjacent stalls in an open barn having visual, olfactory, and auditory contact with ewes outdoors. Both jugular veins of each ewe are cannulated—one for sampling peripheral blood and one for infusing heparin to prevent coagulation. The caps are removed from the collection apparatus and a Silastic tube is coupled to the hub of the sampling (lower) needle. The ewe is then heparinized by systemic infusion, and the stylet for cutting the portal vasculature is passed through the upper needle of the collection apparatus (Fig. 15.1, dark line extending from needle tip). To initiate portal flow, a cut is made at a depth of 1 mm into the pituitary, based on measurements at the time of surgery, with further cuts advancing by 1 mm until a collection rate of approximately 0.1 ml/min is established (cut usually extends 2–3 mm into the pituitary). Only a portion of the portal vasculature is cut, with care being taken to minimize portal-blood loss such that pituitary function is not unduly compromised. The portal and jugular collection lines, and the heparin infusion line, are led across the back of the sheep and into a separate room housing peristaltic pumps (for blood withdrawal/heparin infusion) and a fraction collector for automated dispensing of sequential samples into tubes in an ice bath. The room has an observation window allowing the ewes to be monitored visually without being disturbed. The animals require little attention such that the investigator generally need not be present except for feeding and watering.

This remote and automated collection procedure allows simultaneous sampling of portal blood for measurement of GnRH and jugular blood for measurement of LH in sheep that are fully conscious and behaving normally. It is readily possible to obtain samples with little or no apparent disturbance to the animal. With this technique, sequential portal and jugular samples have been obtained for up to 48 continuous hours and, in some instances, from the same sheep on two separate occasions. The procedure, therefore, is well suited to monitor the time course of GnRH secretion during the preovulatory or estradiol-induced LH surge.

Preovulatory Surge of GnRH

Before describing our findings on GnRH secretion during the pre-ovulatory LH surge, it is pertinent to review the feedback interplay between pituitary and gonadal hormones that lead to the LH surge of the ewe and to summarize previous observations of GnRH secretory patterns at this time of the cycle. The feedback interactions among estradiol, progesterone, and LH have been well characterized (22–24) and are illustrated schematically in Figure 15.2.

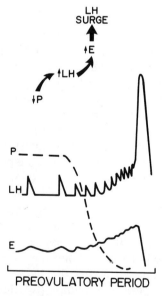

FIGURE 15.2. Sequence of endocrine events that lead to ovulation in the ewe. Modified with permission from Ref. 22.

Prior to regression of the corpus luteum, the pulsatile secretion of LH is held in check by progesterone and, thus, the frequency of LH pulses is low. Once the corpus luteum begins to regress and progesterone secretion wanes, this inhibition is lifted, permitting LH pulse frequency to increase. The resultant rise in circulating LH stimulates the secretion of estradiol from developing ovarian follicles, and the rising tide of circulating estradiol elicits the preovulatory LH surge. This sequence of hormonal events between onset of the decline in progesterone and the preovulatory LH peak occurs within a time span of 2–3 days.

Considerable insight of how GnRH fits into this regulatory interplay has been provided by Clarke and his colleagues. During the luteal phase of the cycle, GnRH is secreted as low-frequency pulses into hypophyseal portal blood (25, 26). This secretory pattern shifts to high-frequency pulses when the corpus luteum regresses at the onset of the follicular phase (25). This shift in GnRH pattern can be accounted for, in large measure, by changes in the secretion of progesterone, which inhibits pulsatile GnRH secretion when present in a high luteal-phase concentration (27). This restraint on GnRH secretion is removed when progesterone plummets at the transition from the luteal to the early follicular phase. During the late follicular phase, however, the regulation of GnRH secretion remains open to question, largely because studies to evaluate the secretory dynamics of GnRH during the preovulatory LH surge have not yielded consistent results. The only previous study that addresses this point revealed a number of different secretory patterns, ranging from a large increase in GnRH to no change at all during the preovulatory LH surge (25).

In our studies, we monitored the time course of GnRH secretion into hypophyseal portal blood during the preovulatory LH surge of two breeds of sheep, Ile de France ewes (France) and Suffolk ewes (Michigan). Since such a study requires proper timing of portal blood collection relative to the preovulatory LH surge, we chose to synchronize the follicular phase of the cycle by means of exogenous progesterone, a procedure commonly used to control the time of ovulation in sheep (28). Constant-release implants containing progesterone were inserted approximately 1 week before luteolysis, such that circulating progesterone was maintained at a luteal-phase level once the corpus luteum regressed (29). Removal of the implants caused a drop in progesterone mimicking that which occurs at luteolysis and initiating the preovulatory endocrine events according to the sequence of steps illustrated in Figure 15.2. Simultaneous collection of jugular and hypophyseal portal blood was initiated 6–12 h prior to the expected onset of the preovulatory LH surge. Sampling continued at 6–10-min intervals for up to 48 h, depending on when the LH surge actually began. Onset of the LH surge was determined by a rapid LH assay performed on selected jugular samples during the course of portal blood collection.

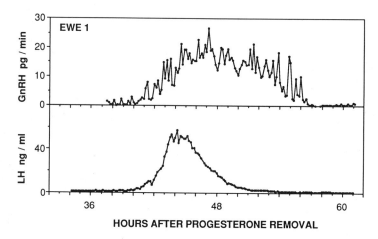

FIGURE 15.3. Time course of GnRH in hypophyseal portal blood (top) and LH in jugular blood (bottom) throughout the preovulatory LH surge of a representative Suffolk ewe. Samples were obtained at 10-min intervals. The preovulatory sequence was initiated by removal of progesterone implants at hour 0. Reprinted with permission from Ref. 30. © by The Endocrine Society, 1991.

Overall, we monitored the secretion of GnRH into hypophyseal portal blood in 19 ewes at the expected time of the preovulatory LH surge. Of these 19 animals, our sampling period actually spanned all or part of the LH surge in 11 ewes (8 Suffolk and 3 Ile de France). In each ewe sampled during the LH discharge, we obtained evidence for a robust surge of GnRH. Representative patterns in one ewe are illustrated in Figure 15.3. The GnRH increase of some ewes was massive, with peaks more than 100-fold greater than the presurge baseline. In other ewes, the GnRH increase was smaller, but unmistakable, ranging from 4- to 20-fold above baseline.

Several characteristics of the preovulatory GnRH surge are noteworthy, as illustrated by the example in Figure 15.3. The onsets of the GnRH and LH surges occurred at approximately the same time, with the increase in both hormones continuing over the course of several hours. The ends of the surges of the two hormones, however, did not coincide. In this regard, the GnRH surge outlasted the LH surge and, in some instances, LH values had returned nearly to baseline at the time the GnRH surge was near its peak (e.g., Fig. 15.3; 50–54 h). Finally, the GnRH values in contiguous 10-min samples exhibited a high degree of variability, raising the possibility of pulsatile secretion of GnRH during the surge. This possibility will be considered in the next section, on the estradiol-induced GnRH surge.

Our findings provide definitive evidence for an unambiguous discharge of GnRH at the time of the preovulatory LH surge of the ewe. This is consonant with the hypothesis that estradiol induces the LH surge, in part, by stimulating GnRH release. Despite the clarity of our results, this study also disclosed a complication of the experimental approach; specifically, an LH surge did not occur during the observation period in approximately 40% of our animals. In this regard, we have preliminary evidence to suggest that the collection procedure, itself, caused an attenuation of the estradiol rise in some ewes, thus reducing the requisite ovarian signal for LH-surge induction and precluding, in those animals, analysis of the very phenomenon we sought to examine. Therefore, having determined that a preovulatory GnRH surge actually exists, our further studies are being conducted with a physiological endocrine model in which a follicular-phase level of estradiol is produced exogenously following the withdrawal of progesterone.

Estradiol-Induced GnRH Surge

Initial descriptions of the pattern of GnRH secretion during the LH surge of sheep were obtained in the mid-1980s on ovariectomized ewes treated with bolus injections of estradiol. Those studies provided evidence that the positive feedback action of estrogen was associated with increased GnRH release in some animals but not in others (31, 32). This raised the possibility that heightened secretion of GnRH is not an obligatory LH-surge-inducing stimulus. This possibility, however, was not borne out by more recent studies in which increased release of GnRH was consistently observed during the LH surge induced by bolus injections of estradiol (20, 33). To facilitate our investigation of the GnRH surge, we have used an endocrine model in which the steroidal milieu of the follicular phase of the estrous cycle is mimicked experimentally, and in which the resulting changes in reproductive neuroendocrine activity are precisely timed.

Endocrine Model

Our model for the follicular phase, illustrated in Figure 15.4, is designed to reproduce physiological patterns and levels of estradiol and progesterone in the approximate time-frame of the estrous cycle (34). On days 6–10 after natural estrus (ovulation day 1), ewes are ovariectomized, treated with subcutaneous Silastic implants that maintain luteal-phase levels of estradiol and progesterone, and equipped with the apparatus for portal blood collection. One week later, the progesterone implants are removed to simulate luteolysis and the estradiol treatment is adjusted according to the objectives of the specific experiment. In the study described here, estradiol implants were added to one group of ewes 16 h after with-

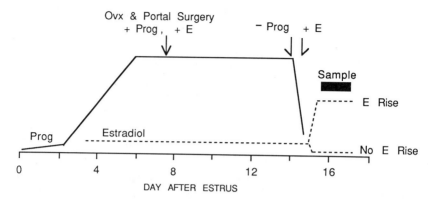

FIGURE 15.4. Model for follicular phase of estrous cycle. Ovx depicts ovariectomy; Prog indicates progesterone; E is estradiol; black rectangle indicates time of portal blood collection. Modified with permission from Ref. 21. © by The Endocrine Society, 1990.

drawing progesterone to produce a rise in circulating estradiol to a peak follicular-phase level of 8 pg/ml (E Rise group in Fig. 15.4). In control ewes, the estradiol implant that was placed at ovariectomy was removed such that a surge-inducing signal was not provided (No E Rise, Fig. 15.4). In this model, a "preovulatory-like" LH surge begins 20–24 h after the addition of estradiol implants in the E Rise group (34). Simultaneous samples of portal and jugular blood were obtained every 5–10 min for 25–30 h bracketing this LH surge.

Induction of the GnRH Surge

The time courses of GnRH in portal blood and LH in jugular blood are shown in Figure 15.5 for one representative control ewe and one receiving the increase in estradiol. In each of 6 controls, concurrent pulses of GnRH and LH were observed, but there was no evidence of sustained surge-like secretion of either hormone. GnRH pulses consisted of one or two elevated values between which the level was virtually undetectable. The estradiol rise caused a profound change in the GnRH secretory pattern. Initially, there was a clear suppression of the pulsatile pattern of GnRH in all ewes receiving the increase in estradiol (Fig. 15.5, right; 28–34 h). This suppression was followed by an unambiguous surge of GnRH. This surge was remarkably similar to that generated endogenously during the estrous cycle in terms of its time course and amplitude, and its temporal relationship to the LH discharge. For example, the GnRH surges we have observed in the model for the follicular phase are robust, exceeding the presurge baseline by as much as 500-fold. Further, the

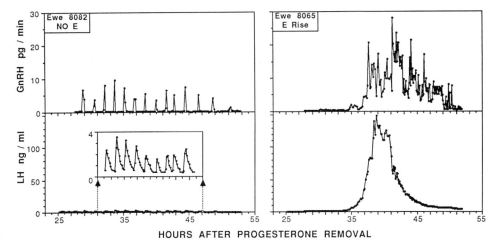

HOURS AFTER PROGESTERONE REMOVAL

FIGURE 15.5. Time course of GnRH in hypophyseal portal blood (top) and LH in jugular blood (bottom) in representative Suffolk ewes either not given an increase in estradiol (left) or provided with estradiol (right) in the endocrine model for the follicular phase (see Fig. 15.4). The estradiol rise was initiated 16 h after removal of progesterone implants at hour 0. Inset on left is expanded y-axis plot to disclose pulsatile LH pattern otherwise obscured by the scale. Modified with permission from Ref. 21. © by The Endocrine Society, 1990.

onsets of the GnRH and LH surges are coincident, but the GnRH surge outlasts that of LH, persisting nearly twice as long in some instances. To date, we have monitored GnRH secretion in 26 ewes treated with the increase in estradiol; a high-amplitude GnRH surge occurred without exception. This includes observations during both the breeding season and anestrus (21).

Our findings using this animal model, which was developed to allow physiological steroid treatments, permits two conclusions concerning the regulation of GnRH secretion by estradiol during the follicular phase of the estrous cycle of the ewe. First, estradiol acts centrally to inhibit pulsatile release of GnRH and thus evoke a negative feedback suppression of gonadotropin secretion in the interval between luteolysis and onset of the LH surge. Second, the follicular phase increase in circulating estradiol induces a massive surge of GnRH. The extended duration of this GnRH surge, relative to that of LH, provides evidence that the preovulatory gonadotropin surge ends for reasons other than a lack of GnRH. Factors that could contribute to the end of the LH surge include a depletion of releasable stores of LH in the pituitary (35–37), a desensitization of gonadotropes to GnRH by the sustained elevation of the decapeptide (38, 39), and the secretion of a gonadotropin-inhibiting factor into hypophyseal portal blood (40, 41).

Moment-to-Moment Pattern of GnRH During the Surge

An interesting question arising from the time course of GnRH in portal blood during the surge is whether or not its secretion is strictly pulsatile and, if it is, whether the surge is composed of increased pulse frequency or amplitude. This is not a trivial issue, for the nature of the change in GnRH release would likely disclose important clues concerning the mode of activation of the GnRH-neuronal network. Pulsatile secretion, on the one hand, is suggested by the high degree of variability among GnRH values in adjacent samples of portal blood during the surge induced in the model (Fig. 15.5, right) as well as during the preovulatory surge (Fig. 15.3). An increased frequency of pulsatile GnRH release has, in fact, been suggested to occur during the estradiol-induced LH surge in the ovariectomized ewe (20, 31). On the other hand, continuous release is suggested by our finding that the lowest GnRH values observed in portal blood obtained during the surge are far in excess of the presurge baseline. It is important to point out in this regard that our procedure monitors only GnRH that has just been released, on its sole pass down the portal vasculature. Once diluted in peripheral blood, GnRH is no longer detectable in our system. That is why GnRH values between pulses are virtually undetectable under conditions in which secretion of the decapeptide is strictly pulsatile (e.g., Fig. 15.5, left). The persistent elevation throughout the surge, therefore, is not due to recirculation from the periphery but reflects GnRH actually released as the sample is obtained.

We are currently performing experiments to assess whether the GnRH surge is generated by an increase in frequency or amplitude of pulses, by a switch to a continuous mode of release, or by a combination of these phenomena (42). Our approach has been to monitor GnRH secretion at extremely frequent intervals, as frequently as once every 30 sec during several "windows" of the GnRH surge. Thus far, we have obtained no evidence for a rhythmic pulsatile secretion of GnRH in 16 of 17 sessions in which 30-sec samples were taken. In one 30-sec window near the end of the GnRH surge, a regular oscillatory pattern was observed with a period of 6 min. In all other cases, GnRH remained continuously elevated and far in excess of the presurge baseline. There were, however, variations around this heightened secretion which could not be attributed to error within our GnRH assay.

Although our study is not complete, it provides preliminary evidence that the GnRH surge may not be composed entirely of discrete synchronous bouts of hormone release. One action of estradiol in eliciting the GnRH surge, therefore, may be to switch the mode of activity of the GnRH neuronal system from a discrete synchronous bursting pattern to one allowing a continuous elevation of GnRH in hypophyseal portal blood. This possibility is particularly intriguing in light of the observation that hypothalamic multi-unit electrical activity in the rhesus monkey switches from a distinctly pulsatile pattern to a nonpulsatile pattern during both the estradiol-induced and the preovulatory LH surge (43, 44). It should be pointed out, however, that in the rhesus monkey, heightened secretion of GnRH may not be necessary for generation of the LH surge; in that species a stimulatory action of estradiol upon the pituitary appears to be sufficient for LH-surge induction (16, 45–47). This raises the question of whether or not, in the ewe, the GnRH surge is necessary to elicit the preovulatory LH discharge, an issue considered briefly in the next section.

Importance of the GnRH Surge

The observations discussed thus far provide compelling evidence that, in the ewe, the follicular-phase rise in estradiol elicits a GnRH surge, but they do not address the importance of this surge in triggering the preovulatory LH discharge. That such an increase in GnRH is indeed essential is documented by studies in which GnRH was administered in various patterns to ewes in which GnRH secretion was abolished (14, 48, 49), or by studies in which a GnRH analog was administered to ewes in which endogenous GnRH was immunoneutralized (50). In all cases, a sudden large increase in GnRH in combination with estradiol was found to be necessary for full expression of a preovulatory-like surge of LH; pulsatile administration of GnRH at a presurge frequency was not an effective stimulus. Moreover, observations by Clarke and colleagues (48, 49) suggest that an acute increase of GnRH (referred to as a "signal" pattern) can trigger onset of the LH surge, but a sustained hypophyseotropic stimulus is needed to achieve a full preovulatory-like LH surge in terms of amplitude and duration. The secretory pattern of GnRH that we have observed, as described above, would seem to fulfill both of these requirements for LH-surge induction, providing the "signal" pattern as well as the sustained stimulus.

Earlier studies in our laboratory, in which the hormonal requirements for the LH surge were evaluated by systemic application of GnRH and estradiol, have revealed that an abrupt increment in GnRH constitutes an effective surge-inducing signal, but a gradual rise to the same level spanning several days does not (14). The LH surge induced by the abrupt GnRH increment, however, could not be prolonged beyond its normal course by maintaining the GnRH stimulus. This fits nicely with the actual secretory dynamics of the two hormones, specifically our finding that the LH surge ends while the GnRH surge is ongoing. This provides a solid empirical basis for the conclusion that the onset of the preovulatory LH surge is triggered by a marked increase in GnRH secretion. The end of the LH surge, however, is not due to termination of this GnRH signal.

Conclusions

It is perhaps most useful to end by returning to the question posed at the start: Does estradiol induce the preovulatory LH surge by eliciting an increased secretion of GnRH into hypophyseal portal blood? From our studies in the sheep, a strong case can be mounted that the follicular-phase rise in estradiol, be it in the normal setting of the estrous cycle or in a physiological endocrine model, elicits a profound increase in GnRH release at the time of the LH surge in virtually all ewes studied. Such an increase in GnRH constitutes an obligatory hypothalamic signal for generation of the LH surge of the ewe. It should be stressed that this conclusion does not exclude an important pituitary site of action of estradiol, for such an action is needed to induce the LH surge in the ewe (14), nor does this conclusion necessarily extend to all other mammals, as species differences in the LH-surge system are clearly extant (51).

As is so often the case, our quest to provide answers has disclosed many new questions. What is the nature of the suppressive effect of estradiol on pulsatile GnRH secretion prior to onset of the preovulatory GnRH surge? Is it true that a strictly pulsatile pattern of GnRH gives way to a continuous elevation in portal blood during the surge and, if it does, what neural mechanisms account for this phenomenon? What causes the preovulatory LH surge to end while the GnRH surge is still in progress, and what is the functional significance of this apparent excess of GnRH? Thus, in the process of documenting the existence of the preovulatory surge of GnRH, the present studies have also pointed to fertile avenues for future research.

Acknowledgments. This work was supported by grants from the NIH (R01-HD-18337, P30-HD-18258, T32-HD-07048), the Institut National de la Recherche Agronomique, and the Office of the Vice-President for Research at the University of Michigan, and by a Rackham Predoctoral Fellowship from the University of Michigan. We thank the Autosyringe Division of Baxter Travenol for travel funds to allow our collaboration.

References

1. Sarkar DK, Chiappa SA, Fink G. Gonadotropin-releasing hormone surge in pro-oestrus rats. Nature 1976;264:461–3.
2. Sarkar DK, Fink G. Effects of gonadal steroids on output of luteinizing hormone releasing factor into pituitary stalk blood in the female rat. J Endocrinol 1979;80:303–13.
3. Levine JE, Ramirez VD. Luteinizing hormone-releasing hormone release during the rat estrous cycle and after ovariectomy, as estimated with push-pull cannulae. Endocrinology 1982;111:1439–48.

4. Sarkar DK, Mitsugi N. Correlative changes of the gonadotropin-releasing hormone and gonadotropin-releasing-hormone-associated peptide immunoreactivities in the pituitary portal plasma in female rats. Neuroendocrinology 1990;52:15–21.
5. Kalra SP, Kalra PS. Neural regulation of luteinizing hormone secretion in the rat. Endocr Rev 1983;4:311–51.
6. Freeman ME. The ovarian cycle of the rat. In: Knobil E, Neill J, et al., eds. The physiology of reproduction. New York: Raven Press, 1988:1893–928.
7. Everett JW, Sawyer CH. A 24-hour periodicity in the "LH-release apparatus" of female rats, disclosed by barbiturate sedation. Endocrinology 1950;47:198–218.
8. Weick RF, Dierschke DJ, Karsch FJ, Butler WR, Hotchkiss J, Knobil E. Periovulatory time courses of circulating gonadotropic and ovarian hormones in the rhesus monkey. Endocrinology 1973;93:1140–7.
9. Hauger RL, Karsch FJ, Foster DL. A new concept for control of the estrous cycle of the ewe based on the temporal relationships between luteinizing hormone, estradiol and progesterone in peripheral serum and evidence that progesterone inhibits tonic LH secretion. Endocrinology 1977;101:807–17.
10. Gordon JH, Reichlin S. Changes in pituitary responsiveness to luteinizing hormone-releasing factor during the rat estrous cycle. Endocrinology 1974;94:974–8.
11. Aiyer MS, Fink G, Greig F. Changes in the sensitivity of the pituitary gland to luteinizing hormone releasing factor during the oestrous cycle of the rat. J Endocrinol 1974;60:47–64.
12. Reeves JJ, Arimura A, Schally AV. Changes in pituitary responsiveness to luteinizing hormone-releasing hormone (LH-RH) in anestrous ewes pretreated with estradiol benzoate. Biol Reprod 1971;4:88–92.
13. Clarke IJ, Cummins JT. Direct pituitary effects of estrogen and progesterone on gonadotropin secretion in the ovariectomized ewe. Neuroendocrinology 1984:267–74.
14. Kaynard AH, Malpaux B, Robinson JE, Wayne NL, Karsch FJ. Importance of pituitary and neural actions of estradiol in induction of the LH surge in the ewe. Neuroendocrinology 1988;48:296–303.
15. Adams TE, Norman RL, Spies HG. Gonadotropin-releasing hormone receptor binding and pituitary responsiveness in estradiol-primed monkeys. Science 1981;213:1388–90.
16. Knobil E. The neuroendocrine control of the menstrual cycle. Recent Progr Horm Res 1981;36:53–88.
17. Clarke IJ, Cummins JT. The temporal relationship between gonadotropin releasing hormone (GnRH) and luteinizing hormone (LH) secretion in ovariectomized ewes. Endocrinology 1982;111:1737–9.
18. Levine JE, Pau K-YF, Ramirez VD, Jackson GL. Simultaneous measurement of luteinizing hormone-releasing hormone and luteinizing hormone-release in unanesthetized, ovariectomized sheep. Endocrinology 1982;111:1449–55.
19. Caraty A, Locatelli A. Effect of time after castration on secretion of LHRH in the ewe. J Reprod Fertil 1988;82:263–9.
20. Caraty A, Locatelli A, Martin GB. Biphasic response in the secretion of gonadotropin-releasing hormone in ovariectomized ewes injected with oestradiol. J Endocrinol 1989;123:375–82.

21. Moenter SM, Caraty A, Karsch FJ. The estradiol-induced surge of gonadotropin-releasing hormone in the ewe. Endocrinology 1990;127: 1375–84.
22. Karsch FJ, Goodman RL, Legan SJ. Feedback basis of seasonal breeding: test of an hypothesis. J Reprod Fertil 1980;58:521–35.
23. Karsch FJ, Bittman EL, Foster DL, Goodman RL, Legan SJ, Robinson JE. Neuroendocrine basis of seasonal reproduction. Recent Prog Horm Res 1984;40:185–232.
24. Goodman RL. Neuroendocrine control of the ovine estrous cycle. In: Knobil E, Neill J, et al., eds. The physiology of reproduction. New York: Raven Press, 1988:1929–69.
25. Clarke IJ, Thomas GB, Yao B, Cummins JT. GnRH secretion throughout the ovine estrous cycle. Neuroendocrinology 1987;46:82–8.
26. Horton RJE, Cummins JT, Clarke IJ. Naloxone evokes large-amplitude GnRN pulses in luteal-phase ewes. J Reprod Fertil 1987;81:277–86.
27. Karsch FJ, Cummins JT, Thomas GB, Clarke IJ. Steroid feedback inhibition of pulsatile secretion of gonadotropin releasing hormone in the ewe. Biol Reprod 1987;36:1207–18.
28. Dziuk PJ, Cook B, Niswender GD, Kaltenbach CC, Doane BB. Inhibition and control of estrus and ovulation in ewes with a subcutaneous implant of silicone rubber impregnated with a progestagen. Am J Vet Res 1968;29: 2415–7.
29. Karsch FJ, Foster DL, Legan SJ, Ryan KD, Peter GK. Control of the preovulatory endocrine events in the ewe: interrelationships of estradiol, progesterone and luteinizing hormone. Endocrinology 1979;105:421–6.
30. Moenter SM, Caraty A, Locatelli A, Karsch FJ. Pattern of gonadotropin-releasing hormone (GnRH) secretion leading up to ovulation in the ewe: existence of a preovulatory GnRH surge. Endocrinology 1991;129:1175–82.
31. Clarke IJ, Cummins JT. Increased gonadotropin-releasing hormone pulse frequency associated with estrogen-induced luteinizing hormone surges in ovariectomized ewes. Endocrinology 1985;116:2376–82.
32. Schillo KK, Leshin LS, Kuehl D, Jackson GL. Simultaneous measurement of luteinizing hormone-releasing hormone and luteinizing hormone during estradiol-induced luteinizing hormone surges in the ovariectomized ewe. Biol Reprod 1985;33:644–52.
33. Clarke IJ. Gonadotropin-releasing hormone secretion (GnRH) in anoestrous ewes and the induction of GnRH surges by oestrogen. J Endocrinol 1988; 117:355–60.
34. Goodman RL, Legan SJ, Ryan KD, Foster DL, Karsch FJ. Importance of variations in behavioural and feedback actions of oestradiol to the control of seasonal breeding in the ewe. J Endocrinol 1981;89:229–40.
35. Roche JF, Foster DL, Karsch FJ, Cook B, Dziuk PJ. Levels of luteinizing hormone in sera and pituitaries of ewes during the estrous cycle and anestrus. Endocrinology 1970;86:568–72.
36. Landefeld TD, Kepa J, Karsch FJ. Estradiol feedback effects on the alpha-subunit mRNA in the sheep pituitary gland: correlation with serum and pituitary luteinizing hormone concentrations. Proc Natl Acad Sci USA 1984;81:1322–6.
37. Crowder ME, Nett TM. Pituitary content of gonadotropins and receptors for gonadotropin-releasing hormone (GnRH) and hypothalamic content of

GnRH during the periovulatory period of the ewe. Endocrinology 1984; 114:234–9.

38. Nett TM, Crowder ME, Moss GE, Duello TM. GnRH-receptor interaction: V. Down-regulation of pituitary receptors for GnRH in ovariectomized ewes by infusion of homologous hormone. Biol Reprod 1981;24:1145–55.

39. McIntosh RP, McIntosh JEA. Dynamic characteristics of luteinizing hormone release from perifused sheep anterior pituitary cells by combined pulsatile and continuous gonadotropin-releasing hormone. Endocrinology 1985;117: 169–79.

40. Hwan J-C, Freeman ME. Partial purification of a hypothalamic factor that inhibits gonadotropin-releasing hormone-stimulated luteinizing hormone release. Endocrinology 1987;120:483–90.

41. Hwan J-C, Freeman ME. A physiological role for luteinizing hormone release-inhibiting factor of hypothalamic origin. Endocrinology 1987;121: 1099–103.

42. Moenter SM, Brand RC, Karsch FJ. Pattern of GnRH secretion during the LH surge in the ewe. In: Program and abstracts, 73rd annual meeting of the Endocrine Society, November 1991.

43. Kesner JS, Wilson RC, Kaufman J-M, et al. Unexpected responses of the hypothalamic gonadotropin-releasing hormone "pulse generator" to physiological estradiol inputs in the absence of the ovary. Proc Natl Acad Sci USA 1987;84:8745–9.

44. O'Byrne K, Thalabard J-C, Williams CL, et al. An unexpected decline in GnRH pulse generator frequency in the late follicular phase of the rhesus monkey menstrual cycle. In: Program and abstracts, 72nd annual meeting of the Endocrine Society, 1990 (abstract 1058).

45. Ferin M, Rosenblatt H, Carmel PW, Antunes JL, Vande Wiele RL. Estrogen-induced gonadotropin surges in female rhesus monkeys after pituitary stalk section. Endocrinology 1979;104:50–2.

46. Wildt L, Hausler A, Hutchinson JS, Marshall G, Knobil E. Estradiol as a gonadotropin releasing hormone in the rhesus monkey. Endocrinology 1981; 108:2011–3.

47. Nakai Y, Plant TM, Hess DL, Keogh EJ, Knobil E. On the sites of negative and positive feedback actions of estradiol in the control of gonadotropin secretion in the rhesus monkey. Endocrinology 1978;102:1008–14.

48. Clarke IJ, Cummins JT, Jenkin M, Phillips DJ. The oestrogen-induced surge of LH requires a "signal" pattern of gonadotrophin-releasing hormone input to the pituitary gland in the ewe. J Endocrinol 1989;122:127–34.

49. Phillips DJ, Cummins JT, Clarke IJ. Effects of modifying gonadotrophin-releasing hormone input before and after the oestrogen-induced LH surge in ovariectomized ewes with hypothalamo-pituitary disconnection. J Endocrinol 1990.

50. Herman ME, Adams TE. Gonadotropin secretion in ovariectomized ewes: effect of passive immunization against gonadotropin-releasing hormone (GnRH) and infusion of a GnRH agonist and estradiol. Biol Reprod 1990; 42:273–80.

51. Karsch FJ. Central actions of ovarian steroids in the feedback regulation of pulsatile secretion of luteinizing hormone. Annu Rev Physiol 1987;49: 365–82.

16

Regulation of Pulsatile LHRH Release in Primates

Ei Terasawa and Andrea C. Gore

LHRH is the single most important molecule involved in the regulation of reproduction. This neurohormone is synthesized in cell bodies as a 92 amino acid precursor peptide, and subsequently cleaved to form the decapeptide (1, 2). LHRH and fragments of its prohormone are subsequently transported down the axon and released into the portal circulation from neuroterminals in the median eminence-pituitary stalk (3, 4), where they act on gonadotropes to regulate the synthesis and release of the gonadotropins. It has been well documented now that the release of LHRH and the release of LH are both pulsatile (5–8) and that changes in this pulsatile pattern govern gamete maturation, steroid hormone secretion, ovulation, and maintenance of luteal function (9–13). An abnormality in the pulsatile pattern of LH secretion (and presumably pulsatile LHRH secretion) is associated with reproductive disorders such as polycystic ovarian syndrome, anorexia nervosa, and amenorrhea (14, 15). Therefore, it is important to study the regulation of pulsatile LHRH release in primates. In this article the control of pulsatile LHRH release will be reviewed, with special emphasis on developmental studies.

Developmental Changes in Pulsatile LHRH Release

Since puberty is defined as the developmental stage during which reproductive function is attained, establishment of an adult pattern of pulsatile LHRH release may occur during puberty. Initially we documented the developmental changes in LHRH release in conscious monkeys. Using a push-pull perfusion method, we obtained samples from the stalk-median eminence of prepubertal (<20 months of age, no signs of puberty apparent), early pubertal (22–30 months of age, some signs of puberty evident, but before menarche), and midpubertal (33–48 months of age, after menarche but before first ovulation) monkeys, and measured LHRH levels in these samples. We found that increases in pulsatile LHRH release occur during the pubertal period to levels and frequency similar to those observed during adulthood (16).

In prepubertal monkeys LHRH release was very low. Mean LHRH levels, basal LHRH release, pulse amplitude, and pulse frequency were all lower than in early and midpubertal monkeys. In early pubertal monkeys, mean LHRH levels, basal LHRH release, pulse amplitude, and pulse frequency increased significantly. In midpubertal animals, mean LHRH release and pulse amplitude further increased, while basal LHRH release and pulse frequency remained unchanged from levels at the early pubertal stage. These data indicate that an increase in LHRH release occurs between the prepubertal and the early pubertal stage, prior to menarche, and that the increase continues through the midpubertal stage. The data further suggest that an increase in LHRH pulse frequency and pulse amplitude occurs prior to the initiation of puberty. Once the pulse frequency reaches an adult level prior to menarche, however, only the pulse amplitude continues to increase through the midpubertal stage. These results demonstrating an increase in LHRH release at the onset of puberty have been predicted from clinical studies measuring LH release (17, 18), as well as from studies in nonhuman primates (19, 20).

Effects of Ovariectomy and Negative Feedback Effects of Estradiol on LHRH Release in Pubertal Monkeys

A body of evidence indicates that in primates, levels of circulating LH are low before puberty independent of the feedback influence of ovarian steroids, and are presumably due to low levels of LHRH release. During the juvenile period LH levels in patients with gonadal dysgenesis are as low as those in normal children (21, 22). Similarly, ovariectomy during the neonatal period does not result in an LH elevation until the age of puberty (23, 24), and ovariectomy before the pubertal age induces a delayed elevation of LH (25). Recently, we have examined the effects of ovariectomy on LHRH and LH release in prepubertal, early pubertal, and midpubertal monkeys. Ovariectomy altered neither LHRH (Fig. 16.1) nor LH release in prepubertal monkeys (26). In contrast, ovariectomy resulted in the elevation of both LHRH (Fig. 16.1) and LH release in early pubertal and midpubertal monkeys (27). Interestingly, the time course of the castration-induced LH increase in early pubertal monkeys was slower than that in midpubertal monkeys. Therefore, low levels of LHRH release prior to the onset of puberty and a subsequent increase in LHRH release at the onset of puberty are independent of the presence of the ovary.

To further determine whether the response of the LHRH neuronal

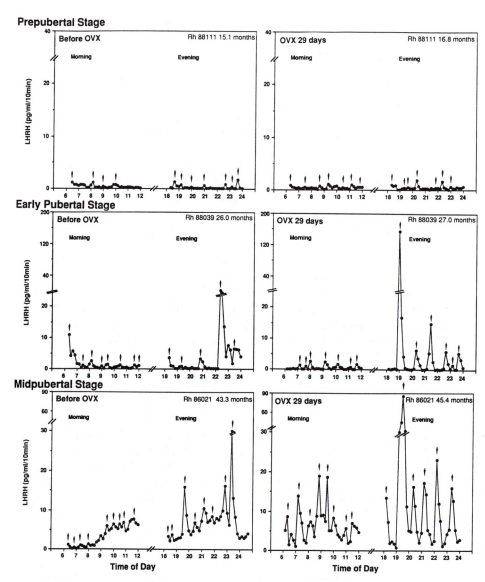

FIGURE 16.1. Effects of ovariectomy on LHRH release at the prepubertal, early pubertal, and midpubertal stages. A representative case from each age group before and 29 days after ovariectomy is shown. LHRH release from the stalk-median eminence was measured by push-pull perfusion for 6h in the morning and 6h in the evening. Ovariectomy did not alter LHRH release in prepubertal monkeys, while LHRH release increased following ovariectomy in early and midpubertal monkeys. An arrowhead indicates an LHRH pulse reported by the PULSAR algorithm (Merriam GR, Wachter KW. Am J Physiol 1982;243: E310–8). From Chongthammakun S, Claypool LE, Terasawa E, unpublished.

system to ovariectomy is due to the ovarian steroid estrogen, the effects of estradiol benzoate on LHRH and LH release were examined in prepubertal, early pubertal, and midpubertal monkeys that were ovariectomized several months earlier. While estrogen caused no effects on LHRH (Fig. 16.2) and LH release in prepubertal monkeys, it significantly suppressed both LHRH and LH release in early and midpubertal monkeys (Fig. 16.2; 27). These results clearly indicate (1) that during the prepubertal stage the LHRH neuronal system is insensitive to estrogen and (2) that negative feedback effects of estrogen first occur after animals undergo the onset of puberty. Therefore, low LHRH release in prepubertal monkeys is due to causes other than the feedback effects of the ovarian steroid estrogen. Perhaps the immaturity of the hypothalamic neuronal circuitry, in which proper stimulatory mechanisms for LHRH release are absent and/or inhibitory neuronal mechanisms influencing LHRH release are predominant (28), is responsible for low levels of LHRH release prior to the onset of puberty.

Limiting Factors for an Increase in LHRH Release Before Puberty

Compelling evidence indicates that the onset of puberty is not limited by ovarian-adenohypophyseal competence or maturation of LHRH neurons themselves, but by mechanisms that regulate the hypothalamic LHRH neurosecretory system: (1) pulsatile infusion of LHRH induced menarche followed by ovulatory cycles in sexually immature monkeys (29); (2) the distribution and number of LHRH neurons in prepubertal monkeys are similar to those observed in adult monkeys (30); (3) the expression of LHRH mRNA was found well before birth (31) and was similar to that of the adult monkey (32); and (4) the administration of the excitatory amino acid analog, N-methyl-D,L-aspartic acid (NMA) in prepubertal monkeys elicited LH (33) and LHRH release (34). Similarly, application of electrical stimulation to the medial-basal hypothalamus of prepubertal monkeys resulted in a large increase in LHRH release (Fig. 16.3; 35). Under electrical stimulation, the pattern of LHRH release in prepubertal monkeys was quite comparable to that observed in early and midpubertal monkeys (35) indicating that the LHRH neurosecretory system is fully competent at the prepubertal stage, even though spontaneous LHRH release is minimal. The low levels of LHRH output in prepubertal monkeys must then be due to an immaturity of the mechanisms controlling pulsatile LHRH release. It is therefore hypothesized that puberty will occur when the adult type of regulatory mechanism for LHRH release is established. It may be useful at this time to review how pulsatile LHRH release is regulated in adult monkeys.

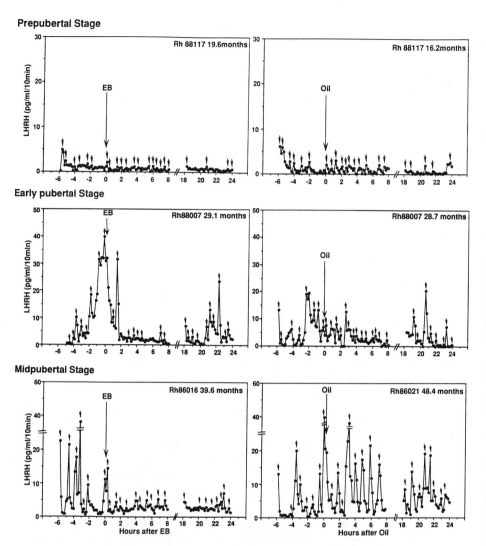

FIGURE 16.2. Negative feedback effects of estradiol benzoate (EB) on LHRH release at the prepubertal, early pubertal, and midpubertal stages. A representative case from each stage with EB or oil injection in shown. In prepubertal monkeys, neither EB nor oil caused any significant effects on LHRH release. In contrast, in early pubertal and midpubertal monkeys, EB injection suppressed LHRH release, while oil injection had no effect. An arrowhead indicates LHRH pulses reported by the PULSAR algorithm, and large arrows indicate the time of EB or oil injection. From Chongthammakun S, Terasawa E, unpublished.

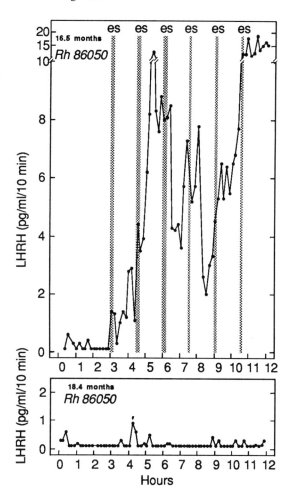

FIGURE 16.3. Effects of electrical stimulation (es) of the stalk-median eminence on LHRH release in a prepubertal monkey. Electrical stimulation was applied to the MBH at 90-min intervals (upper panel) in a monkey at 16.5 months of age. Approximately 2 months later, a control experiment without es was conducted on the same monkey. A shaded vertical bar indicates applications of es. Note that LHRH release was significantly enhanced by es, while spontaneous LHRH release during the control experiment was quite low. Modified with permission from Ref. 35. © by The Endocrine Society, 1990.

Control of Pulsatile LHRH Release in the Adult Monkey

The Endogenous Pulse-Generating Mechanism of LHRH Neurons

We propose the following hypothesis in this article: There is an endogenous pulse-generating mechanism within LHRH neurons, which is controlled by synaptic input of neurotransmitters and/or neuromodulators from other neurons.

There are several reasons to believe that LHRH neurons possess an endogenous pulse-generating mechanism: (1) complete deafferentation of the medial basal hypothalamus, i.e., elimination of a large amount of synaptic input to LHRH neurons, does not abolish pulsatile LH release in the monkey (36), while lesions of the arcuate nucleus-median eminence, where most of the LHRH neurons are distributed (37–39), eliminate it (40, 41); (2) pulsatile LHRH release is also observed in rat hypothalami after complete deafferentation (42) as well as in hypothalamic slices from guinea pigs (43, 44), a species that shares many neuroendocrine characteristics with primates (45, 46); (3) intracellular recordings from magnocellular neurosecretory cells in rat hypothalamic slices indicate that neurosecretory neurons appear to have an intrinsic regenerative mechanism for phasic discharges (47, 48), which is well correlated with neurosecretion (49); and (4) electron microscopic studies suggest that glia at neuroterminals may facilitate contact between neuroendocrine cells and thereby allow synchronization of their firing (50, 51). However, these results are primarily based upon studies using hypothalamic deafferentation in vivo, or in vitro hypothalamic slices that are only useful for considering elimination of extrahypothalamic input, namely from the brainstem and limbic structures, in regulating neural input to the hypothalamic neuroendocrine cells. Therefore, the possibility that synaptic input to LHRH neurons from within the hypothalamus contributes to pulsatile LHRH release is not excluded.

Perhaps the most convincing evidence for an endogenous mechanism of LHRH pulse generation was provided by studies on a neuronal cell line that contains the pro-LHRH gene. Recently, Weiner and colleagues (52) produced an LHRH cell line, GT-1, that expressed neuron-specific, but not glial-specific, characteristics (52). These cells released LHRH into the incubation media in a pulsatile manner at 22-min intervals (53). This pulse frequency is similar to that of LH pulses (20-min intervals) in the rat, a species similar to the mouse, from which the cell line was derived (54), although much faster than that of primates. We need to examine LHRH cells from primates, especially in primary LHRH cultures. Presently, therefore, the question of whether LHRH neurons in primates possess endogenous pulsatility remains unanswered.

Control of LHRH Pulse Generation by Other Neuronal Inputs

Numerous neuroactive substances have been implicated as neurotransmitters and neuromodulators controlling LHRH release (55–59). However, to designate a neuroactive substance as a true regulator of pulsatile LHRH release, the following criteria must be fulfilled. First, the neuroactive substance must be present endogenously, and its release must be pulsatile. If the neuroactive substance is stimulatory to LHRH release, pulses of this substance must occur simultaneously with or shortly before pulses of LHRH. If the neuroactive substance is inhibitory, the release may occur out of phase with LHRH pulses. Second, agonists of the neuroactive substance or the substance itself must stimulate LHRH release. In the case of inhibitory neuroactive substances, agonists must inhibit LHRH release. Third, antagonists of the neuroactive substance must block the action of the endogenous ligand or agonist. Antagonists of a stimulatory neuroactive substance should suppress pulsatile LHRH release, while antagonists of an inhibitory neuroactive substance stimulate LHRH release. To date, we have examined the role of adrenergic neurons and neuropeptide Y (NPY) neurons in the control of pulsatile LHRH release in adult monkeys. To avoid complications of the influence of the ovarian steroid hormones, ovariectomized monkeys were used.

Norepinephrine Neurons

Norepinephrine (NE) neurons in rodents have been implicated in the control of pulsatile LHRH and LH release and in the ovarian steroid-stimulated gonadotropin surge (55–58). In primates as well, adrenergic input modulates pulsatile LH and LHRH release (60–62). In our studies, it was found that the release of norepinephrine from the stalk-median eminence measured by HPLC was pulsatile and synchronous with LHRH pulses (63). Infusion of norepinephrine itself, as well as methoxamine, an α_1-adrenergic stimulant through a push cannula during continuous collection of perfusates, stimulated LHRH release (63, 64). In contrast, prazosin, an α_1-adrenergic blocker, suppressed LHRH pulses (63, 65) and eliminated LH pulses (66). Interestingly, prazosin suppressed LHRH pulse amplitude but did not change LHRH pulse frequency (63, 65). Neither rauwolscine, an α_2-adrenergic blocker nor propranolol, a β-adrenergic blocker, had any effects on LH/LHRH release (65, 66). These results indicate that pulsatile release of LHRH is modulated by adrenergic input, namely norepinephrine neurotransmission through α_1-adrenoreceptors.

NPY Neurons

It has been shown that neurons containing NPY, a 36 amino acid peptide, are involved in the control of gonadotropin release (67–70). Recent studies in our laboratory suggest that NPY release in the stalk-median eminence was pulsatile (71, 72). Moreover, NPY pulses measured in aliquots of the same perfusate samples used for LHRH measurement occurred synchronously with or 10 min preceding LHRH pulses (Fig. 16.4a; Woller and Terasawa, unpublished). NPY infusion to the stalk-median eminence through the push cannula resulted in an increase in LHRH release in a dose-dependent manner (Fig. 16.4b; 73). These results suggest that NPY released at LHRH neuroterminals in the stalk-median eminence may stimulate LHRH release. To support this hypothesis, infusion of antiserum to NPY at 1:100 or 1:1000 concentration suppressed LHRH pulses (72), while similar treatments with vehicle (normal rabbit serum) caused no effects. Therefore, input from NPY neurons also modulates pulsatile LHRH release in adult monkeys.

Other Possible Candidates

Galanin, a 29 amino acid peptide, has been proposed as a modulator of the release of anterior pituitary hormones (74, 75). Galanin was found to be colocalized with LHRH in rats (76) and galanin measured in portal circulation in ovariectomized rats was reported to be pulsatile (77). Although similar studies remain to be done in primates, we have tested the effects of administration of galanin on LHRH release from the stalk-median eminence in vitro and in vivo. Preliminary data indicate that galanin stimulates LHRH release at doses as low as 10^{-10} M (Palmer, Nychis-Florence, and Terasawa, unpublished). It is possible, therefore, that galanin may also be a modulator of LHRH pulses.

In contrast to the facilitatory role of NE and NPY, GABAergic neurons appear to be inhibitory to pulsatile LHRH release: GABA and the GABA agonist, muscimol, when injected into the third ventricle, inhibited LH pulses (78), and GABA release in the preoptic area occurred reciprocally with LH pulses (79). Although opioidergic neurons are also inhibitory to LHRH and LH release, their action appears to be linked to the presence of gonadal steroids (80, 81).

It is quite possible that the LHRH pulse generator is driven by more than a single source. There may be endogenous rhythms in LHRH neurons, which are modulated by synaptic input from other neurons. Such a mechanism exists in the invertebrate oscillating neuron, in which synaptic input plays a role in depolarizing the membrane potential to the critical threshold that generates action potentials (82, 83). Perhaps

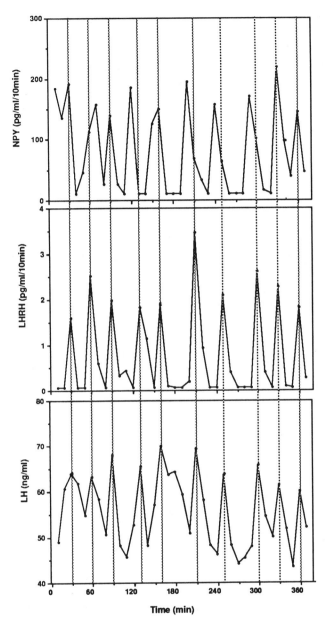

FIGURE 16.4. Release of NPY (upper panel) and LHRH (middle panel) measured in aliquots of the same push-pull perfusate samples collected from the stalk-median eminence of an adult castrated monkey. LH levels (bottom panel) in blood samples collected simultaneously with perfusates were also monitored. The release of NPY, LHRH, and LH was pulsatile. Pulses of NPY occurred simultaneously with or 10 min preceding LHRH pulses, and peaks of LHRH and LH release occurred synchronously. Dotted lines are coincident with pulses of LHRH reported by the PULSAR algorithm. From Woller MJ, Terasawa E, unpublished.

synaptic input contributes to maintaining the rhythmicity of LHRH neurons, or, alternatively, keeps the LHRH cells in check from "free run" (84). The relative contribution of the several sources may vary under different physiological conditions including various gonadal steroid environments. A similar concept has recently been proposed by Rasmussen (85).

What Triggers the Increase in LHRH Release at the Onset of Puberty?

It is quite possible that an inhibitory neuronal system suppresses LHRH release in prepubertal monkeys, and that removal of this inhibition results in the onset of puberty (28). However, despite extensive efforts so far, a neuroactive substance that inhibits the onset of puberty has not been found. Therefore, this chapter will focus on the maturation of a facilitatory neuronal system that would be responsible for the onset of puberty. The first question to be addressed is whether there are any developmental changes in adrenergic and NPY neurons that occur prior to the onset of puberty.

We found that norepinephrine release increased concomitantly with the elevation of LHRH release during puberty (Gore and Terasawa, unpublished). Moreover, methoxamine stimulated LHRH release in prepubertal monkeys (86) as well as early and midpubertal monkeys, although the response in prepubertal monkeys was much larger than that in midpubertal monkeys. These results indicate (1) that α_1-adrenoreceptors are present in the hypothalamus of prepubertal monkeys and (2) that LHRH neurons or interneurons in prepubertal monkeys may be more sensitive to norepinephrine because of the presence of a very small amount of norepinephrine in the stalk-median eminence. It is known that when little or no norepinephrine is present, receptors are up-regulated (i.e., "denervation hypersensitivity"), which appears to occur during the prepubertal period. Although it is unknown whether α_1-adrenergic blockers affect LHRH release in pubertal monkeys, or if norepinephrine release is pulsatile prior to the onset of puberty or undergoes developmental changes, it is clear that maturational changes in the α_1-adrenergic neuronal system occur before the onset of puberty.

Release of NPY in the stalk-median eminence also increased with age (Fig. 16.5; 87). When NPY and LHRH release were measured in aliquots of the same perfusate samples, mean release, basal release, pulse amplitude, and pulse frequency all increased with the progress of puberty. Interestingly, the pulse frequencies of NPY in the 3 respective developmental groups were identical to those of LHRH (Fig. 16.5; 87). It is possible that developmental changes in the LHRH and NPY neuronal systems occur simultaneously. Moreover, while NPY infusion

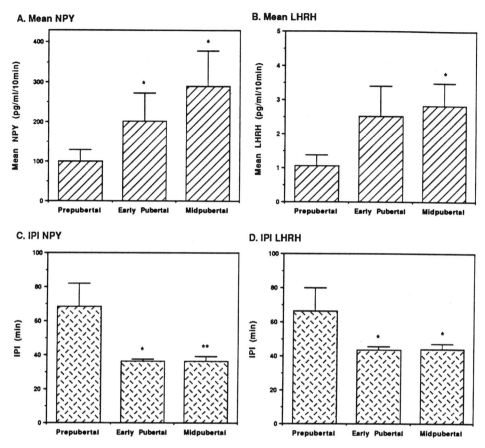

FIGURE 16.5. Developmental changes in the release of NPY (panels A and C) and LHRH (panels B and D) measured in aliquots of the same perfusate samples from 9 prepubertal, 7 early pubertal, and 8 midpubertal monkeys. Data were analyzed by the PULSAR algorithm and changes in mean release (A and B) and interpulse interval (IPI; C and D) are shown. Both mean NPY and LHRH release increased from the prepubertal through the midpubertal stage, while IPI of both NPY and LHRH release decreased significantly between the prepubertal and early pubertal stages. (*P < 0.05 vs. prepubertal stage; **P < 0.01 vs. prepubertal stage.) From Gore AC, Terasawa E, unpublished.

to the stalk-median eminence in prepubertal monkeys did not stimulate LHRH release, it significantly facilitated LHRH pulses in peripubertal monkeys (Fig. 16.6; 87), and infusion of a specific antibody to NPY suppressed LHRH release in midpubertal monkeys (Gore and Terasawa, unpublished). These studies suggest that the pubertal increase in NPY release may result in a further increase in LHRH release. Taken together, changes in stimulatory input to the LHRH neurosecretory system from

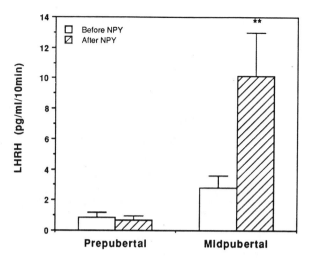

FIGURE 16.6. Effects of direct infusion of NPY to the stalk-median eminence on LHRH release in 5 prepubertal and 7 midpubertal monkeys. Open bars indicate mean LHRH levels prior to NPY infusion; hatched bars indicate mean LHRH levels 10 min after infusion of NPY. Note that infusion of NPY stimulated significant increases in LHRH release in midpubertal monkeys, while it did not cause any significant effects in prepubertal monkeys. (**$P < 0.01$ vs. before NPY.) From Gore AC, Terasawa E, unpublished.

adrenergic and NPY neurons contribute to the pubertal increase in LHRH release. It is possible that many more neuronal systems play a similar role during puberty.

Conclusion

It appears that the LHRH neuron possesses an endogenous pulse-generating mechanism. However, the endogenous pulse generation of the LHRH neuron is undoubtedly controlled by synaptic input of neuro-transmitters and/or neuromodulators, the secretory activity of which is also oscillatory. In this chapter the role of NE neurons and NPY neurons in control of LHRH pulsatility is examined. The questions of whether any particular neuron or neuronal systems are responsible for a common pulse-generating mechanism, or whether there is a master pulse generator for hypothalamic peptidergic/catecholaminergic neurons, or whether any network is formed between them, remain to be determined. Nevertheless, before sexual maturation inputs from NE neurons and NPY neurons are small and insufficient for stimulating pulsatile LHRH release. Puberty occurs when these neurons undergo maturational changes and thereby contribute to the increased release of pulsatile LHRH release.

Perhaps these maturational changes are normally regulated by genes, although hormonal and environmental factors could influence the course of preprogrammed genomic expression.

References

1. Adelman JP, Mason AJ, Hayflick JS, Seeburg PH. Isolation of the gene and hypothalamic cDNA for the common precursor of gonadotropic-releasing hormone and prolactin release-inhibiting factor in human and rat. Proc Natl Acad Sci USA 1986;283:179-83.
2. Phillips HS, Nikolics K, Branton D, Seeburg PH. Immunocytochemical localization in the rat brain of a prolactin release-inhibiting sequence of gonadotropin-releasing hormone. Nature 1985;316:542-5.
3. Sarkar DK, Fink G. Effects of gonadal steroids on output of luteinizing hormone releasing factor into pituitary stalk blood in the female rat. J Endocrinol 1979;80:303-13.
4. Clarke IJ, Cummins JT. The temporal relationship between gonadotropin releasing hormone (GnRH) and luteinizing hormone (LH) secretion in the ovariectomized ewe. Endocrinology 1982;111:1737-9.
5. Gay VL, Sheth NA. Evidence for a periodic release of LH in castrated male and female rats. Endocrinology 1972;90:158-62.
6. Dierschke DJ, Bhattacharya AN, Atkinson LE, Knobil E. Circhoral oscillations of plasma LH levels in the ovariectomized rhesus monkey. Endocrinology 1970;87:850-3.
7. Levine JE, Pau K-YF, Ramirez VD, Jackson GL. Simultaneous measurement of luteinizing hormone-releasing hormone and luteinizing hormone release in unanesthetized, ovariectomized sheep. Endocrinology 1982;111:1449-55.
8. Gearing M, Terasawa E. Luteinizing hormone releasing hormone (LHRH) neuroterminals mapped using the push-pull perfusion method in the rhesus monkey. Brain Res Bull 1988;21:117-21.
9. Knobil E. The neuroendocrine control of the menstrual cycle. Recent Prog Horm Res 1980;36:53-88.
10. Belchetz PE, Plant TM, Nakai Y, Keogh EJ, Knobil E. Hypophysial responses to continuous and intermittent delivery of hypothalamic gonadotropin-releasing hormone. Science 1978;202:631-3.
11. Crowley WF, Filicori M, Spratt DT, Santoro NF. The physiology of gonadotropin-releasing hormone (GnRH) secretion in men and women. Recent Prog Horm Res 1985;41:473-531.
12. Hutchinson JS, Kubik CJ, Nelson PB, Zeleznik AJ. Estrogen induces premature luteal regression in rhesus monkeys during spontaneous menstrual cycles, but not in cycles driven by exogenous gonadotropin-releasing hormone. Endocrinology 1987;121:466-74.
13. Knobil E, Hotchkiss J. The menstrual cycle and its neuroendocrine control. In: Knobil E, Neill J, eds. The physiology of reproduction. New York: Raven Press, 1988:1971-94.
14. Yen SSC. Neuroendocrine regulation of the menstrual cycle. In: Krieger DT, Hughes JC, eds. A hospital practice book. Massachusetts: Sinauer Associates, 1980:259-72.

15. Marshall LA, Monroe SE, Jaffe RB. Physiologic and therapeutic aspects of GnRH and its analogs. In: Martini L, Ganong WF, eds. Frontiers in neuro-endocrinology. New York: Raven Press, 1988:239–78.

16. Watanabe G, Terasawa E. In vivo release of luteinizing hormone-releasing hormone increases with puberty in the female rhesus monkey. Endocrinology 1989;125:92–9.

17. Reiter EO, Grumbach MM. Neuroendocrine control mechanisms and the onset of puberty. Annu Rev Physiol 1982;44:595–613.

18. Delemarre-van de Waal HA, Wennink JMB, Odink RJH. Gonadotropin secretion during puberty in man. In: Delmarre-van de Waal HA, Plant TM, van Rees GP, Schoemaker J, eds. Control of the onset of puberty, III. Amsterdam: Excerpta Medica, 1989:151–81.

19. Terasawa E, Nass TE, Yeoman RR, Loose MD, Schultz NJ. Hypothalamic control of puberty in the female rhesus macaque. In: Norman RL, ed. Neuroendocrine aspects of reproduction. New York: Academic Press, 1983:149–82.

20. Plant TM. Puberty in primates. In: Knobil E, Neill J. eds. The physiology of reproduction. New York: Raven Press, 1988:1763–88.

21. Winter JSD, Faiman C. Serum gonadotropin concentrations in agonadal children and adults. J Clin Endocrinol Metab 1972;35:561–4.

22. Ross JL, Loriaux DL, Culter GB Jr. Developmental changes in neuro-endocrine regulation of gonadotropin secretion in gonadal dysgenesis. J Clin Endocrinol Metab 1983:288–93.

23. Terasawa E, Bridson WE, Nass TE, Noonan JJ, Dierschke DG. Developmental changes in the luteinizing hormone secretory pattern in peripubertal female rhesus monkeys: comparison between gonadally intact and ovariectomized animals. Endocrinology 1984;115:2233–40.

24. Wilson M. Relationship between growth and puberty in the rhesus monkey. In: Delemarre-van de Waal HA, Plant TM, van Rees GP, Schoemaker J, eds. Control of the onset of puberty. Amsterdam: Excerpta Medica 1989:137–49.

25. Dierschke DJ, Karsch FJ, Weick RF, Weiss G, Hotchkiss J, Knobil E. Hypothalamic pituitary regulation of puberty: feedback control of gonadotropin secretion in the rhesus monkey. In: Grumbach MM, Graves GD, Mayer FE, eds. Control of the onset of puberty, I. New York: John Wiley & Sons, 1974:104–14.

26. Chongthammakun S, Claypool LE, Terasawa E. Ovariectomy increases in vivo LHRH release in peripubertal, but not prepubertal female rhesus monkeys [Abstract]. In: Proceedings of the seventy-second annual meeting of The Endocrine Society, Atlanta, GA, 1990:1477.

27. Chongthammakun S, Claypool LE, Terasawa E. Developmental changes in in vivo GnRH release in response to estrogen in the female rhesus monkey [Abstract]. Neuroendocrinology 1990;52(S1):134.

28. Terasawa E, Claypool LE, Gore AC, Watanabe G. The timing of the onset of puberty in the female rhesus monkey. In: Delemarre-van de Waal HA, Plant TM, van Rees FP, Schoemaker J, eds. Control of the onset of puberty, III. Amsterdam: Excerpta Medica, 1989:123–36.

29. Wildt L, Marshall G, Knobil E. Experimental induction of puberty in the infantile rhesus monkey. Science 1980;207:1373–5.

30. Cameron JL, McNeill TH, Fraser HM, Bremmer WJ, Clifton DK, Steiner RA. The role of endogenous gonadotropin-releasing hormone neurons in the control of luteinizing hormone and testosterone secretion in the juvenile male monkey, *Macaca fascicularis*. Biol Reprod 1985;33:147–56.
31. Ronnekleiv OK, Resko JA. Ontogeny of gonadotropin-releasing hormone-containing neurons in early fetal development of rhesus macaques. Endocrinology 1990;126:498–511.
32. Adams LA, Vician L, Clifton DK, Steiner RA. Gonadotropin-releasing hormone (GnRH) mRNA content in GnRH neurons is similar in the brain of juvenile and adult male monkeys, *Macaca fascicularis* [Abstract]. In: Proceedings of the sixty-ninth annual meeting of The Endocrine Society, Indianapolis, IN, 1987:64.
33. Gay VL, Plant TM. N-methyl-D,L-aspartate (NMA) elicits hypothalamic GnRH release in prepubertal male rhesus monkeys (*Macaca mulatta*). Endocrinology 1987;120:2289–96.
34. Claypool LE, Terasawa E. N-methyl-D,L-aspartate (NMA) induces LHRH release as measured by in vivo push-pull perfusion in the stalk-median eminence of pre- and peripubertal female monkeys [Abstract]. Biol Reprod 1989;40:83.
35. Claypool LE, Watanabe G, Terasawa E. Effects of electrical stimulation of the medial basal hypothalamus on the in vivo release of luteinizing hormone-releasing hormone in the prepubertal and peripubertal female monkey. Endocrinology 1990;127:3014–22.
36. Krey LC, Butler WR, Knobil E. Surgical disconnection of the medial basal hypothalamus and pituitary function in the rhesus monkey, I. Gonadotropin secretion. Endocrinology 1975;96:1073–87.
37. Silverman AJ, Antunes JL, Abrams GM, et al. The luteinizing hormone-releasing hormone pathways in rhesus (*Macaca mulatta*) and pigtailed (*Macaca nemestrina*) monkeys: new observation on thick, unembedded sections. J Comp Neurol 1982;211:309–16.
38. Goldsmith PC, Lamberts R, Bregina LR. Gonadotropin-releasing hormone neurons and pathways in the primate hypothalamus and forebrain. In: Norman RL, ed. Neuroendocrine aspects of reproduction. New York: Academic Press, 1983:7–45.
39. King JC, Anthony ELP, Fitzgerald DM, Stopa EG. Luteinizing hormone-releasing hormone neurons in human preoptic/hypothalamus: differential interneuronal localization of immunoactive forms. J Clin Endocrinol Metab 1985;60:88–96.
40. Plant TM. Pulsatile LH secretion in the male rhesus monkey (*Macaca mulatta*): an index of the activity of the hypothalamic GnRH pulse generator. In: Leyendecker G, Wildt L, eds. Brain and pituitary peptides, II. Basel: Karger, 1983:125–39.
41. Plant TM, Krey LC, Moossy J, McCormack JT, Hess DL, Knobil E. The arcuate nucleus and the control of gonadotropin and prolactin secretion in the female rhesus monkey (*Macaca mulatta*). 1978;102:52–62.
42. Phelps CP, Kalra PS. Pulsatile LHRH release in vitro after surgical disconnection of the mediobasal hypothalamus (MBH) in vivo [Abstract]. In: Proceedings of the seventieth annual meeting of The Endocrine Society, New Orleans, LA, 1988:16.

43. Kelly MJ, Condon TP, Levine JE, Ronnekleiv OK. Combined electro-physiological, immunocytochemical and peptide release measurements in the hypothalamic slice. Brain Res 1985;345:264–70.
44. McKibbin PE, Belchetz PE. Prolonged pulsatile release of gonadotropin-releasing hormone from the guinea pig hypothalamus in vivo. Life Sci 1986;38:2145–50.
45. Terasawa E, Weigand SJ. Effects of hypothalamic deafferentation on ovulation and estrous cyclicity in the female guinea pig. Neuroendocrinology 1978;26:229–48.
46. Terasawa E, Yeoman RR, Schultz NJ. Factors influencing the progesterone-induced luteinizing hormone surge in rhesus monkeys: diurnal influence and time interval after estrogen. Biol Reprod 1984;31:732–41.
47. Andrew RD, Dudek FE. Burst discharge in mammalian neuroendocrine cells involves an intrinsic regenerative mechanism. Science 1983;221:1050–2.
48. Andrew RD. Oscillatory activity in supraoptic nucleus. In: Jacklet JW, ed. Neuronal and cellular oscillators. New York: Dekker, 1989:121–47.
49. Dreifuss JJ, Tribollet E, Baertschi A, Lincoln DW. Mammalian endocrine neurones: control of phasic activity by antidromic action potentials. Neurosci Lett 1976;3:281–6.
50. Hatton GI. Reversible synapse formation and modulation of cellular relationships in the adult hypothalamus under physiological conditions. In: Cotman CW, ed. Synaptic plasticity. New York: Guilford Press, 1985: 373–404.
51. Kozlowski GP, Coates PW. Ependymoneuronal specializations between LHRH fibers and cells of the cerebroventricular system. Cell Tissue Res 1985;242:301–11.
52. Mellon PL, Windle JJ, Goldsmith PC, Padula CA, Roberts JL, Weiner RI. Immortalization of hypothalamic GnRH neurons by genetically targeted tumorigenesis. Neuron 1990;5:1–10.
53. Weiner RI, Goldsmith PC, Windle JJ, Mellon PL. Cell biology and regulation of GnRH cell lines derived from transgenic mice [Abstract]. Neuroendocrinology 1990;52(S1):20.
54. Steiner RA, Bremmer WJ, Clifton DK. Regulation of luteinizing hormone pulse frequency and amplitude by testosterone in the adult male rat. Neuroendocrinology 1982;111:2055–61.
55. Barraclough CA, Wise PM, Selmanoff MK. A role for hypothalamic catecholamines in the regulation of gonadotropin secretion. Recent Prog Horm Res 1984;40:487–529.
56. Kalra SP. Neural circuitry involved in the control of LHRH secretion: a model for preovulatory LH release. In: Martini L, Ganong WR, eds. Frontiers in neuroendocrinology, vol. 9. New York: Raven Press, 1986: 31–75.
57. Ramirez VD, Feder HH, Sawyer CH. The role of brain catecholamines in the regulation of LH secretion: a critical inquiry. In: Ganong WF, ed. Frontiers in neuroendocrinology, vol. 7. New York: Raven Press, 1984:27–84
58. Sawyer CH. Some recent developments in brain-pituitary-ovarian physiology. Neuroendocrinology 1975;17:97–124.
59. Lincoln DW. LHRH pulse generation. In: Leng G, ed. Pulsatility in neuroendocrine systems. Boca Raton, FL: CRC Press, 1988:35–60.

60. Bhattacharya AN, Dierschke, DJ, Yamaji T, Knobil E. The pharmacologic blockade of the circhoral mode of LH secretion in ovariectomized rhesus monkeys. Endocrinology 1972;90:778–86.
61. Plant TM, Nakai Y, Belchetz P, Keogh E, Knobil E. The sites of action of estradiol and phentolamine in the inhibition of the pulsatile, circhoral discharges of LH in the rhesus monkey (*Macaca mulatta*). Endocrinology 1978;102:1015–8.
62. Kaufman J-M, Kesner JS, Wilson RC, Knobil E. Electrophysiological manifestation of luteinizing hormone-releasing hormone pulse generator activity in the rhesus monkey: influence of α-adrenergic blocking agents. Endocrinology 1985;116:1327–33.
63. Terasawa E, Krook C, Hei DL, Gearing M, Schultz NJ, Davis GA. Norepinephrine is a possible neurotransmitter stimulating pulsatile release of luteinizing hormone-releasing hormone in the rhesus monkey. Endocrinology 1989;123:1808–16.
64. Gearing M, Terasawa E. The stimulatory effect of methoxamine on in vivo LHRH release is mediated by prostaglandin E_2 (PGE_2) in ovariectomized unprimed monkeys [Abstract]. In: Proceedings of the twentieth annual meeting of the Society for Neuroscience, St. Louis, MO: 1990:126.11.
65. Gearing M, Terasawa E. The α_1-adrenergic neuronal system is involved in pulsatile release of luteinizing hormone-releasing hormone (LHRH) in the ovariectomized female monkey. Neuroendocrinology 1991;93:373–81.
66. Gearing M, Terasawa E. Suppression of luteinizing hormone (LH) release by the α_1-adrenergic receptor antagonist prazosin in the ovariectomized female rhesus monkey. Am J Primatol 1991.
67. Crowley WR, Hassid A, Karla SP. Neuropeptide Y enchances the release of luteinizing hormone (LH) induced by LH-releasing hormone. Endocrinology 1987;120:941–5.
68. McDonald JK. NPY and related substances. In: Nelson J, ed. Critical review in neurobiology, vol 4. Boca Raton, FL: CRC Press, 1987:97–135.
69. Khorram O, Pau K-YF, Spies HG. Bimodal effects of neuropeptide Y on hypothalamic release of gonadotropin-releasing hormone in conscious rabbits. Neuroendocrinology 1987;45:290–7.
70. Sabatino FD, Collins P, McDonald JK. Neuropeptide-Y stimulation of luteinizing hormone-releasing hormone secretion from the median eminence in vivo by estrogen-dependent and extracellular Ca^{2+}-independent mechanisms. Endocrinology 1989;124:2089–98.
71. Woller MJ, McDonald JK, Terasawa E. In vivo release of neuropeptide Y in the stalk-median eminence of castrated rhesus monkeys is pulsatile [Abstract]. In: Proceedings of the nineteenth annual meeting of the Society for Neuroscience, Phoenix, AZ, 1989:82.4.
72. Terasawa E, Woller MJ, Gearing M, Gore AC. Role of neuropeptide Y and norepinephrine in control of pulsatile GnRH release in ovariectomized monkeys [Abstract]. Neuroendocrinology 1990;52(S1):88.
73. Woller MJ, Terasawa E. Infusion of neuropeptide Y into the stalk-median eminence stimulates in vivo release of luteinizing hormone releasing hormone in gonadectomized rhesus monkeys. Endocrinology 1991;128:1144–50.
74. Beal MF, Gabriel SM, Swartz KJ, MacGarvey UM. Distribution of galanin-like immunoactivity in baboon brain. Peptides 1988;9:847–51.

75. Gabriel S, Koenig JI, Kaplan LM. Galanin-like immunoactivity is influenced by estrogen in peripubertal and adult rats. Neuroendocrinology 1990;51: 168–73.
76. Merchenthaler I, Negro-Vilar A. Sexual dimorphism in the co-expression of luteinizing hormone-releasing hormone (LHRH) and galanin in the preoptic region of the rat brain [Abstract]. In: Proceedings of the seventy-second annual meeting of The Endocrine Society, Atlanta, GA, 1990:465.
77. Lopez FJ, Merchenthaler I, Ching M, Wisniewski MG, Negro-Vilar A. Galanin: a hypothalamic-hypophysiotropic hormone modulating reproductive function [Abstract]. In: Proceedings of the seventy-second annual meeting of The Endocrine Society, Atlanta, GA, 1990:464.
78. Lamberts R, Vijayan E, Graf M, Mansky T, Wuttke W. Involvement of preoptic-anterior hypothalamic GABA neurons in the regulation of pituitary LH and prolactin release. Exp Brain Res 1983;52:356–62.
79. Jarry H, Perschl A, Wuttke W. Further evidence that preoptic anterior hypothalamic GABAergic neurons are part of the GnRH pulse and surge generator. Acta Endocrinol 1988;118:573–9.
80. Kalra SP, Kalra PS. Neural regulation of luteinizing hormone secretion in the rat. Endocr Rev 1983;4:311–51.
81. Ferin M, van Vugt D, Wardlaw S. The hypothalamic control of the menstrual cycle and the role of endogenous opioid peptides. Recent Prog Horm Res 1984;40:441–85.
82. Barker JL, Smith TG Jr. Bursting pacemaker activity in a peptidergic and peptide-sensitive neuron. In: Baker JL, Smith TG Jr, eds. The role of peptides in neuronal function. New York: Dekker, 1980:189–228.
83. Marder E, Hooper SL. Neurotransmitter modulation of the stomatogastric ganglion of decapod crustaceans. In: Selverston AI, ed. Model neural networks and behavior. New York: Plenum, 1985:319–37.
84. Terasawa E. What is the LHRH pulse generator? A hypothesis. In: Sagara Y, Seto K, eds. Pheromones and reproduction. Lancs: The Parthenon Publishing Group, 1990:77–87.
85. Rasmussen DD. The interaction between mediobasohypothalamic dopaminergic and endorphinergic neuronal systems as a key regulator of reproduction: a hypothesis. J Endocrinol Invest 1991;14.
86. Gore AC, Terasawa E. Methoxamine (MTX), an α_1-adrenergic agonist, stimulates in vivo LHRH release in pre- and peripubertal female rhesus monkeys [Abstract]. In: Proceedings of the nineteenth annual meeting of the Society for Neuroscience, Phoenix, AZ, 1989:528.7.
87. Gore AC, Terasawa E. Evidence that neuropeptide Y (NPY) plays a role in the pubertal increase in LHRH release in the female monkey [Abstract]. In: Proceedings of the twentieth annual meeting of the Society for Neuroscience, St. Louis, MO, 1990:393.2.

Part IV

GnRH Antagonists

17

An Overview of GnRH Antagonist Development: Two Decades of Progress

Marvin J. Karten

The first 13 years following the structural elucidation of porcine GnRH, $<\text{Glu}^1\text{-His}^2\text{-Trp}^3\text{-Ser}^4\text{-Tyr}^5\text{-Gly}^6\text{-Leu}^7\text{-Arg}^8\text{-Pro}^9\text{-Gly}^{10}\text{-NH}_2$ (1), witnessed the development of potent GnRH antagonists ([2] and references therein). D-arginine was introduced in position 6 primarily to improve water solubility and resulted in the potent antiovulatory analog, $[\text{Ac-DCpa}^{1,2},\text{DTrp}^3,\text{DArg}^6,\text{DAla}^{10}]\text{GnRH}$ (3). Modifications of this prototype provided two GnRH antagonists, Nal-Arg, $[\text{Ac-DNal}^1,\text{DFpa}^2,\text{DTrp}^3,\text{DArg}^6]\text{GnRH}$, (4) and Detirelix, $[\text{Ac-DNal}^1,\text{DCpa}^2,\text{DTrp}^3\text{-DhArg-}(\text{Et}_2)^6,\text{DAla}^{10}]\text{GnRH}$ (5, 6), for clinical investigation. It also provided, unfortunately, a class of peptides that ranks among the most potent in vitro histamine releasers known (7). The first indication of its potent histamine-releasing properties was discovered by Schmidt et al. (8), who reported that Nal-Arg produced transient edema of the face and extremities at $1.25\,\text{mg/kg}$, sc, in rats ($100\times$ the antiovulatory dose in rats). Nal-Arg and Detirelix were subsequently withdrawn from clinical trials because of histamine-mediated systemic side effects (9, 10). With the recognition of the potent histamine-releasing properties of these antagonists came the realization that a redesign of the Nal-Arg generation of GnRH antagonists was necessary. The goals were to maintain or increase the gonadotropin-suppressive potency of the Nal-Arg generation of antagonists while drastically reducing or eliminating its histamine-releasing potency. After a brief summary of the development of GnRH antagonists through 1984, including Nal-Arg and Detirelix, this review will focus on efforts to achieve these goals from 1985 to the present time.

Development of GnRH Antagonists (1971–1984)

A comprehensive review of the development of GnRH analogs through the middle of 1985 was presented by Karten and Rivier (2). A more recent review, including a compilation of the antiovulatory potencies of 364 GnRH antagonists, is available (11). A primarily empirical approach dominated the quest for potent GnRH antagonists. Early antagonistic modifications of GnRH focused on positions 2; 2, 6; and 2, 3, 6 of GnRH. [Des-His[2]]GnRH was the first competitive antagonist of GnRH to be reported (12). Structural features of the weakly active [DPhe[2]]GnRH (13) were combined with those of the agonist [DAla[6]]GnRH to provide [DPhe[2]-DAla[6]]GnRH, the first antagonist to inhibit ovulation in the rat, albeit at high doses (14). A variety of trisubstituted derivatives of GnRH at positions 2, 3, and 6 followed with [DPhe[2],Pro[3],DTrp[6]]GnRH (15) being one of the (relatively) more potent GnRH antagonists discovered at this point in time with an antiovulatory ED_{100} = 750 µg/rat. Momany's semi-empirical conformational energy calculations on GnRH and its analogs provided a working model (16) to explore further structure-activity relationships of GnRH analogs. These studies gave rise to [D<Glu[1],DPhe[2],DTrp[3,6]]GnRH, a tetrasubstituted and position 1-modified antagonist, exhibiting complete inhibition of ovulation in the rat at 250 µg/rat (17). Further dramatic enhancement of antagonist potency arose with other tetrasubstituted derivatives with position 1 and, simultaneously, position 2 modifications—e.g., [Ac-DPhe[1],DCpa[2], DTrp[3,6]]GnRH (18) and [Ac-dehydro-Pro[1],DCpa[2]-DTrp[3,6]]GnRH (19), the latter showing complete inhibition of ovulation at 7.5 µg/rat. GnRH antagonists were now displaying significant hydrophobic properties at positions 1 and/or 2, 3, and 6, as well as increased resistence to proteolysis. This hydrophobic trend continued unabated with the incorporation of 3-(2-naphthyl)-D-alanine into positions 3 and 6 resulting in [Ac-dehydro-Pro[1], DFpa[2]-Nal[3,6]]GnRH, which completely inhibited ovulation at a dose of 2.5 µg/rat (19). Similarly, the use of DAla at position 10 provided another potent, hydrophobic, antagonist, [Ac-DCpa[1,2],DTrp[3],DPhe[6], DAla[10]]GnRH (20). This trend toward increasing hydrophobicity (and insolubility in water) was reversed somewhat by the introduction of basic D-amino acids such as DArg at position 6, providing very potent analogs with increased water solubility (21). The most potent of these analogs, [Ac-DNal[1],DCpa[2],DTrp[3],DArg[6],DAla[10]]GnRH (22), exhibited complete inhibition of ovulation in the 1 µg/rat range and was the prototype for the equipotent antagonist, Nal-Arg, [Ac-DNal[1],DFpa[2],DTrp[3],DArg[6]]GnRH, (4), which was eventually withdrawn from clinical trials because of histamine-mediated systemic side effects (9). The prolonged duration of action of the DArg[6] analogs (21) was suggested to be the result of a hydrophilic depot effect and hypothesized to be due to electrostatic binding of the DArg[6] group to phospholipid cell membranes (5). On this basis another potent, long-acting antagonist, [Ac-DNal[1],DCpa[2],DTrp[3]-DhArg(Et2)[6],DAla[10]]GnRH, Detirelix, was designed with the potential for both electrostatic binding and additional hydrophobic interactions between the DhArg(Et2)[6] moiety and the bilayer (5, 6, 23). Detirelix was

also withdrawn from clinical trials due to histamine-mediated systemic effects (6, 10).

Histamine Release Studies

Even before the discovery of clinically adverse effects with Nal-Arg and Detirelix, the observation that Nal-Arg produced transient edema in rats (8) necessitated a new approach to the design of the potent GnRH antagonists if they were to have any clinical utility. This observation also suggested that the release of histamine and other inflammatory mediators from cells might be triggered by GnRH analogs and, subsequently, accounts of in vitro histamine release were reported relating the structural parameters of GnRH analogs that were responsible for potent histamine release (24–28). The experimental methods for in vitro histamine release, the characteristics of the histamine release reaction, and the reproducibility of the assay have been described (27). Initial data (24–26) indicated that the most potent in vitro histamine-releasing GnRH analogs, such as Nal-Arg (with ED_{50} = 0.17 μg/ml), had structural features consisting of a basic D-amino acid side chain in position 6, in close proximity to the naturally occurring basic arginine side chain in position 8, and a cluster of hydrophobic aromatic amino acids at the N-terminus. This was subsequently confirmed by more extensive observations on structure-activity relationships (27, 28). The least potent in vitro histamine releasers were the superagonists (ED_{50} = 46–108 μg/ml) and GnRH (ED_{50} = 150–300 μg/ml) that have no basic amino acid at position 6 and have a relatively hydrophilic N-terminus. It was noteworthy that one relatively potent GnRH antagonist, [Ac-dehydro-Pro^1,DFpa^2-DTrp^{3,6}]GnRH, previously found to be inactive in the rat edema assay (8) also had low in vitro histamine-releasing potency (ED_{50} = 39 μg/ml). This analog lacks DArg^6 and has somewhat lesser hydrophobic character at the N-terminus than does Nal-Arg. In vitro histamine release data generally correlate well with in vivo rat edema assay results (7). It was also apparent that the release of histamine by GnRH analogs (as well as other peptides) appeared to be a function of structural characteristics that were independent of other biological properties—e.g., gonadotropin-suppressive potency of the GnRH antagonists (7, 27).

General Strategies Utilized for the Development of Safer GnRH Antagonists

With the above knowledge of structure-activity relationships, and the emphasis placed on reducing histamine-releasing potency while maintaining high gonadotropin-suppressive potency, structural modifications of the antagonists focused primarily on position 6 and/or 8 (a) to reduce (or eliminate) basicity at position 6, and/or (b) to reduce basicity at position 8, and/or (c) to shield the positive charge at position 6 and/or 8. Elimination of basicity at both positions 6 and 8 drastically reduced gonadotropin-suppressive potency. Introduction of hydrophilic character at the N-terminus could be tolerated at position 3 with retention of high gonadotropin-suppressive potency, and, in fact, DPal^3 substitutions generally became the rule. On the other hand, introduction of amino acids with greater hydrophilic character than DNal in position 1 reduced both histamine-releasing and gonadotropin-suppressive potency, and this approach was rarely employed.

Clinically Relevant GnRH Antagonists (1985–1990)

The clinically relevant GnRH antagonists developed during the period 1985–1990 are listed in Table 17.1 and reflect those strategies that have resulted in GnRH antagonists with high gonadotropin-suppressive potency and significantly reduced histamine-releasing potency relative to Nal-Arg or Detirelix. Table 17.1 also provides a convenient order in which to review the chronological development of GnRH antagonists that are in various phases of clinical investigation or are anticipated to undergo clinical evaluation.

Nal-Glu

Roeske et al. (29, 30) found that a transposition of residues 5 and 6 (Tyr^5,DArg^6 → Arg^5,DTyr^6) produced an antagonist, [Ac-DNal^1,

TABLE 17.1. Clinically relevant GnRH antagonists.

Nal-Glu (Rivier, 1985)
[AcDNal^1,DCpa^2,DPal^3,Arg^5,DGlu(AA)^6,DAla^{10}]GnRH (31)^a

Antide (Folkers, 1987)
[AcDNal^1,DCpa^2,DPal^3,Lys(Nic)^5,DLys(Nic)^6,Lys(Ipr)^8,D-Ala^{10}]GnRH (42)

SB-75 (Bajusz, 1988)
[AcDNal^1,DCpa^2,DPal^3,DCit^6,DAla^{10}]GnRH (54)^b

RS-26306 (Nestor, 1988)
[AcDNal^1,DCpa^2,DPal^3,DhArg(Et$_2$)^6,hArg(Et$_2$)^8,DAla^{10}]GnRH (58)

HOE 013 (Konig, 1988)
[AcDNal^1,DCpa^2,DTrp^3,DSer(Rha)^6,AzaGly^{10}]GnRH (63)

^{a} Reference numbers are indicated in parentheses.
^{b} [AcDNal^1,DCpa^2,DPal^3,D,L-Cit^6,DAla^{10}]GnRH was first reported by Folkers et al. (52).
Note: Abbreviations: AA = anisole adduct; D-Glu(AA) = D-4-(p-methoxy-benzoyl)-2-aminobutyric acid; DSer(Rha) = O-(α-L-rhamnopyranosyl)-D-serine.

D4ClαMePhe^2-DTrp^3,Arg^5,DTyr^6,DAla^{10}]GnRH, with antiovulatory potency equivalent to that of Nal-Arg and 22-fold less histamine-releasing potency. Rivier et al. (31) explored this transposition further with other amino acid substitutions in position 6 while simultaneously modifying the hydrophobic N-terminus with DPal^3, a concept first introduced by Folkers et al. (32). One of the most potent of this series of analogs was [Ac-DNal^1,DCpa^2,DPal^3,Arg^5,DGlu(AA)^6,DAla^{10}]GnRH, Nal-Glu, with antiovulatory potency $\geq$ Nal-Arg, but with 10-fold less histamine-releasing potency in vitro, ED$_{50}$ = 1.6 µg/ml (31), and at least 10-fold less potent than Nal-Arg in an in vivo edema assay (7).

Short-term clinical studies in males (33–35) and females (36, 37) with Nal-Glu disclosed local reactions at the injection site, but no systemic toxicity was reported. Ninety-day toxicology studies in rats and rabbits showed no evidence of systemic toxicity (38). In long-term studies, observations of a mild systemic reaction in one female (39) and in one male (40) have been made. Azoospermia has been achieved in men by the daily injection of 7.5–10 mg of Nal-Glu plus administration of testosterone enanthate (40, 41). No loss of libido has been observed.

Antide (Nal-Lys)

An extensive study of the use of DLys(Nic) in position 6 as well as Lys(Nic) in positions 5 and 8, and particularly Lys(Ipr) in position 8, was undertaken by Ljungqvist et al. (42) in an effort to obtain antagonists with greatly reduced histamine-release potency. It had already been observed that the use of DPal in positions 3 and 6 had a substantial effect on reducing histamine-releasing potency (43). Furthermore, Roeske et al. (30) had explored the use of DLys(Ipr) in position 6 and Lys(Ipr) in positions 5 and 8, hoping to enhance the oral activity of the GnRH antagonists. (Hocart et al. [44, 45] extended this latter work using a variety of N-epsilon-alkylated lysine derivatives for the purpose of reducing histamine-releasing potency [see below].)

Several important points emerge from the study of Ljungqvist et al. (42): First, there is no longer any lack of information to enable one to design GnRH analogs with in vitro histamine-releasing potencies 100–1000 times less than that of Nal-Arg while retaining gonadotropin-suppressive potencies equal to or greater than that of Nal-Arg. Second, although histamine-releasing potency can be readily eliminated by removing strongly basic character at positions 6 and 8—e.g., [Ac-DNal^1, DCpa^2,DPal^3-DLys(Nic)^6,Lys(Nic)^8,DAla^{10}]GnRH had an in vitro histamine release ED$_{50}$ > 300 µg/ml—this weakly basic DLys(Nic)^6, Lys(Nic)^8 combination severely reduced antiovulatory potency. Third, weakly basic groups such as DLys(Nic) can be accommodated at position 6 provided that the counterbalancing strongly basic amino acid required at position 8, to retain high gonadotropin-suppressive potency, has a sterically hindered cationic charge, to reduce histamine-releasing potency. Thus, [Ac-DNal^1,DCpa^2,DPal^3,Lys(Nic)^5,DLys(Nic)^6,Lys(Ipr)^8, DAla^{10}]GnRH, Antide, completely inhibited ovulation at 1.0 µg/rat and had an in vitro histamine release ED$_{50}$ > 300 µg/ml (or in the same range as GnRH). It is interesting to note that the Tyr^5 derivative of Antide had a somewhat higher in vitro histamine-release potency (ED$_{50}$ = 133 µg/ml), while the more basic Lys(Ipr)^5 derivative had a markedly higher in vitro histamine-release potency (ED$_{50}$ = 20 µg/ml). It was also found that the corresponding Lys(Pic)^5, DLys(Pic)^6 derivative (Pic = picolyl) had an in vitro histamine release ED$_{50}$ = 93 µg/ml, while the Lys(INic)^5-DLys(INic)^6 derivative (INic = isonicotinoyl) had an in vitro histamine release ED$_{50}$ = 15 µg/ml, reflecting the fact that subtle changes in the spatial orientation of the pyridine ring in the side chains of positions 5 and 6 produce large effects on histamine-releasing potency. The latter two analogs also had high antiovulatory potency.

Antide showed no edema reaction in rats at 12.5 mg/kg (7). Antide has been compared with Nal-Glu and Nal-Arg in other in vivo histamine-related studies and appears to possess a greater safety margin with respect to the histamine-releasing potential of these antagonists (46). Azoospermia was achieved between weeks 9 and 13 in cynomolgus monkeys treated daily with 450 µg/kg of Antide for 18 weeks with delay of testosterone supplementation until week 6 (47). Phase I clinical studies with Antide are scheduled to begin shortly.

Prolonged duration of action of Antide has been reported in monkeys. In adult male monkeys, a single dose of 10 mg/kg, sc, of Antide inhibited testosterone production for more than 60 days in some males, whereas in others testosterone recovery began in 1 week (48). This finding coincides with previous observations of prolonged suppression of gonadotropin levels in ovariectomized monkeys (49, 50). The explanation for the variations in testosterone suppression is not clear, but among the reasons postulated (48) are variable depot effects at the injection site, differences in levels of serum binding proteins, individual variations in initial testosterone levels, and the contribution of the propylene glycol and water (1:1) vehicle to the variable responses.

The duration of action of a single injection of 225, 625, and 1200 µg/kg of Antide and other potent antagonists was evaluated in orchidectomized monkeys over a period of 96 h (51). All of the antagonists lowered gonadotropin levels within 3–6 h postinjection, with pronounced suppression occurring at 12–24 h. The major difference was in duration of suppression and, classified according to duration of action, Antide and SB-75 (see below) were the most potent with SB-75 > Antide = Detirelix > Nal-Glu as inhibitors of gonadotropin secretion.

SB-75

Another approach to reducing the histamine-releasing properties of the Nal-Arg class of antagonists was the introduction of ureidoalkylamino acids such DL-Cit^6 by Folkers et al. (52) and DCit^6 and DHci^6 (Hci = homocitrulline) by Bajusz et al. (53). These amino acids were regarded by both groups of investigators as neutral residues. Folkers et al. (52) have synthesized only one analog, [Ac-DNal^1-DCpa^2,DPal^3,DL-Cit^6, DAla^{10}]GnRH (a mixture of two peptides), and noted that it was unique that the "neutral DL-Cit^6 moiety and the basic D-NicLys^6 moiety provided peptides that are equivalent in (antiovulatory) activity." Histamine release, as measured by wheal areas, was higher for the DL-Cit^6 analog than for the corresponding D-NicLys^6 analog. Bajusz et al. (53) subsequently reported on a larger series of DCit^6 and DHci^6 analogs with [Ac-DNal^1,DCpa^2,DTrp^3,DCit^6-DAla^{10}]GnRH being a potent antiovulatory analog, showing no edema effects at 1.5 mg/kg in rats and having an in vitro histamine release ED$_{50}$ = 3.5 µg/ml compared with an ED$_{50}$ = 1.0 µg/ml for [Ac-DCpa^{1,2},DTrp^3,DArg^6,DAla^{10}]GnRH. Subsequently, [Ac-DNal^1,DCpa^2,DPal^3,DCit^6,DAla^{10}]GnRH (SB-75) was synthesized as a single substance by Bajusz et al. (54). The replacement of the less hydrophobic DPal^3 for DTrp^3, to give SB-75, decreased in vitro histamine release 2-fold, but had only marginal effects on antagonistic potency. SB-75 displayed no edema effects at 1.5 mg/kg in rats. Pharmacokinetic studies in rats with microcapsules consisting of SB-75 acetate (55) and SB-75 pamoate (56) in poly-DL-lactide-co-glycolide, a biodegradable polymer, have been reported. SB-75 pamoate appears to have a longer duration of release than SB-75 acetate.

SB-75 and other antagonists have been compared in 4-day duration of action studies in orchidectomized monkeys ([51]; see Antide, above).

In clinical studies with SB-75, no histamine-mediated systemic effects were observed at doses up to 1.2 mg (single injection) in climacteric women or doses of 300 micrograms b.i.d. (every 12 h, sc) for 6 weeks in two patients with advanced prostate cancer (57).

RS-26306

The presence of Arg^8 was considered by Nestor et al. (58) to be a critical factor in causing mast cell degranulation (MCD) by GnRH analogs. This was suggested by the fact that neuropeptides cause MCD with release of histamine and that a structural feature common to neuropeptides was the presence of an Arg-Pro sequence. With this as the rationale and, in order to circumvent the histamine-releasing problem associated with Detirelix, [Ac-DNal^1,DCpa^2,DTrp^3,DhArg(Et$_2$)^6-DAla^{10}]GnRH (6), Nestor et al. (58) studied the effect of increased steric hindrance in the guanidino function in position 8 on histamine-releasing and antiovulatory potency. Shielding of this positive charge would hopefully inhibit the presumed electrostatic interaction between the guanidino group of the GnRH antagonist and the mast cell membranes that trigger histamine release.

(Sundaram et al. [59] found that some potent histamine-releasing GnRH antagonists bind specifically to rat mast cells and concluded that histamine release is mediated by specific binding of these antagonists to cell membranes.) Interestingly, the effect of this steric hindrance $[hArg(Et_2)^8]$ on reducing histamine release in vitro was much more pronounced when coupled with $DPal^6$ (ED_{50} = 200 µg/ml for $[Ac-DNal^1, DCpa^2, DPal^{3,6}, hArg(Et_2)^8, DAla^{10}]$GnRH, RS-15378) than with $DhArg(Et_2)^6$ (ED_{50} = 13 µg/ml for $[Ac-DNal^1, DCpa^2, DPal^3, DhArg(Et_2)^6, hArg(Et_2)^8, DAla^{10}]$GnRH, RS-26306) (58). By comparison, Detirelix displayed an in vitro histamine release ED_{50} = 0.18 µg/ml. Nevertheless, RS-26306 was selected for clinical trials because of its superior physical properties (for formulation purposes) and its greater therapeutic index in vivo with respect to antiovulatory and hypotensive potencies when compared with RS-15378 (58, 60). With respect to antigonadotropic potency, relatively high oral bioavailability (1.8%) was found for RS-26306 administered in gelatin capsules to dogs, compared with the subcutaneous route (61).

Phase I clinical studies have been initiated in men and women (62). No systemic histamine-mediated reactions were observed in three groups of 5 women each treated with 1, 3, and 6 mg of RS-26306 (single, sc doses at 2-week intervals) or in four groups of 4 men each treated with 1, 3, 6, and 12 mg of RS-26306 (single, sc doses). Mean gonadotropin levels were still maximally suppressed (by 60–70% for LH and by 20–30% for FSH) after 24 h in women receiving ≥3 mg of RS-26306. Mean serum testosterone levels remained suppressed by at least 75%, 24 h after dosing, in men receiving ≥3 mg of RS-26306.

HOE-013

As a consequence of the finding that $[DSer(Rha)^6, Pro^9NHEt]$GnRH, which contains the hydrophilic O-(α-L-rhamnopyranosyl)-D-serine in position 6, had GnRH agonist potency comparable to that of Buserelin, $[DSer(tBu)^6, Pro^9NHEt]$GnRH, a series of GnRH antagonists were synthesized using the nonbasic, but hydrophilic DSer(Rha) in position 6 by Konig et al. (63). $AzaGly^{10}$ analogs were more potent then $DAla^{10}$ analogs with respect to decreasing prostate weight in adult male rats. One of the most potent antagonists in this series, $[Ac-DNal^1, DCpa^2, DTrp^3, DSer(Rha)^6, AzaGly^{10}]$GnRH, HOE-013, showed no symptoms of histamine release in dogs at 0.5 mg/kg, IV. The receptor affinity for HOE-013 was 10-fold higher than that found for Buserelin using rat pituitary membranes, and no effects on blood pressure were observed in monkeys, dogs, and rats at doses of 100 µg/kg, IV (64). Intravenous and subcutaneous doses of 0.5–1.0 mg/kg of HOE-013 were well tolerated by rabbits, guinea pigs, mice, and rats. HOE-013 is reported to have a long duration of action, and clinical studies with HOE-013 can be expected to be initiated shortly.

Exploration of Other Approaches in the Development of GnRH Antagonists (1985–1990)

During the past 5 years, a wide variety of other linear GnRH antagonists as well as truncated and cyclic antagonists have been designed, synthesized, and tested in animal models. The rationale for these explorations and the results and status of these endeavors are presented below.

GnRH Antagonists with DLys(alkyl)[6] and/or Lys(alkyl)[8] Modifications

Using [Ac-DNal[1],DPhe[2,3],DArg[6],Phe[7],DAla[10]]GnRH as the model peptide, Hocart et al. studied the effect of alterations in the basic side chains in position 6 (44) and in positions 6 and 8 or 8 alone (45) in an attempt to reduce histamine-releasing potency (in vitro) and retain high antiovulatory potency. N-epsilon-alkylated lysine derivatives with varying basicities, hydrophobicities, and size were substituted in the model peptide in position 6 and/or 8. It was concluded that (a) providing that the position 6 side chain retains a high degree of basicity, alterations in the hydrophobic character of the side chain have little effect on antiovulatory potency or histamine-releasing potency; (b) similar changes in position 8 alone (with DArg[6]) resulted in more than a 10-fold decrease in histamine-releasing potency; (c) aralkyl-lysine derivatives in position 6 or 8 caused the greatest reduction in histamine-releasing potency along with a reduction in antiovulatory potency in either series of analogs; (d) [Ac-DNal[1],DPhe[2,3],DLys(1-butylpentyl)[6], Phe[7],Lys(1-butylpentyl)[8], DAla[10]]GnRH, an analog with the largest N-epsilon-alkyl-lysine group in positions 6 and 8, afforded the greatest reduction in both histamine-releasing potency ($ED_{50} > 300\,\mu g/ml$) and antiovulatory potency (completely inactive at $6\,\mu g/rat$).

Similar to these results, Rivier et al. (65) also found that the biopotency (as determined by antiovulatory assays, in vitro measurements, and binding affinity studies) is inversely proportional to the size of the alkyl substituent in [Ac-DNal[1],DCpa[2],DTrp[3],DLys(alkyl)[6],Lys(alkyl)[8], DAla[10]]GnRH analogs.

CH$_2$NH and CH$_2$NAc Peptide Bond Isosteres

Using [Ac-DNal[1],DPhe[2,3],DArg[6],Phe[7],DAla[10]]GnRH as the model peptide, Hocart et al. (66) investigated the effect of CH$_2$NH and

CH$_2$NHAc peptide bond isosteres on histamine-releasing potency and antiovulatory potency. All of the reduced peptide bond analogs showed lower antiovulatory potencies than the model peptide, particularly those with replacements at positions 1–2, 2–3, 3–4, and 7–8. The effect on in vitro histamine release was generally slight, although substitutions at positions 1–2 and 5–6 gave an ED$_{50}$ = 1.5 µg/ml compared with 0.11 µg/ml for the parent analog.

Org 30850

The biological properties of [Ac-DCpa^{1,2},DBta^3,DLys^6,DAla^{10}]GnRH, Org 30850, were reported by Deckers et al. (67). Bta, benzothienylalanine, is an isostere of Trp. Comparisons with [Ac-DCpa^{1,2},DTrp^3,DArg^6, DAla^{10}]GnRH, Org 30276, were made and it was concluded that Org 30850 was about 4 times as potent as Org 30276 in inhibiting ovulation in rats. Org 30850 did not induce edema in rats. No in vitro histamine releasing data were reported. However, the structure of Org 30850 is related to that of Org 30276, which was previously reported (27) to have high in vitro histamine-releasing potency (ED$_{50}$ = 0.26 µg/ml). It was also previously reported that two other closely related antagonists, [Ac-DCpa^{1,2},DBta^3,DArg^6-DAla^{10}]GnRH and [Ac-DCpa^{1,2},DTrp^3,DLys^6, DAla^{10}]GnRH, have high in vitro histamine-releasing potencies, with ED$_{50}$ = 0.52 and 0.19 µg/ml, respectively (27).

Single doses of 1.0 and 3.0 mg/kg of Org 30850 administered to ovariectomized monkeys produced a persistent suppression (35 ± 10 days) of LH levels (68).

Further Modifications of Antide

Subsequent modifications of Antide with variations in positions 5–8 including Lys(Nic)^5 and Lys(Pic)^5, cis- and trans-D-acylated-aminocyclohexyl-alanine^6, and Lys(Ipr)^8 or Orn(Ipr)^8 have been reported by Ljungqvist et al. (69). The most potent of these variations was [Ac-DNal^1,DCpa^2, DPal^3,Lys(Pic)^5-cisDAla(PzAC)^6,Lys(Ipr)^8,DAla^{10}]GnRH, wherein Ala-(PzAC) is 3-(4-pyrazinyl-carbonylaminocyclohexyl)alanine. This analog was approximately twice as potent as Antide in inhibiting ovulation but had considerably higher histamine-releasing potency than Antide. In an effort to improve on the gonadotropin-suppressive potency of these analogs, Ljungqvist et al. (70) investigated a series of acylated amino-cyclohexylalanines in position 5 or 6 as well as acylated Lys^5 and/or DLys^6 residues. In neither series did any of the modifications show any improvement in antiovulatory potency compared with the potency of the parent antagonists, [Ac-DNal^1,DCpa^2,DPal^3,Lys(Pic)^5,cisDAla(PzAC)^6 or DLys(Pic)^6-Lys(Ipr)^8,DAla^{10}]-GnRH. The use of the very weakly basic pyrimidine group in positions 5 and 6 [e.g., Lys(Pmc)^5, DLys(Pmc)^6

(Pmc = 4-pyrimidylcarbonyl) in place of Lys(Pic)^5-DLys(Pic)^6] was particularly detrimental to antiovulatory potency.

Dialkylaminomethyl-Phe^6 Analogs of GnRH

Based upon the parent GnRH antagonist, [Ac-DNal^1,DCpa^2,DPal^3, Arg^5,DPal^6-DAla^{10}]GnRH (43), Liu et al. (71) synthesized several dialkylamino-(and cyclic amino)-methyl-Phe^6 derivatives. The most potent, the D-4-(morpholino-methyl)-Phe^6 derivative, completely blocked ovulation in rats at 1.0 µg (saline vehicle), compared with the parent, which completely blocked ovulation at 0.5 µg (corn oil vehicle). Histamine releasing data were not reported.

Position Ten Explorations

Feng et al. (72) evaluated the effect of C-terminal changes on inhibition of ovulation in rats. With various substitutions in positions 5, 6, and 8, it was generally found that replacing DAla^{10} with Sar^{10}, DSer^{10} (desGly^{10},Pro^{9}NHEt), Abu^{10}, Gly^{10}, and 3-difluoro-Ala^{10} led to reduced antiovulatory potency. One analog with Sar^{10}, [Ac-DNal^1,DCpa^2,DPal^3, cisAla(PzAC)^5,DLys(Pic)^6,Lys(Ipr)^8-Sar^{10}]GnRH, showed complete inhibition of ovulation at 0.5 µg/rat, or potency equivalent to that of the DAla^{10} parent analog.

Azaline

A novel approach to reducing the histamine release of certain potent GnRH antagonists was reported by Theobald et al. (73, 74). The guanidino group of various arginine and homoarginine residues was replaced with the considerably less basic N^w-cyanoguanidino function, while the basicity of the distal amino groups of lysine, ornithine, and p-aminophenylalanine was modified by the incorporation of the N^w-triazolyl function. Such modifications generally led to large reductions in the in vitro histamine release potency of the analogs. One of the more interesting antagonists to emerge from this study was Azaline, [Ac-DNal^1, DCpa^2, DPal^3, Lys(atz)^5, DLys(atz)^6, Lys(Ipr)^8, DAla^{10}]GnRH—[Lys(atz) = N-epsilon-5'-(3'-amino-1H-1',2',4'-triazolyl)-lysine], with ED$_{50}$ = 139 µg/ml in the rat mast cell assay, comparable to that of GnRH. In addition, Azaline showed potent gonadotropin suppression with 90% inhibition of ovulation at 2.0 µg per rat. [Ac-DNal^1,DCpa^2, DLys(atz)^{3,6},Lys(Ipr)^8,DAla^{10}]GnRH had a biological profile similar to that of Azaline.

Hexapeptide Analogs of GnRH

A series of hexapeptide analogs was synthesized by Haviv et al. (75) containing residues corresponding to positions 4–9 of GnRH with a

C-terminal Pro[9]NHEt group and an N-terminus consisting of a carboxylic acid designed to mimic the Trp[3] residue. One antagonist, 3-(1-naphthyl)-propionyl-Ser-Tyr-D2Nal-Leu-Arg-ProNHEt, had a binding affinity exceeding, by 4-fold, that of GnRH itself but still 10-fold less than that of the antagonist, [Ac-DCpa[1,2],DTrp[3]-DArg[6],DAla[10]]GnRH. This hexapeptide also had in vivo activity (castrate male rats), but antiovulatory activity was not reported. These analogs, with hydrophobic amino acids in position 6, appear to have very short half-lives. Rather uniquely, within this series of analogs, the size, length, and shape of the side chain substituent in position 3 determine antagonist or agonist activity. In addition, depending upon the nature of the residues in positions 4 (Ser or Ser[O-Bzl]) and 6 (e.g., DLeu, DTrp, or DNal), interconversions between agonist and antagonist activity are observed. The effect of size and physicochemical properties on the bioavailability of a series of hexapeptides in which the properties of the side chain in position 6 varied from highly hydrophobic to highly hydrophilic was further studied (76). Whereas highly hydrophobic amino acids such as DNal or DTrp in position 6 had a beneficial effect on binding affinity of these analogs, they had adverse pharmacokinetic effects as reflected in shorter duration of action of the analogs. Conversely, highly hydrophilic amino acids such as DLys and DArg prolonged the half-life of the analogs and improved pharmacokinetics. Computer-assisted molecular modeling has also been used to study the consequences of the modifications on the conformation of these analogs (77).

Cyclic Antagonists of GnRH

Although several thousand linear analogs of GnRH have been synthesized, little information has been available with regard to the nature of the physicochemical interaction of GnRH with its pituitary receptor. This is due to the facts that (a) the GnRH pituitary receptor has not been structurally characterized and (b) mammalian GnRH appears to have a random coil conformation in aqueous solution. This situation, described by Rivier et al. (78), led them to embark on a pioneering effort to define the "bioactive conformation" of GnRH using a multidisciplinary approach involving peptide synthesis and biological testing (79), computer simulation studies (80, 81), and nuclear magnetic resonance spectroscopy (82). After extensive studies, it was found (79) that a monocyclic analog, cyclo(4–10)[Ac-DNal[1],DFpa[2],DTrp[3],Asp[4],DArg[6], Dpr[10]]GnRH, showed biological potencies (antiovulatory, in vitro, and receptor binding assays) of approximately one-half that of the corresponding linear analog, [Ac-DNal[1],DFpa[2],DTrp[3],DArg[6]]-GnRH, Nal-Arg. This observation was significant with respect to the ligand's assumed conformation during receptor binding (79). Interestingly, this cyclic analog also showed histamine-releasing potency at least equivalent to that of its linear counterpart. Further conformational constraints were imposed on the GnRH antagonists by the introduction of a second bridge between residues 5 and 8 to produce bicyclic GnRH antagonists (78). (Dutta et al. [83] had previously reported on the antiovulatory potency of the monocyclic (Glu^5-Lys^8)-GnRH antagonists, with the most potent having an ED_{50} = 92 µg/kg in rats.) Nevertheless, by combining the Glu^5-Lys^8 constraint with an Asp^4-Dpr^{10} constraint, Rivier et al. (78) produced a bicyclic GnRH antagonist, bicyclo(4/10, 5/8)[Ac-$DNal^1$, $DCpa^2$-$DTrp^3$,Asp^4,Glu^5,$DArg^6$,Lys^8,Dpr^{10}]GnRH, which showed 80% inhibition of ovulation (2 of 10 rats ovulated) at 5 µg/rat. The corresponding $DPal^3$,$DNal^6$ cyclic analog was about 10-fold less potent but, it was noted, this latter cyclic analog was the first GnRH analog that had no positive charge but nevertheless had significant GnRH receptor affinity. However, the much lower antiovulatory potency of this $DPal^3$,$DNal^6$ cyclic analog reflects the need for a strongly basic amino acid at either position 6 or position 8 for the retention of high antiovulatory potency. It has been suggested (79) that the greater compact conformation of the cyclic antagonist compared with that of the linear antagonist would increase its potential for relatively higher oral potency, since its effectiveness at crossing the stomach lining into the blood stream may increase. There has not been a realization of this potential as yet. In order to obtain a fairly rigid analog, additional conformational constraints will have to be introduced (78).

Summary and Conclusions

Much effort has gone into the development of GnRH antagonists. Initially, the focus was on increasing the potency of GnRH analogs that displayed only weak in vitro antagonist potency. During the latter part of this initial period (1971–1975), antagonists were synthesized that exhibited antiovulatory activity at high doses. During the next long phase (1976–1984), potent antagonists were gradually obtained, but the achievement was somewhat offset by the finding that the potent $DArg^6$ class of antagonists also had very potent histamine-releasing properties. Redesign of the antagonists has been successful (1985–1990) in that potent GnRH antagonists are now available with greatly reduced histamine-releasing properties. With the ability now to design antagonists with very low histamine-releasing properties (in the range of GnRH itself), it is difficult to justify pursuing the commercial development of future antagonists that do not possess this characteristic. The prudent course of action would dictate that only GnRH antagonists with in vitro histamine-releasing potency of less than 0.1% relative to Nal-Arg be considered for commercial development, providing that the antagonists show no in vivo histamine-releasing properties at high doses in rats.

Other in vivo assays, such as effects on blood pressure, could profitably be added to the screening procedures for initial safety assessment.

Acute antiovulatory potencies (in rats) of the various clinically relevant antagonists (Table 17.1) do not appear to differ by more than a factor of two, although larger potency differences may be observed depending upon the nature of the vehicle employed—e.g, corn oil versus saline solution. It may therefore be advisable to determine acute antiovulatory potencies in both corn oil and saline. Determinations of the potencies of the antagonists in corn oil would be of importance insofar as permitting comparisons with a large antiovulatory data base of results from corn oil experiments, whereas determinations of potencies in saline would be pertinent for extrapolation to clinical use. It is also important to recognize that acute antiovulatory potencies in rats do not necessarily parallel potencies as determined by suppression of gonadotropin levels in duration of action (short or long) studies with primates.

High oral bioavailability of GnRH antagonists would obviously be a very desirable property, particularly for indications or regimens requiring long-term (daily) administration of the peptide. Good oral bioavailability (1.8%), compared with the subcutaneous route, was reported for RS-26306 in dogs, but no direct comparison with other antagonists was reported. Previous indications of oral bioavailability for other GnRH antagonists can be gleaned from general observations that the oral:sc acute antiovulatory activity ratio in rats is approximately 1000:1. Considering the present costs of the agonists and the subcutaneous potencies of the current antagonists and their potential cost, the cost of oral administration of any antagonist showing less than 10% oral bioavailabilty would be prohibitive.

The finding that the subcutaneous administration of large doses of some potent GnRH antagonists results in a prolonged (albeit inconsistent) duration of suppression of gonadotropin levels in ovariectomized monkeys and testosterone levels in male monkeys warrants further comment. One of the primary reasons for their prolonged duration of action is probably the fact that the antagonist forms a gel (depot) at the injection site. It is also probable that the observed inconsistent results in these duration of action studies is due to the inability to obtain consistent gel characteristics at the injection site, and the inability, therefore, to obtain consistent release rates. This situation, then, raises some question as to the wisdom of relying on such depots to produce long-lasting effects. The alternative, and probably wiser, course of action is to incorporate the antagonist into an appropriate drug delivery system to produce the desired duration of action. Additionally, the successful commercialization of these antagonists may very well depend upon the development of improved formulations, to enhance the solubility of these antagonists for subcutaneous administration, by the pharmaceutical industry.

Currently available GnRH antagonists may have sufficient gonadotropin-suppressive potency and/or duration of action to be useful in the treatment of certain indications such as prostatic cancer, endometriosis, and polycystic ovarian disease, and for predictable ovulation induction for the purpose of in vitro fertilization. However, these antagonists are not sufficiently potent to be considered as practical male contraceptive agents, although their potential in this direction has been demonstrated. Thus, an important goal for the near future is to design GnRH antagonists with a minimum of a ten-fold increase in gonadotropin-suppressive potency, compared with those currently available. Additionally, although azoospermia has been achieved, another important goal for the near future will be the clinical demonstration that azoospermia can be consistently achieved within practical time limits—i.e., within approximately 12 weeks of initial treatment with the antagonist. The quest for more potent antagonists is predicated primarily on using these peptides for male contraception or any other indications where long-term therapy is required. With much more potent antagonists, the cost of such applications may be more realistically addressed.

Two decades of progress in the development of GnRH antagonists have been reviewed above. It should be clear that the antagonists have now reached the stage of development wherein their potential therapeutic use is receiving serious consideration by the pharmaceutical industry. Although the current antagonists do not have sufficient potency to warrant their consideration as male contraceptive agents, we are nevertheless hopeful that through further chemical modifications the desired potency of the antagonists can be achieved and that the first male contraceptive agent may be available before the year 2000.

Acknowledgment. I wish to express my appreciation to Dr. Jean Rivier of the Salk Institute for his helpful comments and suggestions pertaining to this review.

References

1. Matsuo H, Baba Y, Nair RM, Arimura A, Schally AV. Structure of the porcine LH- and FSH-releasing hormone: I. The proposed amino acid sequence. Biochem Biophys Res Commun 1971;43:1334–9.
2. Karten MJ, Rivier JE. Gonadotropin-releasing hormone analog design: structure-function studies toward the development of agonists and antagonists: rationale and perspective. Endocr Rev 1986;7:44–66.
3. Coy DH, Horvath A, Nekola MV, Coy EJ, Erchegyi J, Schally AV. Peptide antagonists of LH-RH: large increases in antiovulatory activities produced by basic D-amino acids in the six position. Endocrinology 1982;110:1445–7.

4. Rivier J, Rivier C, Perrin M, Porter J, Vale WW. LHRH analogs as antiovulatory agents. In: Vickery BH, Nestor JJ Jr, Hafez ESE, eds. LHRH and its analogs. Lancaster, UK: MTP Press, 1984:11–22.

5. Nestor JJ Jr, Ho TL, Tahilramani R, et al. LHRH agonists and antagonists containing very hydrophobic amino acids. In: Vickery BH, Nestor JJ Jr, Hafez ESE, eds. LHRH and its analogs. Lancaster, UK: MTP Press, 1984: 23–33.

6. Nestor JJ Jr, Tahilramani R, Ho TL, McRae GI, Vickery BH. Potent, long-acting luteinizing hormone-releasing hormone antagonists containing new synthetic amino acids: N,N'-dialkyl-D-homoarginines. J Med Chem 1988; 31:65–72.

7. Karten MJ, Hoeger CA, Hook WA, Lindberg MC, Naqvi RH. The development of safer GnRH antagonists: strategy and status. In: Bouchard P, Haour S, Franchimont P, Schatz B, eds. Recent progress on GnRH and gonadal peptides. Amsterdam: Elsevier, 1990:147–58.

8. Schmidt F, Sundaram K, Thau RB, Bardin CW. [Ac-D-Nal(2)^1,4FD-Phe^2,D-Trp^3,D-Arg^6]LHRH, a potent antagonist of LHRH, produces transient edema and behavioral changes in rats. Contraception 1984;29:283–9.

9. Hall JE, Brodie TD, Badger TM, et al. Evidence of differential control of FSH and LH secretion by gonadotropin-releasing hormone (GnRH) from the use of a GnRH antagonist. J Clin Endocrinol Metab 1988;67:524–31.

10. Monroe S. Personal communication.

11. Dutta AS. Luteinizing hormone-releasing hormone (LHRH) antagonists. Drugs Fut 1988;13:761–87.

12. Vale W, Grant G, Rivier J, et al. Synthetic polypeptide antagonists of the hypothalamic luteinizing hormone releasing factor. Science 1972;176:933–4.

13. Rees WAR, Foell TJ, Chai SY, Grant N. Synthesis and biological activities of analogs of the luteinizing hormone-releasing hormone (LH-RH) modified in position 2. J Med Chem 1974;17:1016–9.

14. Corbin A, Beattie CW. Inhibition of the pre-ovulatory proestrous gonadotropin surge, ovulation and pregnancy with a peptide analogue of luteinizing hormone releasing hormone. Endocr Res Commun 1975;2:1–23.

15. Humphries J, Wan YP, Folkers K, Bowers CY. Presence of proline in position 3 for potent inhibition of the activity of the luteinizing hormone releasing hormone and of ovulation. Biochem Biophys Res Commun 1976; 72:939–44.

16. Momany FA. Conformational analysis of the molecule luteinizing hormone-releasing hormone: 3. Analog inhibitors and antagonists. J Med Chem 1978; 21:63–8.

17. Rivier JE, Vale WW. [D-p-Glu^1,DPhe^2,D-Trp^{3,6}]-LRF: a potent luteinizing hormone releasing factor antagonist *in vitro* and inhibitor of ovulation in the rat. Life Sci 1978;23:869–76.

18. Coy DH, Mezo I, Pedroza E, et al. LH-RH antagonists with potent antiovulatory activity. In: Gross E, Meinhofer J, eds. Peptides: structure and biological function: proceedings of the Sixth American Peptide Symposium. Rockford, IL: Pierce Chemical Co., 1979:775–9.

19. Rivier J, Rivier C, Perrin M, Porter J, Vale WW. GnRH analogs: structure activity relationships. In: Zatuchni GI, Shelton JD, Sciarra JJ, eds. LHRH

peptides as female and male contraceptives. Philadelphia: Harper & Row, 1981:13–23.

20. Erchegyi J, Coy DH, Nekola MV, et al. Luteinizing hormone-releasing hormone analogs with increased antiovulatory activity. Biochem Biophys Res Commun 1981;100:915–20.

21. Coy DH, Horvath A, Nekola MV, Coy EJ, Erchegyi J, Schally AV. Peptide antagonists of LH-RH: large increases in antiovulatory activities produced by basic D-amino acids in the six position. Endocrinology 1982;110:1445–7.

22. Horvath A, Coy DH, Nekola MV, Coy EJ, Schally AV, Teplan I. Synthesis and biological activity of LH-RH antagonists modified in position 1. Peptides 1982;3:969–71.

23. Nestor JJ Jr, Tahilramani R, Ho TL, McRae GI, Vickery BH, Bremner WJ. New luteinizing hormone-releasing factor antagonists. In: Hruby VJ, Rich DH, eds. Peptides: structure and function: proceedings of the Eighth American Peptide Symposium. Rockford, IL: Pierce Chemical Co., 1983: 861–4.

24. Nekola, MV, O'Neil C, Morgan J, Coy D. Antagonists of luteinizing hormone releasing hormone (LHRH): potent releasers of histamine in rats [Abstract]. Clin Res 1984;32:865A.

25. Hook WA, Karten M, Siraganian RP. Histamine release by structural analogs of LHRH [Abstract]. Fed Proc 1985;44:1323.

26. Morgan JE, O'Neil CE, Coy DH, Hocart SJ, Nekola MV. Antagonistic analogs of luteinizing hormone-releasing hormone are mast cell secretagogues. Int Arch Allergy Appl Immunol 1986;80:70–5.

27. Karten MJ, Hook WA, Siraganian RP, et al. In vitro histamine release with LHRH analogs. In: Vickery BH, Nestor JJ Jr, eds. LHRH and its analogs: contraceptive and therapeutic applications, part 2. Lancaster, UK: MTP Press, 1987:179–90 (and references therein).

28. Roeske RW, Chaturvedi NC, Hrinyo-Pavlina T, Kowalczuk M. LHRH antagonists with low histamine releasing activity. In: Vickery BH, Nestor JJ Jr, eds. LHRH and its analogs: contraceptive and therapeutic applications, part 2. Lancaster, UK: MTP Press, 1987:17–24.

29. Roeske RW, Chaturvedi NC, Rivier J, Vale W, Porter J, Perrin M. Substitution of Arg^5 for Tyr^5 in GnRH antagonists. In: Deber CM, Hruby VJ, Kopple KD, eds. Peptides: structure and function: proceedings of the Ninth American Peptide Symposium. Rockford, IL: Pierce Chemical Co., 1985: 561–4.

30. Roeske RW, Chaturvedi NC, Hrinyo-Pavlina T, Kowalczuk M. LHRH antagonists with low histamine releasing activity. In: Vickery BH, Nestor JJ Jr, eds. LHRH and its analogs: contraceptive and therapeutic applications, part 2. Lancaster, UK: MTP Press, 1987:17–24.

31. Rivier JE, Porter J, Rivier CL, et al. New effective gonadotropin releasing hormone antagonists with minimal potency for histamine release in vitro. J Med Chem 1986;29:1846–51.

32. Folkers K, Bowers CY, Kubiak T, Stepenski J. Antagonists of the luteinizing hormone releasing hormone with pyridyl-alanines which completely inhibit ovulation at nanogram dosage. Biochem Biophys Res Commun 1983;111: 1089–95.

33. Bagatell CJ, McLachlan RI, DeKretser DM, et al. A comparison of the suppressive effects of testosterone and a potent new gonadotropin-releasing hormone antagonist on gonadotropin and inhibin levels in normal men. J Clin Endocrinol Metab 1989;69:43–8.
34. Pavlou SN, Wakefield GB, Schlechter NL, et al. Mode of suppression of pituitary and gonadal function after acute or prolonged administration of a luteinizing hormone-releasing hormone antagonist in normal men. J Clin Endocrinol Metab 1989;68:446–54.
35. Salameh W, Bhasin S, Steiner BS, et al. Marked suppression of gonadotropins and testosterone by an antagonist analog of gonadotropin-releasing hormone in men. Fertil Steril (in press).
36. Hall JE, Whitcomb RW, Rivier J, Vale W, Crowley WF Jr. Differential regulation of LH, FSH, and free alpha-subunit secretion from the gonadotroph by GnRH: evidence from the use of two GnRH antagonists. J Clin Endocrinol Metab 1989;70:328–35.
37. Mortola JF, Sathanandan M, Pavlou S, et al. Suppression of bioactive and immunoreactive follicle-stimulating hormone and luteinizing hormone levels by a potent gonadotropin-releasing hormone antagonist: pharmacodynamic studies. Fertil Steril 1989;51:957–63.
38. Sundaram K, Didolkar A, Keizer-Zucker A, et al. A 90-day subcutaneous toxicity and fertility study of a LHRH antagonist in rats. Fundam Appl Toxicol 1990;14:734–44.
39. Bouchard P. Personal communication.
40. Swerdloff RS, Bhasin S, Salameh W, Tom L, Peterson M, Steiner B. Combined GnRH antagonist and testosterone enanthate for experimental male contraception [Abstract]. In: Gynecological endocrinology, vol 4, suppl No. 2, International Symposium on GnRH Analogues in Cancer and Human Reproduction, Geneva, November 7–10, 1990:#35.
41. Pavlou SN, Brewer K, Lindner J, et al. Complete suppression of spermatogenesis without loss of libido by administering a GnRH antagonist plus testosterone [Abstract]. Presented at the 72nd annual meeting of The Endocrine Society, Atlanta, GA, June 20–23, 1990:#443.
42. Ljungqvist A, Feng D-M, Tang P-FL, et al. Design, synthesis and bioassays of antagonists of LHRH which have high antiovulatory activity and release negligible histamine. Biochem Biophys Res Commun 1987;148:849–56.
43. Folkers K, Bowers C, Xiao S, Tang P-FL, Kubota M. Increased potency of antagonists of the luteinizing hormone releasing hormone which have D-3-Pal in position 6. Biochem Biophys Res Commun 1986;137:709–15.
44. Hocart SJ, Nekola MV, Coy DH. Effect of reductive alkylation of D-lysine in position 6 on the histamine-releasing activity of luteinizing hormone-releasing hormone antagonists. J Med Chem 1987;30:739–43.
45. Hocart SJ, Nekola MV, Coy DH. Effect of reductive alkylation of lysine in positions 6 and/or 8 on the histamine-releasing activity of luteinizing hormone-releasing hormone antagonists. J Med Chem 1987;30:1910–4.
46. Phillips A, Hahn DW, McGuire JL, et al. Evaluation of the anaphylactoid activity of a new LHRH antagonist. Life Sci 1988;43:883–8.
47. Weinbauer GF, Khurshid S, Fingscheidt U, Nieschlag E. Sustained inhibition of sperm production and inhibin secretion induced by a gonadotropin-

releasing hormone (GnRH) antagonist and delayed testosterone substitution in non-human primates (*Macaca fascicularis*). J Endocrinol 1989;123:303–10.

48. Edelstein MC, Gordon K, Williams RF, Danforth DR, Hodgen GD. Single dose long-term suppression of testosterone secretion by a gonadotropin-releasing hormone antagonist (Antide) in male monkeys. Contraception 1990;42:209–14.

49. Leal JA, Williams RF, Danforth DR, Gordon K, Hodgen GD. Prolonged duration of gonadotropin inhibition by a third generation GnRH antagonist. J Clin Endocrinol Metab 1988;67:1325–7.

50. Danforth DR, Gordon K, Leal JA, Williams RF, Hodgen GD. Extended presence of Antide (Nal-Lys GnRH antagonist) in circulation: prolonged duration of gonadotropin inhibition may derive from Antide binding to serum proteins. J Clin Endocrinol Metab 1990;70:554–6.

51. Weinbauer GF, Nieschlag E. Evaluation of the antigonadotropic activity of different GnRH antagonists in the non-human primate [Abstract]. In: Gynecological endocrinology, vol 4, suppl No. 2, International Symposium on GnRH Analogues in Cancer and Human Reproduction, Geneva, November 7–10, 1990:#21.

52. Folkers K, Bowers C, Xiao S, et al. Activities of antagonists of the luteinizing hormone releasing hormone with emphasis on positions 1, 5 and 6 and on positions 1, 2 and 3. Z Naturforsch 1987;42b:101–6.

53. Bajusz S, Kovacs M, Gazdag M, et al. Highly potent antagonists of luteinizing hormone-releasing hormone free of edematogenic effects. Proc Natl Acad Sci USA 1988;85:1637–41.

54. Bajusz S, Csernus VJ, Janaky T, Boker L, Fekete M, Schally AV. New antagonists of LHRH, II. Inhibition and potentiation of LHRH by closely related analogues. Int J Peptide Protein Res 1988;32:425–35.

55. Csernus VJ, Szende B, Groot K, Redding TW, Schally AV. Development of radioimmunoassay for a potent luteinizing hormone-releasing hormone antagonist. Arzneim-Forsch/Drug Res 1990;40:111–8.

56. Bokser L, Bajusz S, Groot K, Schally AV. Prolonged inhibition of luteinizing hormone and testosterone levels in male rats with the luteinizing hormone-releasing hormone antagonist SB-75. Proc Natl Acad Sci USA 1990;87:7100–4.

57. Gonzalez-Barcena D, Vadillo-Buenfil M, Guerra-Arquero L, Carreno J, Comaru-Schally AM, Schally AV. Potent antagonistic analog of LH-RH (SB-75) inhibits LH, FSH and testosterone levels in human beings [Abstract]. Presented at the 72nd annual meeting of The Endocrine Society, Atlanta, GA, June 20–23, 1990:#1318.

58. Nestor JJ Jr, Tahilramani R, Ho TL, Goodpasture JC, Vickery BH Ferrandon P. Design of luteinizing hormone releasing hormone antagonists with reduced potential for side effects. In: Jung G, Bayer E, eds. Peptides 1988: proceedings of the 20th European Peptide Symposium. Berlin: Walter de Gruyter & Co., 1989:592–4.

59. Sundaram K, Didolkar A, Thau R, Chaudkuri M, Schmidt F. Antagonists of luteinizing hormone releasing hormone bind to rat mast cells and induce histamine release. Agents Actions 1988;25:307–13.

60. Lee C-H, VanAntwerp D, Hedley L, Nestor JJ Jr, Vickery BH. Comparative studies on the hypotensive effect of LHRH antagonists in anesthetized rats. Life Sci 1989;45:697–702.

61. Vickery BH, McRae G, Lee C-H, Nerenberg CA, Ferrandon P, Nestor J. A new highly potent LHRH antagonist with low histamine releasing activity has unusually high oral bioavailability [Abstract]. Presented at the 72nd annual meeting of The Endocrine Society, Atlanta, GA, June 20–23, 1990:#1375.

62. Rothman P, Rabinovici J, Jaffe R, Gaitan D, Pavlou S, Monroe S. Effects of a new GnRH antagonist (RS-26306) on the secretion of LH, FSH, and testosterone in postmenopausal women or men [Abstract]. In: Gynecological endocrinology, vol 4, suppl No. 2, International Symposium on GnRH Analogues in Cancer and Human Reproduction, Geneva, November 7–10, 1990:addendum.

63. Konig W, Sandow J, Jerabek-Sandow G, Kolar C. Glycosylated gonadoliberin antagonists. In: Jung G, Bayer E, eds. Peptides 1988: proceedings of the 20th European Peptide Symposium. Berlin: Walter de Gruyter & Co., 1989: 334–6.

64. Sandow J, Jerabek-Sandow G, Stockemann K, Fraser HM, Konig W, Lill N. A new antagonist of luteinizing hormone-releasing hormone [Abstract]. Acta Endocrinologica 1990;122(suppl 1):122.

65. Rivier J, Rivier C, Perrin M, et al. GnRH antagonists: N-alkylation of primary amino functions generate new potent analogs. Coll Soc Fr Etudes Fertil 1988;26:25–31.

66. Hocart SJ, Nekola MV, Coy DH. Effect of the CH_2NH and CH_2NAc peptide bond isosteres on the antagonistic and histamine releasing activities of a luteinizing hormone-releasing hormone analogue. J Med Chem 1988;31: 1820–4.

67. Deckers GHJ, Kloosterboer HJ, Loozen HJJ. Properties of a new LHRH-antagonist (Org 30850) [Abstract]. Presented at the 71st annual meeting of The Endocrine Society, Seattle, WA, June 21–24, 1989:#923.

68. Scott RT Jr, Gordon K, Williams RF, et al. New long-acting GnRH antagonist: accelerated GnRH test response in primates [Abstract]. Presented at the 71st annual meeting of The Endocrine Society, Seattle, WA, June 21–24, 1989:#216.

69. Ljungqvist A, Feng D-M, Hook W, Shen Z-X, Bowers C, Folkers K. Antide and related antagonists of luteinizing hormone release with long action and oral activity. Proc Natl Acad Sci USA 1988;85:8236–40.

70. Ljungqvist A, Feng D-M, Bowers C, Hook W, Folkers K. Antagonists of LHRH superior to Antide: effective sequence/activity relationships. Tetrahedron 1990;46:3297–304.

71. Liu K, He B, Xiao S, Xia Q, Fang X, Wang Z. Antagonists of luteinizing hormone releasing hormone with novel unnatural amino acids at position six. Int J Peptide Protein Res 1990;35:157–60.

72. Feng DM, Ljungqvist A, Hook WA, Bowers CY, Folkers K. Position 10 is critical for antagonists of the luteinizing hormone-releasing hormone and for inhibition of ovulation in rats. Z Naturforsch [B] (in press).

73. Theobald P, Porter J, Hoeger C, Rivier J. A general method for incorporation of modified N^w-cyanoguanidino moieties on selected amino functions during SPPS. J Am Chem Soc 1990;112.

74. Theobald P, Porter J, Rivier C, et al. Novel gonadotropin releasing hormone antagonists: peptides incorporating an N^w-cyano modified guanidine moiety. J Med Chem (in press).
75. Haviv F, Palabrica CA, Bush EN, et al. Active reduced-size hexapeptide analogs of luteinizing hormone-releasing hormone. J Med Chem 1989;32: 2340–4.
76. Haviv F, Fitzpatrick TD, Bush EN, et al. Structure-activity relationships, pharmacokinetics, and bioavailability studies for reduced size analogs of gonadotropin-releasing hormone (GnRH). In: Rivier JE, Marshall GR, eds. Peptides: chemistry, structure and biology: Eleventh American Peptide Symposium. Leiden, The Netherlands: ESCOM Science, 1990:192–4.
77. Haviv F, Fitzpatrick TD, Nichols CJ, et al. The effect of size and physico-chemical properties on activity and bioavailability of GnRH analogs [Abstract]. In: Gynecological endocrinology, vol 4, suppl No. 2, International Symposium on GnRH Analogues in Cancer and Human Reproduction, Geneva, November 7–10, 1990:#3.
78. Rivier JE, Rivier C, Vale W, et al. Bicyclic gonadotropin releasing hormone (GnRH) antagonists. In: Rivier J, Marshall G, eds. Peptides: chemistry, structure and biology: proceedings of the Eleventh American Peptide Symposium. Leiden, The Netherlands: ESCOM Science, 1990:33–7.
79. Rivier J, Kupryszewski G, Varga J, et al. Design of potent cyclic gonadotropin releasing hormone antagonists. J Med Chem 1988;31:677–82.
80. Struthers RS, Hagler AT, Rivier J. Theoretical simulation of conformation, energetics, and dynamics in the design of peptide analogs. In: Vida JA, Gordon M, eds. Conformationally directed drug design: peptides and nucleic acids as templates or targets. Washington, DC: American Chemical Society, 1984:239–61.
81. Struthers RS, Rivier J, Hagler AT. Molecular dynamics and minimum energy conformations of GnRH and analogs: a methodology for computer-aided drug design. In: Venkataraghavan B, Feldman RJ, eds. Macromolecular structure and specificity: computer assisted modeling and applications. Ann NY Acad Sci 1985;459:81–96.
82. Baniak EL, Gierasch LM, Rivier JE, Hagler A. NMR analysis and con-formational characterization of cyclic antagonists of gonadotropin-releasing hormone. In: Marshall GR, ed. Proceedings of the Tenth American Peptide Symposium. Leiden, The Netherlands: ESCOM Science, 1988:457–58.
83. Dutta AS, Gormley JJ, McLachlan PF, Woodburn JR. Conformationally restrained cyclic peptides as antagonists of luteinizing hormone-releasing hormone. Biochem Biophys Res Commun 1989;159:1114–20.

18

GnRH Antagonists in Men

Spyros N. Pavlou

GnRH is a decapeptide, secreted from the hypothalamus in a pulsatile fashion, that regulates the synthesis and secretion of pituitary gonado-tropins (1–9). In contrast, synthetic GnRH agonists or antagonists inhibit gonadotropin secretion and subsequently gonadal function (10, 11). Since synthetic agonist analogs were shown to suppress gonadotropin secretion after an initial phase of stimulation (12–17), several studies were performed aiming toward modulation of androgen secretion and the development of a male contraceptive (18–24). GnRH agonists can effectively suppress secretion of gonadal steroids (25–28), but during the initial 2–3-week period of administration a transient stimulation of LH release occurs, resulting in an increase in gonadal steroid levels, which can in some cases induce a flare of the underlying disease. Agonists failed, however, to effectively and consistently suppress spermatogenesis (29–32). Oligospermia was achieved by most men in these studies, but only very few men reached azoospermia (33). This failure of GnRH agonists can be attributed to incomplete suppression of serum FSH immunoreactivity and bioactivity (34) and to the fact that, during long-term agonist administration, FSH serum levels tend to return toward baseline (35).

Antagonist analogs of GnRH inhibit pituitary and gonadal function by competing with endogenous GnRH for binding to gonadotrope receptors and suppressing mRNA levels of both α- and β-subunits of gonadotropins (36–40). Induction of suppression is potentiated by a decrease in the biological potency of the FSH and LH molecules (41–46). Administration of GnRH antagonists induces rapid and sustained pituitary and gonadal suppression in humans (46–53), with no initial stimulatory phase as is the case with GnRH agonists. Therefore, antagonists should be the agents of choice for all clinical situations that require rapid and effective induction of gonadal suppression. Development of GnRH antagonists, however, has been slow because of low potency of early analogs (54), and histamine-like side-effects caused by more potent analogs (55–57). A potent GnRH antagonist, synthesized by Drs. J. Rivier and W. Vale

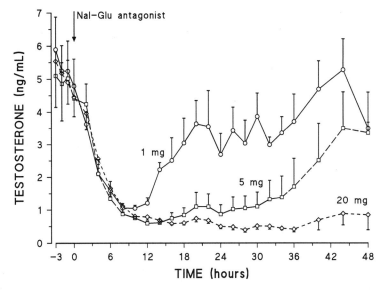

FIGURE 18.1. Mean (±SEM) serum testosterone levels in five normal men who were given 1, 5, and 20 mg Nal-Glu sc at time zero (arrow).

at the Salk Institute, and relatively free of side effects (48, 58), has permitted us to study the pharmacology of GnRH antagonists in men and evaluate their antigonadal and antispermatogenic properties.

Clinical Pharmacology

In the first studies the Nal-Glu antagonist, [Ac-D2Nal[1], 4ClDPhe[2], D3Pal[3], Arg[5], DGlu[6] (AA), DAla[10]]GnRH, was given as single doses to normal men, and immunoreactive FSH, LH, and bioactive LH decreased significantly after all doses of the antagonist. Testosterone levels, shown in Figure 18.1, decreased with the same rate after all doses of Nal-Glu, reaching nadirs of 78.5 ± 4.0%, 86.8 ± 2.6%, and 90.9 ± 2.8% after the 1-, 5-, and 20-mg doses, respectively. The duration of T suppression rather than the nadir reached was dose-dependent. Estradiol levels also decreased from mean baseline levels of 17.6 ± 2.0 pg/mL to a nadir of 4.2 ± 1.4 pg/mL 36 h after Nal-Glu administration. Serum FSH decreased by 28.9 ± 5.4%, 38.2 ± 7.9%, and 44.5 ± 3.6%, while IR-LH decreased by 39 ± 13.8%, 53.2 ± 10%, and 53.1 ± 14.4% after the 1-, 5-, and 20-mg doses, respectively. Bioactive LH levels, shown in Figure 18.2, decreased significantly after the 20-mg dose and reached a nadir of only 12.2% of baseline 16 h after Nal-Glu administration. The B/I ratio of LH (Fig. 18.2) decreased from 0.93 ± 0.026 during baseline to a nadir of 0.2 ± 0.02 at 16 h, where it remained for at least 36 h.

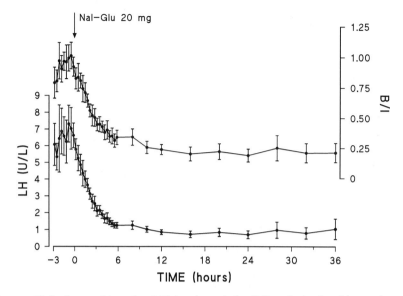

FIGURE 18.2. Serum bioactive LH levels and the B/I ratio in 5 subjects given a 20-mg Nal-Glu dose.

In order to determine the mechanism of suppression of gonadotropin secretion, we studied the effects of a single dose of the antagonist on the pulsatile activity of serum bio-LH, IR-LH, alpha subunit, and testosterone for 24 h in normal men (46). Following administration of 5 mg of the Nal-Glu antagonist (Fig. 18.3), IR-LH levels decreased (P < 0.001) from 2.81 ± 0.06 at baseline to a nadir of 0.75 ± 0.02 U/L. Bio-LH levels followed the same pattern, decreasing by 89% (P < 0.001) from 4.54 ± 0.13 to a nadir of 0.51 ± 0.13 U/L, 6.8 h after injection of Nal-Glu. In contrast, serum α-subunit levels did not change (P > 0.05) during the 14-h period after antagonist administration—being 0.85 ± 0.01 and 0.75 ± 0.01 μg/L before and after Nal-Glu, respectively. Serum testosterone levels decreased by more than 80%, from 17.6 ± 0.2 at baseline to a mean nadir of 3.3 ± 0.7 nmol/L, 12.8 h after Nal-Glu administration. Pulse frequency and the number of significant pulses remained the same for all the measured hormones during the 10-h baseline period and the 14 h following Nal-Glu administration. In contrast, pulse amplitude of IR-LH, bio-LH, and testosterone decreased significantly after injection of the antagonist. Pulse amplitude of the α-subunit also declined, albeit not significantly. Coincidence analysis revealed that both during the 10-h baseline and the 14-h post-Nal-Glu period there was a highly significant nonrandom synchrony between peaks of IR-LH, bio-LH, α-subunit, and testosterone. These results suggested that coordinate pulsatile secretion of IR-LH, bio-LH, and testosterone persists following administration of

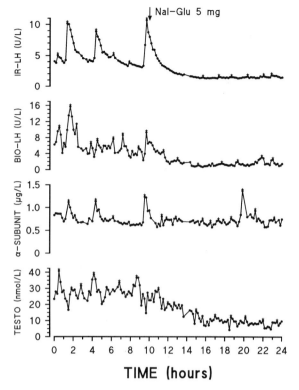

FIGURE 18.3. Serum IR-LH, bio-LH, α-subunit, and testosterone levels in one subject given a 5-mg Nal-Glu dose at 10 h (arrow). The stars denote significant pulses.

5 mg Nal-Glu LHRH antagonist. The decrease in LH and testosterone seems to result from the suppression of pulse amplitude rather than pulse frequency of these hormones.

We then postulated that a 5-mg dose of Nal-Glu given daily should result in sustained gonadal suppression, since that dose had been shown to suppress serum testosterone levels for more than 24 h. We administered 5 mg Nal-Glu daily for 3 weeks to normal men, and—contrary to expectation—serum testosterone levels were not consistently suppressed (48). After initial suppression (Fig. 18.4), serum testosterone increased between days 2 and 8, though not to baseline values, and then progressively declined to the castrate range toward the end of the study period. This fluctuating suppression of serum testosterone was similar to that we had previously found using a less potent LHRH antagonist, given to normal men for 7 days (54). When a 5-mg dose of Nal-Glu was administered twice daily, LH and testosterone levels decreased promptly after the first Nal-Glu dose and remained suppressed throughout the

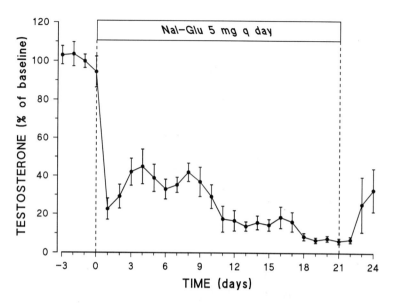

FIGURE 18.4. Mean (±SEM) serum testosterone, expressed as percentages of mean baseline levels, in seven normal men given 5 mg Nal-Glu sc daily for 21 days.

study period. In contrast, serum free α-subunit decreased slowly to only 50% of baseline levels on day 8 (59).

Meanwhile, newer antagonists, free of histamine-like adverse reactions, are being developed, such as that recently synthesized at Syntex Research by Drs. J. Nestor and B. Vickery (60). Twenty-two men were given increasing doses, from 0.03 to 12 mg, of the RS-26306 GnRH antagonist, [Ac-D2Nal[1],DpClPhe[2],D3Pal[3],DhArg(Et$_2$)[6],LhArg(Et$_2$)[8], DAla[10]]GnRH, by a single sc injection, as shown in Figure 18.5. Furthermore, groups of 4 men received 1-, 3-, 6-, and 12-mg doses. Serum FSH, LH, and testosterone levels were measured before administration, at frequent intervals for 48 h, and at 72 h and 168 h after administration of the antagonist. Mean serum FSH levels decreased by 30 ± 3.5%, 50 ± 11%, 39 ± 4.7%, and 55 ± 2.3% after the doses of 1, 3, 6, and 12 mg, respectively. LH levels decreased faster than those of FSH, by 80 ± 4.7%, 89 ± 2.8%, 86 ± 4.6%, and 91 ± 2.7% after the same doses, respectively. Testosterone levels followed those of LH and decreased by 71 ± 3.2%, 81 ± 8.6%, 89 ± 5%, and 90 ± 3.1% after the same doses, respectively. FSH levels remained significantly suppressed ($P < 0.05$) for 8 h (from 12 h to 20 h post antagonist administration) after the 1-mg dose, 40 h (8 to 48 h) after the 3-mg dose, 32 h (16 to 48 h) after the 6-mg dose, and 36 h (12 to 48 h) after the 12-mg dose. LH levels remained suppressed for 26 h (2 to 28 h) after the 1-mg dose, and for at least 47 h (1 to 48 h)

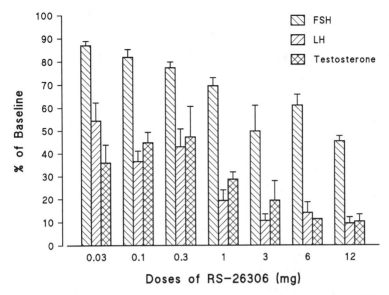

FIGURE 18.5. Maximum decrease (mean ± SEM) of serum FSH, LH, and testosterone, expressed as percentages of mean baseline levels, in normal men given increasing doses of RS-26306.

after the doses of 3, 6, and 12 mg; frequent sampling ended at 48 h. Testosterone levels were suppressed for 24 h (4 to 28 h) after the 1-mg dose, and for at least 44 h (4 to 48 h) after the doses of 3, 6, and 12 mg. No side effects were associated with the administration of this GnRH antagonist, other than occasional minimal erythema at the injection site. These results indicated that RS-26306 is a safe and potent GnRH antagonist and that the properties of this new antagonist could be of high clinical utility for suppression of gonadal function.

Development of a Male Contraceptive

The antispermatogenic effects of combined GnRH antagonist and testosterone administration in men were evaluated in a protocol simulating a prototype of a likely male contraceptive regimen. Nal-Glu was given daily (10 mg, sc) for 20 weeks to 8 normal men and a low dose of testosterone enanthate (25 mg, IM) every week. Results on sperm density and serum FSH and LH levels are shown in Figure 18.6. Sperm counts started declining on week 4 and complete azoospermia was reached within 6 to 12 weeks in 6 of the 8 subjects. Subjects 7 and 8, whose sperm counts and serum gonadotropin levels were not suppressed

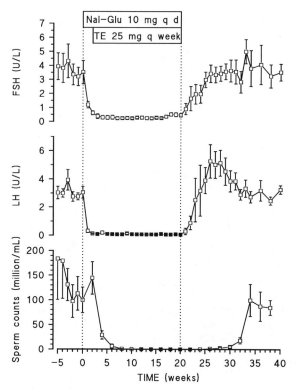

FIGURE 18.6. Mean (±SEM) FSH, LH, and sperm density in six men who received 10 mg Nal-Glu and TE for 20 weeks. Closed symbols denote complete absence of sperm in the ejaculate·of all 6 men or LH values below the 0.1 U/L assay detectability limits.

after 10 weeks, were given 20 mg Nal-Glu starting week 10. One became azoospermic on week 16, while the other's total sperm counts continued declining and reached a nadir of 1.4 million on week 20. Sperm motility and viability in this subject were completely suppressed after week 14. Sperm counts returned to baseline levels 12–14 weeks after the end of Nal-Glu administration. Mean serum LH levels of the first 6 subjects decreased from 3 ± 0.3 U/L at baseline to less than 0.1 U/L until week 20, and then levels returned to baseline. FSH levels similarly decreased from a combined mean of 3.6 ± 0.9 U/L at baseline to below 0.3 U/L after 4 weeks of Nal-Glu administration. Serum mean testosterone levels between weekly injections of TE ranged from 27.4 ± 5.9 to 4.8 ± 1.4 nmol/L, but remained in the hypogonadal range, below 10 nmol/L, for 4 of the 7 days. None of the subjects, however, complained of decreased libido or potency as assessed by a questionnaire. No systemic or significant local side effects were observed other than a minimal reaction at the injection site. These data suggest that complete sustained azoospermia can be achieved in man, without loss of libido, by chronic administration of a GnRH antagonist plus testosterone.

Conclusions

Recent development of potent GnRH antagonists, free of anaphylactoid reactions, has permitted short- and long-term studies to elucidate the clinical pharmacology of these antireproductive agents in man. Larger studies should allow us to determine whether GnRH antagonists will change reproductive medicine to the extent that agonists did a few years ago.

References

1. Conn PM, Crowley WF Jr. Gonadotropin-releasing hormone and its analogues. N Engl J Med 1991;324:93–103.
2. Conn PM, Huckle WR, Andrews WV, McArdle CA. The molecular mechanism of action of gonadotropin releasing hormone (GnRH) in the pituitary. Recent Prog Horm Res 1987;43:29–68.
3. Clayton RN. Mechanism of GnRH action in gonadotrophs. Hum Reprod 1988;3:479–83.
4. Negro Vilar A, Valenca MM, Culler MD. Transmembrane signals and intracellular messengers mediating LHRH and LH secretion. Adv Exp Med Biol 1987;219:85–108.
5. Pfaff DW, Jorgenson K, Kow LM. Luteinizing hormone-releasing hormone in rat brain: gene expression, role as neuromodulator, and functional effects. Ann NY Acad Sci 1987;519:323–33.
6. Seeburg PH, Mason AJ, Stewart TA, Nikolics K. The mammalian GnRH gene and its pivotal role in reproduction. Recent Prog Horm Res 1987;43:69–98.
7. Veldhuis JD. Contemporary insights into the regulation of luteinizing hormone secretion in man. Horm Res 1987;28:126–38.
8. Conn PM, Hsueh AJ, Crowley WF. Gonadotropin-releasing hormone: molecular and cell biology, physiology, and clinical applications. Fed Proc 1984;43:2351–61.
9. Sandow J. The regulation of LHRH action at the pituitary and gonadal receptor level: a review. Psychoneuroendocrinology 1983;8:277–97.
10. Santen RJ, Bourguignon JP. Gonadotropin-releasing hormone: physiological and therapeutic aspects, agonists and antagonists. Horm Res 1987;28:88–103.
11. Karten MJ, Rivier JE. Gonadotropin-releasing hormone analog design: structure-function studies toward the development of agonists and antagonists: rationale and perspective. Endocr Rev 1986;7:44–66.
12. Rabin D, McNeil LW. Pituitary and gonadal desensitization after continuous luteinizing hormone-releasing hormone infusion in normal females. J Clin Endocrinol Metab 1980;51:873–6.

13. McLachlan RI, Healy DL, Burger HG. Clinical aspects of LHRH analogues in gynaecology: a review. Br J Obstet Gynaecol 1986;93:431–54.

14. Shaw RW. LHRH analogues in the treatment of endometriosis—comparative results with other treatments. Baillieres Clin Obstet Gynaecol 1988;2:659–75.

15. Hoffman PG, Henzl MR, Chaplin MD, Nerenberg CA. Clinical development of nafarelin acetate: phase I and phase II studies. J Androl 1987;8:S17–S22.

16. Henzl MR. Gonadotropin-releasing hormone (GnRH) agonists in the management of endometriosis: a review. Clin Obstet Gynecol 1988;31: 840–56.

17. Boepple PA, Mansfield MJ, Wierman ME, et al. Use of a potent, long acting agonist of gonadotropin-releasing hormone in the treatment of precocious puberty. Endocr Rev 1986;7:24–33.

18. Linde R, Doelle GC, Alexander N, et al. Reversible inhibition of testicular steroidogenesis and spermatogenesis by a potent gonadotropin-releasing hormone agonist in normal men: an approach toward the development of a male contraceptive. N Engl J Med 1981;305:663–7.

19. Rabin D, Evans RM, Alexander AN, et al. Heterogeneity of sperm density profiles following 20-week therapy with high-dose LHRH analog plus testosterone. J Androl 1984;5:176–80.

20. Doelle GC, Alexander AN, Evans RM, et al. Combined treatment with an LHRH agonist and testosterone in man: reversible oligozoospermia without impotence. J Androl 1983;4:298–302.

21. Corbin A, Bex FJ, Jones RC. LHRH and analogs: contraceptive and therapeutic considerations. Int J Fertil 1985;30:57–65.

22. Sundaram K. Use of LHRH agonists and antagonists in male contraception: a review. Contraception 1984;29:163–70.

23. Swerdloff RS, Handelsman DJ, Bhasin S. Hormonal effects of GnRH agonist in the human male: an approach to male contraception using combined androgen and GnRH agonist treatment. J Steroid Biochem 1985;23:855–61.

24. Bhasin S, Heber D, Steiner BS, Handelsman DJ, Swerdloff RS. Hormonal effects of gonadotropin-releasing hormone (GnRH) agonist in the human male: III. Effects of long term combined treatment with GnRH agonist and androgen. J Clin Endocrinol Metab 1985;60:998–1003.

25. Monroe SE, Blumenfeld Z, Andreyko JL, Schriock E, Henzl MR, Jaffe RB. Dose-dependent inhibition of pituitary-ovarian function during administration of a gonadotropin-releasing hormone agonistic analog (nafarelin). J Clin Endocrinol Metab 1986;63:1334–41.

26. Vickery BH. Comparisons of the potential utility of LHRH agonists and antagonists for fertility control. J Steroid Biochem 1985;23:779–91.

27. Fraser HM, Baird DT. Clinical applications of LHRH analogues. Baillieres Clin Endocrinol Metab 1987;1:43–70.

28. Folkers K, Bowers C, Xiao SB, Tang PF, Kubota M. Increased potency of antagonists of the luteinizing hormone releasing hormone which have D-3-Pal in position 6. Biochem Biophys Res Commun 1986;137:709–15.

29. Doelle G, Linde R, Alexander N, et al. Intermittent long-term administration of a potent gonadotropin-releasing hormone agonist in normal men. Int J Fertil 1982;27:234–7.

30. Schurmeyer T, Knuth UA, Freischem CW, Sandow J, Akhtar FB, Nieschlag E. Suppression of pituitary and testicular function in normal men by constant

gonadotropin-releasing hormone agonist infusion. J Clin Endocrinol Metab 1984;59:19–24.

31. Pavlou SN, Interlandi JW, Wakefield G, Rivier J, Vale W, Rabin D. Heterogeneity of sperm density profiles following 16-week therapy with continuous infusion of high-dose LHRH analog plus testosterone. J Androl 1986;7:228–33.

32. Bouchard P, Garcia E. Influence of testosterone substitution on sperm suppression by LHRH agonists. Horm Res 1987;28:175–80.

33. Swerdloff RS, Steiner BS, Bhasin S. Gonadotropin releasing hormone (GnRH) agonists in male contraception. Med Biol 1986;63:218–24.

34. Pavlou SN, Dahl KD, Wakefield G, et al. Maintenance of the ratio of bioactive to immunoreactive follicle-stimulating hormone in normal men during chronic luteinizing hormone-releasing hormone agonist administration. J Clin Endocrinol Metab 1988;66:1005–9.

35. Santen RJ, Demers LM, Max DT, Smith J, Stein BS, Glode LM. Long term effects of administration of a gonadotropin-releasing hormone superagonist in men with prostatic carcinoma. J Clin Endocrinol Metab 1984;58:397–400.

36. Rivier C, Vale W, Rivier J. Effects of gonadotropin releasing hormone agonists and antagonists on reproductive functions. J Med Chem 1983;26:1545–50.

37. Rivier C, Rivier J, Perrin M, Vale W. Comparison of the effect of several gonadotropin releasing hormone antagonists on luteinizing hormone secretion, receptor binding and ovulation. Biol Reprod 1983;29:374–8.

38. Perrin MH, Haas Y, Rivier JE, Vale WW. Gonadotropin-releasing hormone binding to rat anterior pituitary membrane homogenates: comparison of antagonists and agonists using radiolabeled antagonist and agonist. Mol Pharmacol 1983;23:44–51.

39. Jennes L, Stumpf WE, Conn PM. Receptor-mediated binding and uptake of GnRH agonist and antagonist by pituitary cells. Peptides 1984;5(suppl 1):215–20.

40. Wierman ME, Rivier JE, Wang C. Gonadotropin-releasing hormone-dependent regulation of gonadotropin subunit messenger ribonucleic acid levels in the rat. Endorcrinology 1989;124:272–8.

41. Dahl KD, Pavlou SN, Kovacs WJ, Hsueh AJ. The changing ratio of serum bioactive to immunoreactive follicle-stimulating hormone in normal men following treatment with a potent gonadotropin releasing hormone antagonist. J Clin Endocrinol Metab 1986;63:792–4.

42. Dahl KD, Bicsak TA, Hsueh AJ. Naturally occurring antihormones: secretion of FSH antagonists by women treated with a GnRH analog. Science 1988;239:72–4.

43. Hsueh AJ, Bicsak TA, Jia XC, et al. Granulosa cells as hormone targets: the role of biologically active follicle-stimulating hormone in reproduction. Recent Prog Horm Res 1989;45:209–73; discussion.

44. Pavlou SN, Debold CR, Island DP, et al. Single subcutaneous doses of a luteinizing hormone-releasing hormone antagonist suppress serum gonadotropin and testosterone levels in normal men [published erratum appears in J Clin Endocrinol Metab 1986 Oct;63:940]. J Clin Endocrinol Metab 1986;63:303–8.

45. Urban RJ, Pavlou SN, Rivier JE, Vale WW, Dufau ML, Veldhuis JD. Suppressive actions of a gonadotropin-releasing hormone antagonist on luteinizing hormone, follicle-stimulating hormone, and prolactin release in estrogen-deficient postmenopausal women. Am J Obstet Gynecol 1990;162: 1255–60.

46. Pavlou SN, Veldhuis JD, Lindner J, et al. Persistence of concordant luteinizing hormone (LH), testosterone, and alpha-subunit pulses after LH-releasing hormone antagonist administration in normal men. J Clin Endocrinol Metab 1990;70:1472–8.

47. Pavlou SN, Wakefield GB, Island DP, et al. Suppression of pituitary-gonadal function by a potent new luteinizing hormone-releasing hormone antagonist in normal men. J Clin Endocrinol Metab 1987;64:931–6.

48. Pavlou SN, Wakefield G, Schlechter NL, et al. Mode of suppression of pituitary and gonadal function after acute or prolonged administration of a luteinizing hormone-releasing hormone antagonist in normal men. J Clin Endocrinol Metab 1989;68:446–54.

49. Jockenhovel F, Bhasin S, Steiner BS, Rivier JE, Vale WW, Swerdloff RS. Hormonal effects of single gonadotropin-releasing hormone antagonist doses in men. J Clin Endocrinol Metab 1988;66:1065–70.

50. Bagatell CJ, McLachlan RI, de Kretser DM, et al. A comparison of the suppressive effects of testosterone and a potent new gonadotropin-releasing hormone antagonist on gonadotropin and inhibin levels in normal men. J Clin Endocrinol Metab 1989;69:43–8.

51. Hall JE, Brodie TD, Badger TM, et al. Evidence of differential control of FSH and LH secretion by gonadotropin-releasing hormone (GnRH) from the use of a GnRH antagonist. J Clin Endocrinol Metab 1988;67:524–31.

52. Mortola JF, Sathanandan M, Pavlou S, et al. Suppression of bioactive and immunoreactive follicle-stimulating hormone and luteinizing hormone levels by a potent gonadotropin-releasing hormone antagonist: pharmacodynamic studies. Fertil Steril 1989;51:957–63.

53. Daneshdoost L, Pavlou SN, Molitch ME, et al. Inhibition of follicle-stimulating hormone secretion from gonadotroph adenomas by repetitive administration of a gonadotropin-releasing hormone antagonist. J Clin Endocrinol Metab 1990;71:92–7.

54. Pavlou SN, Interlandi JW, Wakefield G, et al. Gonadotropins and testosterone escape from suppression during prolonged luteinizing hormone-releasing hormone antagonist administration in normal men. J Clin Endocrinol Metab 1987;64:1070–4.

55. Schmidt F, Sundaram K, Thau RB, Bardin CW. [Ac-D-NAL(2)1, 4FD-Phe2, D-Trp3, D-Arg6]-LHRH, a potent antagonist of LHRH, produces transient edema and behavioral changes in rats. Contraception 1984;29:283–9.

56. Hahn DW, McGuire JL, Vale WW, Rivier J. Reproductive/endocrine and anaphylactoid properties of an LHRH-antagonist, ORF 18260 [Ac-DNAL1(2), 4FDPhe2, D-Trp3, D-Arg6]-GnRH. Life Sci 1985;37:505–14.

57. Sundaram K, Didolkar A, Thau R, Chaudhuri M, Schmidt F. Antagonists of luteinizing hormone releasing hormone bind to rat mast cells and induce histamine release. Agents Actions 1988;25:307–13.

58. Rivier JE, Porter J, Rivier CL, et al. New effective gonadotropin releasing hormone antagonists with minimal potency for histamine release in vitro. J Med Chem 1986;29:1846–51.

59. Lindner J, Rivier JE, Vale WW, Pavlou SN. Regulation of pituitary glycoprotein alpha-subunit secretion after administration of a luteinizing hormone-releasing hormone antagonist in normal men. J Clin Endocrinol Metab 1990;70:1219–24.
60. Nestor JJ Jr, Tahilramani R, Ho TL, McRae GI, Vickery BH. Potent, long-acting luteinizing hormone-releasing hormone antagonists containing new synthetic amino acids: N,N'-dialkyl-D-homoarginines. J Med Chem 1988; 31:65–72.

19

Use of GnRH Antagonists as Physiologic Probes in the Female*

JANET E. HALL AND WILLIAM F. CROWLEY, JR.

The development of GnRH antagonists has provided investigators studying reproductive hormones with unique opportunities that have not been available for the study of other hormonal systems. Although GnRH antagonists have been used to advantage in basic studies and in animal models, they are particularly important tools for clinical investigation because of the relatively restricted number of models with which basic physiologic and pathophysiologic questions can be addressed in the human and the additional opportunities that GnRH antagonists have afforded.

The strength of the antagonists lies in two areas. The first is that, unlike GnRH agonists for example, their mechanism of action is definable. GnRH antagonists are competitive receptor blockers that bind to a single receptor type (1, 2). The second is that, unlike PTH antagonists for example, the potency achieved is now adequate for clinical studies. However, the GnRH antagonists do not bind to the GnRH receptor in a manner absolutely identical to that of GnRH, as evidenced by different dissociation constants than for GnRH (1). In addition, their chemistry is complex (3) and a propensity to histamine release has been an ongoing issue in the development of this series of compounds (3, 4).

We have used GnRH antagonists as physiologic probes in the human to provide insights at the hypothalamic, pituitary, and ovarian levels in women under various physiologic and pathophysiologic circumstances (4–9). All of the studies discussed herein are in women of reproductive age, and the Nal-Glu GnRH antagonist ([Ac-D2Nal^1,D4ClPhe^2,D3Pal^3, Arg^5,DGlu(AA)^6,DAla^{10}]-GnRH) has been used in all of the work reviewed in this chapter. The data presented are from radioimmunoassays previously described (10–12). The LH assay is a β-directed polyclonal assay with a sensitivity of 0.8 IU/L, the FSH assay is a polyclonal assay

* This work was supported by Grants HD-15080, HD-3-2837, and RR-1066 from the NIH.

directed to the intact molecule, also with a sensitivity of 0.8 IU/L, and the assay for free α-subunit (FAS) is a monoclonal assay with virtually no crossreactivity with intact LH, FSH, or TSH and with an assay sensitivity of 30 ng/L.

Differential Control of LH, FSH, and FAS Secretion by GnRH

To examine the degree to which GnRH controls pituitary secretion of LH, FSH, and FAS in normal women (5), studies were performed in euthyroid women in the early follicular phase (EFP). This cycle phase was chosen for this series of investigations because the EFP is the time in the normal menstrual cycle in which gonadal feedback effects are at a nadir. Thus, evaluation of the effects of GnRH receptor blockade on secretion of the gonadotropins and FAS will be relatively unimpeded by direct pituitary feedback and will more directly reflect the effect of GnRH on their secretion.

Blood was sampled at 10-min intervals to assess pulsatility for 4 h before and 8 h following administration of a single dose of the Nal-Glu GnRH antagonist and hourly thereafter for a further 16 h to assess the duration of the antagonist effect. Two additional samples were drawn, at 48 and 72 h after antagonist administration. The antagonist was administered subcutaneously at doses of 15 (n = 6), 50 (n = 5), and 150 μg/kg (n = 6). Mean data were used to assess the overall pattern of response to the antagonist and the duration of its effect. To assess the maximum amount of suppression at each dose, the nadir was calculated using a moving average, and the difference between the mean baseline and the nadir was expressed as a percentage of the baseline value for each study (Fig. 19.1). This allowed comparisons to be made of the response to GnRH receptor blockade between the three hormones measured.

LH decreased promptly in response to the GnRH antagonist at all doses. The duration of the effect of this antagonist was clearly dose-related, with recovery to baseline by 24 h following administration of the 15 μg/kg dose, but not until 72 h following the 150 μg/kg dose. Concordance of pulses of FAS and LH was demonstrated in the baseline sampling portions of the study and, as with LH, FAS levels decreased promptly with anatagonist administration. As with LH, administration of the highest dose of the antagonist resulted in abolition of pulsatile secretion of FAS (Fig. 19.1). FSH responses to the antagonist were less acute, in keeping with the relatively longer half-life of this hormone in comparison with LH and FAS. However, a nadir was clearly reached within the timeframe of this study protocol, and recovery to baseline was demonstrated. Expression of the data as percentages of inhibition permits separation of the maximal amount of suppression from the duration of suppression. Construction of a dose-response curve then permits com-

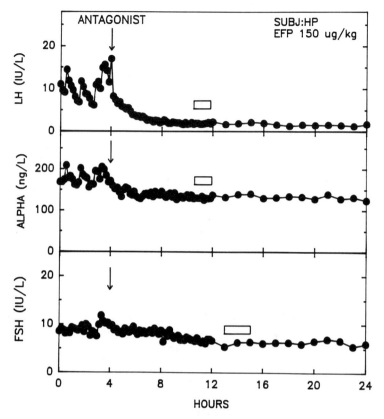

FIGURE 19.1. Response of LH, FAS, and FSH to a single subcutaneous injection of 150 μg/kg of the Nal-Glu GnRH antagonist given at 4 h in a representative subject studied in the EFP. The boxes indicate the nadir as determined by a moving average for LH (6 points), FAS (6 points), and FSH (3 points), which was then used to calculate the percentages of inhibition for each hormone.

parisons to be made of the responses of all three hormones to GnRH receptor blockade (Fig. 19.2). Viewed in this way, the difference in the responses of the three hormones is striking, with a maximum inhibition of 80% for LH, 40% for FSH, and 28% for FAS. For LH, this is very close to the maximum percentage of inhibition possible given the assay sensitivity, but it is considerably less so for FSH and FAS. For all three hormones, the response is not different between the two higher doses. From this flattening of the dose-response curve it can be assumed that the maximum inhibition possible has been achieved for this antagonist in short-term studies.

LH is suppressed 80–90% in women in the EFP in response to GnRH receptor blockade, in keeping with the fact that GnRH is the only known secretagogue for LH. The relatively modest decrease in FAS in response

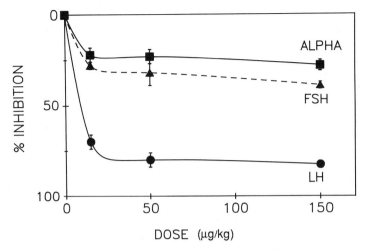

FIGURE 19.2. Percentages of inhibition of LH, FSH, and FAS in response to increasing doses of the Nal-Glu GnRH antagonist. Modified with permission from Ref. 5. © by The Endocrine Society, 1990.

to GnRH receptor blockade is compatible with the known second releasing factor for this glycoprotein hormone subunit—i.e., TRH (13–15). However, the abolition of pulsatile FAS secretion in conjunction with the abolition of LH pulses by the GnRH antagonist provides important information in support of the hypothesis that FAS can be used as a marker of GnRH secretion in the human (5, 15). FSH, like FAS, is incompletely suppressed in response to GnRH receptor blockade, providing support for the presence of other biologically important releasing factors for FSH secretion, such as activin (16) or the putative FSH releasing factor (17), and a model for their investigation in the human. Studies from other investigators have indicated that bioactive FSH, as measured in one of the available bioassays, is suppressed to a somewhat greater degree than is immunoactive FSH in response to GnRH antagonism (18). Although the maximal amount of FSH suppression is still far from complete when assessed by bioassay, this potential effect will need to be considered in further studies of the control of FSH secretion.

Estimation of the Quantity of GnRH Secreted in the Human

While direct assessment of the amount of GnRH is possible in animal studies (19–22), indirect approaches are required in the human. We have proposed that GnRH antagonists can be used to provide an estimate of the overall amount of GnRH secreted under various physiologic and pathophysiologic circumstances in the human (7) in much the same way as naloxone has been utilized to understand the opioid system (23, 24). The general principle that underlies this indirect approach is that the relative amount of an unmeasurable endogenous ligand can be estimated by the susceptibility of a marker of its action to inhibition by a competitive antagonist. In the presence of a constant amount of endogenous ligand, a dose-response curve can be generated for a given antagonist, while a constant submaximal dose of antagonist will produce an effect that is inversely proportional to the amount of endogenous ligand present. Thus, using LH as a marker of GnRH, the overall amount of endogenous GnRH present will be proportional to the degree of inhibition of LH in response to a submaximal dose of a GnRH antagonist. In order to use these concepts, a number of assumptions are made and the data evaluated taking into consideration the degree to which these assumptions may be valid in a given circumstance. The endogenous ligand should be the only secretagogue for the marker of its action, and points need to be established on the linear portion of the dose-response curve, as indicated above. In addition, the affinity and number of GnRH receptors should remain constant, as should postreceptor influences on the response of LH secretion to GnRH. Animal studies have failed to show changes in GnRH receptor affinity over a broad range of conditions (1). However, possible changes in receptor number comparable to those demonstrated during the estrus cycle in the rat (25), as well as potential postreceptor influences on LH in response to GnRH at different times in the cycle, need to be considered in interpretation of the data.

To test the hypothesis that the amount of GnRH secreted changes at different times in the menstrual cycle, studies in the EFP described above were used as the point of reference. Additional studies were performed in the late follicular phase (LFP) in the presence of elevated estradiol (E_2) concentrations, in the early luteal phase (ELP) in the presence of elevated levels of both E_2 and P (7), and at midcycle (MCS; 8). Studies at the MCS are distinguished from the LFP studies by the presence of LH levels greater than 2 SD above the LFP mean (26) and a P level less than 6.4 nmol/L.

Baseline values confirmed the expected differences in E_2 and P between the cycle phases. Results indicated a remarkable degree of precision in the LH response to GnRH receptor blockade. The decrease in LH in response to GnRH receptor blockade was virtually identical in the LFP and ELP in comparison with the EFP "standard" when expressed as a percentage of baseline (7). This was true at the submaximal 15 μg/kg dose as well as at the doses that produced the maximum amount of LH inhibition. In preliminary studies at the MCS, there was no difference in the maximal degree of suppression at the two higher doses, but there was a greater degree of suppression at the 15 μg/kg dose (Fig. 19.3) in

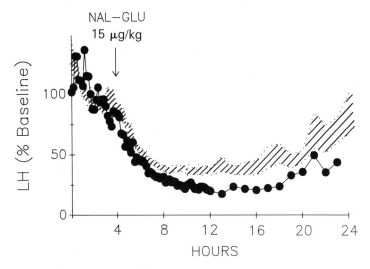

FIGURE 19.3. LH results expressed as percentages of baseline in an individual subject (filled circles) studied at the midcycle using a 15 µg/kg dose of the Nal-Glu GnRH antagonist in comparison with studies in the EFP (±SEM, hatched area). The arrow indicates the time of antagonist administration.

comparison with the EFP (8). These studies suggest that despite the changing frequency of GnRH secretion between the EFP, LFP, and ELP in the normal human menstrual cycle (26), the overall amount of GnRH secreted at these times does not change. However, in contrast to the elevated levels of GnRH in the sheep at the midcycle (22), the overall amount of GnRH secreted in women at the midcycle may not be increased in comparison with other cycle phases. Although the validity of the assumptions underlying this indirect approach must be considered, increases in receptor number and/or augmentation of LH secretion in response to GnRH mediated at a postreceptor level at the time of the surge would both tend to make it more difficult to suppress LH. Therefore, it is unlikely that alterations in either of these factors at the midcycle are responsible for the results observed.

Ovarian Dependence on Gonadotropin Support

The absolute requirement of the developing follicle and corpus luteum for GnRH-induced gonatotropin stimulation is undisputed. However, evidence from primate studies suggests that the dependence of the ovary on gonadotropin support varies as a function of developmental changes within the ovary during the process of folliculogenesis and corpus luteum function (27–29). This hypothesis was investigated in normal women by imposing a 72-h GnRH receptor blockade achieved by administration of 150 μg/kg sc of the Nal-Glu GnRH antagonist for 3 consecutive days (6). For each subject, results were compared with a vehicle control cycle. Studies were performed in the midfollicular phase (MFP), the late follicular phase, or the midluteal phase (MLP).

In studies in the MFP (Fig. 19.4, top), the initial day of antagonist administration was between 5 and 9 days from the onset of menses. Follicular size was 11 ± 2 mm and mean estradiol was 220 ± 40 pmol/L on the first day of antagonist treatment. Antagonist administration resulted in a 76% decrease in LH and a 21% decrease in FSH (not statistically significant). E_2 was suppressed to the limit of assay detection and did not return to the pre-antagonist level for 6 days following the final injection, despite a return of gonadotropin levels within 48 h. Total cycle length was prolonged in the antagonist cycles, entirely because of an increase in follicular phase length. The interval between the final day of antagonist administration and ovulation was 15.1 ± 1 days, and was not different from the follicular phase length in the control cycle. The subsequent preovulatory E_2 peak, the luteal phase length, and the luteal phase progesterone levels were not different from those of the control cycles.

In the LFP studies (Fig. 19.4, middle), antagonist administration was initiated between 3 and 5 days from anticipated ovulation as predicted by serial ultrasound. In this group of studies, follicular size was 16 ± 1 mm ($P < 0.05$ vs. MFP) and the estradiol level was 394 ± 95 pmol/L ($P < 0.05$ vs. MFP) on the first day of antagonist administration. Both LH and FSH were significantly decreased in response to the antagonist in this cycle phase. The decrease in E_2 was more variable than in the MFP group, and E_2 levels returned to pre-antagonist levels within 3 days of the final antagonist injection, just 24 h following the return of LH and FSH to pretreatment levels. Total cycle length was prolonged as a result of an increase in follicular phase length. The interval from the final day of antagonist administration until ovulation was 8.0 ± 1.5 days, significantly less than the control follicular phase length ($P < 0.001$) and also less than this interval in the MFP studies ($P < 0.001$). The subsequent preovulatory E_2 peak, the luteal phase length, and the peak luteal phase progesterone were not different than in the control cycle. When the MFP and LFP studies were combined (Fig. 19.5), the interval from the last antagonist injection until ovulation was inversely correlated with the E_2 level on the first day of antagonist administration ($R = 0.57$; $P < 0.05$).

In the MLP studies (Fig. 19.4, bottom), a corpus luteum was present on ultrasound in all subjects and the Nal-Glu GnRH antagonist was administered on day 4 or 5 from ovulation. Decreases in LH and FSH were accompanied by a prompt decrease in E_2 and P to the limit of sensitivity of the assay. Menstrual bleeding occured within 24 to 48 h of the final day of antagonist administration in all subjects. The total length of the follow-up cycle was slightly longer than the control cycle ($P <$

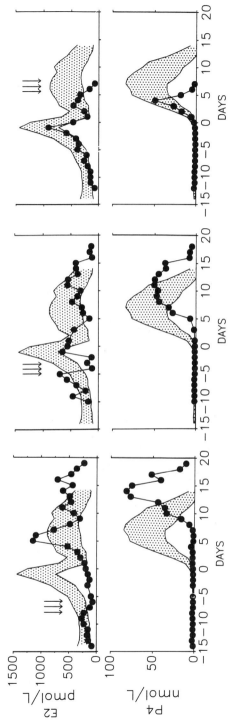

FIGURE 19.4. E_2 and P determinations in representative subjects who received 150 µg/kg of the Nal-Glu GnRH antagonist in the MFP (top), LFP (middle) and the MLP (bottom) graphed in relation to the range (± 1SD) determined from 81 normal cycles. The subject results in the MFP and the LFP are centered to the day of ovulation in the vehicle control cycle, while in the MLP results are centered to the day of ovulation in the antagonist cycle. Reprinted with permission from Ref. 6. © by The Endocrine Society, 1991.

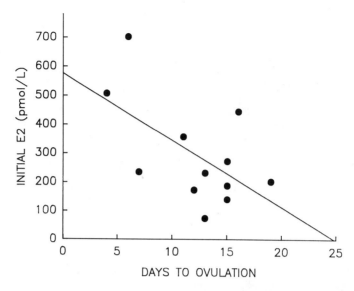

FIGURE 19.5. The relationship of the interval from the day of the final antagonist injection until ovulation to the E_2 level on the initial day of antagonist administration in the subjects studied in the MFP and LFP.

0.05); however, daily hormonal analysis was not available to determine the dynamics of the follow-up cycles, although all were ovulatory.

These studies suggest that this degree of gonadotropin deprivation in the MFP results in demise of the initial dominant follicle and reinitiation of folliculogenesis, while in the LFP the follicle is more resistant and ovulation is delayed from the existing dominant follicle. The relationship of the interval to ovulation with the preexisting E_2 level suggests a continuum of tolerance of the follicle to gonadotropin withdrawal that is dependent on the functional capacity of the developing follicle. In the MLP, the degree of GnRH receptor blockade achieved in these studies resulted in prompt luteolysis. Previous studies have demonstrated variable results with a single injection of a GnRH antagonist (29), but complete luteolysis with a longer duration or more complete suppression of gonadotropins (30, 31), as seen in these studies.

Conclusions

As physiologic probes, GnRH antagonists can provide insights at all levels of the hyothalamic-pituitary-gonadal axis. At the pituitary level, acute responses to maximal GnRH receptor blockade provide a relative quantitation of the contribution of GnRH to secretion of LH, FSH, and free α-subunit, and emphasize the differential effects of GnRH on the secretory control of these three hormones. Evidence from these studies and others confirms the overwhelming importance of GnRH in the control of LH secretion. Because of these observations, the response of LH to a submaximal GnRH antagonist dose can then be used to provide an indirect estimate of the amount of endogenous GnRH secreted by the hypothalamus in the human. At the ovarian level, the effect of varying degrees and duration of GnRH-induced gonadotropin withdrawal on the function of the developing follicle and corpus luteum can be investigated by using GnRH antagonists, and inferences can be drawn regarding the importance of LH, FSH, or other ovarian factors at different cycle stages.

Acknowledgments. These studies were done in collaboration with Drs. J. Rivier and W. Vale of the Salk Institute, La Jolla, CA, who supplied the Nal-Glu GnRH antagonist. The contributions of J. Adams, H. Whitney, R.N., and Drs. K. Martin and A. Taylor to many of the protocols are gratefully acknowledged. Dr. R. Whitcomb collaborated in the study of free α-subunit, and Dr. N. Bhatta collaborated in the studies focusing on the ovary.

References

1. Clayton RN, Catt KJ. Gonadotropin-releasing hormone receptors: characterization, physiological regulation and relationship to reproductive function. Endocr Rev 1981;2:186–209.
2. Wynn PC, Suarez-Quian, Childs GV, Catt KJ. Pituitary binding and internalization of radioiodinated gonadotropin-releasing hormone agonist and antagonist ligands "in vitro" and "in vivo." Endocrinology 1986;119:1852–63.
3. Karten MJ, Rivier JE. Gonadotropin-releasing hormone analog design: structure-function studies toward the development of agonists and antagonists: rationale and perspective. Endocr Rev 1986;7:44–66.
4. Hall JE, Brodie TD, Badger TM, et al. Use of a gonadotropin releasing-hormone antagonist in the early follicular phase of the menstrual cycle: evidence of GnRH-independent FSH secretion. J Clin Endocrinol Metab 1988;67:534–53.
5. Hall JE, Whitcomb RW, Rivier JE, Vale WW, Crowley WF Jr. Differential regulation of LH, FSH and free α-subunit secretion from the gonadotrope by GnRH: evidence from the use of two GnRH antagonists. J Clin Endocrinol Metab 1990;70:328–35.
6. Hall JE, Bhatta N, Adams JM, Rivier JE, Vale WW, Crowley WF Jr. Variable tolerance of the developing follicle and corpus luteum to GnRH antagonist-induced gonadotropin withdrawal in the human. J Clin Endocrinol Metab 1991;72:993–1000.
7. Hall JE, Crowley WF Jr. Use of a GnRH antagonist as a physiologic probe of GnRH secretion in women [Abstract]. In: Program of the 72nd annual meeting of The Endocrine Society, Atlanta, GA, 1990:350.

8. Hall JE. The midcycle surge: quantity of GnRH secretion in the human, estimated by susceptibility to GnRH antagonism [Abstract]. In: Program of the 73rd annual meeting of The Endocrine Society, Washington, DC, 1991.

9. Hall JE, Taylor AE, Martin KA, Crowley WF Jr. Response of patients with polycystic ovarian disease to GnRH antagonist administration [Abstract]. Clin Res 1990;38:342A.

10. Crowley WF Jr, Beitins IZ, Vale WW, et al. The biologic activity of a potent analogue of gonadotropin-releasing hormone in normal and hypogonadotropic men. N Engl J Med 1980;302:1052–7.

11. Filicori M, Butler JP, Crowley WF. Neuroendocrine regulation of the corpus luteum in the human. J Clin Endocrinol Metab 1984;73:1638–47.

12. Whitcomb RW, Sangha JS, Schneyer AL, Crowley WF Jr. Improved measurement of free alpha subunit of glycoprotein hormones by assay with use of a monoclonal antibody. Clin Chem 1988;34:2022–5.

13. Kourides IA, Weintraub BD, Ridgway EC, Maloof F. Pituitary secretion of free alpha and beta subunits of human thyrotropin in patients with thyroid disorders. J Clin Endocrinol Metab 1975;40:872–85.

14. Kourides IA, Re RN, Weintraub BD, Ridgway EC, Maloof F. Metabolic clearance and secretion rates of subunits of human thyrotropin. J Clin Invest 1977;77:508–16.

15. Whitcomb RW, O'Dea LStL, Finkelstein JS, Heavern DM, Crowley WF Jr. Utility of free α-subunit as an alternative neuroendocrine marker of gonadotropin-releasing hormone (GnRH) stimulation of the gonadotroph in the human: evidence from normal and GnRH-deficient men. J Clin Endocrinol Metab 1990;70:1654–61.

16. Schwall RH, Nikolics K, Szonyi E, Gorman C, Mason AJ. Recombinant expression and characterization of human activin A. Mol Endocrinol 1988; 2:1237–42.

17. Lumpkin MD, Moltz JH, Yu WH, Samson WK, McCann SM. Purification of FSH-releasing factor: its dissimilarity from LHRH of mammalian, avian, and piscian origin. Brain Res Bull 1987;18:175–8.

18. Dahl KD, Pavlou SN, Kovacs WJ, Hsueh AJW. The changing ratio of serum bioactive to immunoreactive follicle-stimulating hormone in normal men following treatment with a potent gonadotropin releasing hormone antagonist. J Clin Endocrinol Metab 1986;63:792–4.

19. Clarke I. Exactitude in the relationship between GnRH and LH secretion. In: Crowley WF Jr, Conn PM, eds. Modes of action of GnRH and GnRH analogs. (See Chapter 11, this volume.)

20. Urban JH, Meredith JM, Bauer-Dantoin AC, Strobl FJ, Levine J. Gonadal feedback regulation of LHRH release and actions in the rat. In: Crowley WF Jr, Conn PM, eds. Modes of action of GnRH and GnRH analogs. (See Chapter 13, this volume.)

21. Caraty A, Bouchard P, Blane MR. Studies of LHRH secretion into the hypophyseal portal blood of the ram: gonadal regulation of LH secretion is mainly exerted at the hypothalamic level. In: Crowley WF Jr, Conn PM, eds. Modes of action of GnRH and GnRH analogs. (See Chapter 12, this volume.)

22. Karsch F, Moenter SM, Caraty A. The preovulatory surge of GnRH secretion: characterization and regulation. In: Crowley WF Jr, Conn PM, eds. Modes of action of GnRH and GnRH analogs. (See Chapter 15, this volume.)

23. Cicero TJ, Owens DP, Schmoeker PF, Meyer ER. Morphine-induced supersensitivity to the effects of naloxone on luteinizing hormone secretion in the male rat. J Pharmacol Exp Ther 1983;225:35–41.
24. Ferin M, van Vugt D, Wardlaw S. The hypothalamic control of the menstrual cycle and the role of endogenous opioid peptides. Recent Prog Horm Res 1984;40:441–85.
25. Clayton RN, Solano AR, Garcia-Vela A, Dufau ML, Catt KJ. Regulation of pituitary receptors for gonadotropin-releasing hormone during the rat estrous cycle. Endocrinology 1980:699–706.
26. Filicori M, Santoro N, Merriam GR, Crowley WF Jr. Characterization of the physiological pattern of episodic gonadotropin secretion throughout the human menstrual cycle. J Clin Endocrinol Metab 1986;62:1136–44.
27. Hodgen GD. The dominant ovarian follicle. Fertil Steril 1982;38:281–300.
28. Fraser HM, Abbott M, Laird NC, McNeilly AS, Nestor JJ Jr, Bickery BH. Effects of an LH-releasing hormone antagonist on the secretion of LH, FSH, prolactin and ovarian steroids at different stages of the luteal phase in the stumptailed macaque (Macaca arctoides). J Endocrinol 1986;111:83–90.
29. Hutchison JS, Zeleznik AJ. The corpus luteum of the primate menstrual cycle is capable of recovering from a transient withdrawal of pituitary gonadotropin support. Endocrinology 1985;117:1043–9.
30. Roseff SJ, Bangah ML, Kettel LM, et al. Dynamic changes in circulating inhibin levels during the luteal-follicular transition of the human menstrual cycle. J Clin Endocrinol Metab 1989;69:1033–9.
31. Mortola JF, Sathanandan M, Pavlou S, et al. Suppression of bioactive and immunoreactive follicle-stimulating hormone and luteinizing hormone levels by a potent gonadotropin-releasing hormone antagonist: pharmacodynamic studies. Fertil Steril 1989;51:957–63.
32. McLachlan RI, Cohen NL, Vale WW, et al. The importance of luteinizing hormone in the control of inhibin and progesterone secretion by the human corpus luteum. J Clin Endocrinol Metab 1989;68:1078–85.

20

Gonadotropin Releasing Hormone Antagonist Plus Testosterone: A Potential Male Contraceptive

WILLIAM J. BREMNER, CARRIE J. BAGATELL, AND ROBERT A. STEINER

Although hormonal regimens provide effective, reversible contraception for women, no effective hormonal contraceptive regimen has yet been developed for men. Testosterone decreases gonadotropin secretion by exerting negative feedback at both the hypothalamus and pituitary (1–3), thereby inhibiting spermatogenesis. Administration of exogenous T causes azoospermia in only 50–70% of men, however (4). Agonist analogs of GnRH can inhibit gonadotropin secretion and gonadal function (5), but they do not consistently induce azoospermia in primates when given alone or in combination with androgen (6–9).

GnRH antagonists are synthetic analogs of GnRH that compete with endogenous GnRH for pituitary binding sites, thereby inhibiting the secretion of LH and FSH (5). In short-term studies in humans and in nonhuman primates, these antagonists reversibly suppress plasma levels of LH, FSH, T, and inhibin (10–12). When given without androgen replacement, GnRH antagonists can induce azoospermia in adult monkeys (13–15). An androgen must be administered with a GnRH antagonist in a contraceptive regimen to maintain the normal androgen milieu. However, in previous studies of concomitant antagonist and androgen administration in experimental animals, induction of azoospermia was inconsistent (15, 16). The present study was undertaken to determine the effects of daily injections of the GnRH antagonist, Detirelix, [N-Ac-D-Nal(2)^1-DpCl-Phe^{2}D-Trp^{3}D-hArg(Et2)^6-DAla^{10}] GnRH, alone and in conjunction with simultaneous T replacement, on sperm production and on serum testosterone levels in adult male monkeys.

Experimental Procedures

Adult male monkeys, *Macaca fascicularis*, were housed under controlled conditions of temperature (21 ± 2°C) and light (on at 0600 h, off at 1800 h) in individual cages at the Regional Primate Center at the University of Washington. In addition to monkey chow, the animals received fresh fruit, chewable vitamins, and iron injections. The animals were aged 8 to 15 years (as assessed by dental radiographs). The GnRH antagonist (supplied courtesy of Drs. Brian Vickery and John J. Nestor of the Syntex Corporation, Palo Alto, CA) was dissolved at a concentration of 4 µg/ml in a vehicle containing glacial acetic acid, benzyl alcohol, sodium hydroxide, and sterile water. The vehicle was supplied by the Syntex Corporation and contained 0.02 M sodium acetate buffer, 0.9% benzyl alcohol preservative, and 0.02 M glacial acetic acid. Antagonist was added to this solution and was filtered through a 0.8 µm nucleopore filter. Aliquots of 20 ml were frozen at −20°C until use. During the study period, either the antagonist or the vehicle was injected subcutaneously daily between 0800 h and 1200 h.

All animals in the experimental groups received Silastic capsule implants subcutaneously 5 days prior to the first injection of GnRH antagonist. The capsules were 0.33 cm ID × 0.46 cm OD and were 5.5 cm in length. These implants contained either crystalline testosterone or were empty, depending on the treatment regimen. Capsules were sterilized in Zephiran and rinsed in sterile saline before implantation. Implants were removed when injections of GnRH antagonist were completed.

Serum testosterone was measured by radioimmunoassay, using methods previously described (1). The minimum detectability of the assay was less than 0.35 nmol/L. The intra- and interassay coefficients of variation were 5.1% and 9.8%, respectively. GnRH antagonist levels were measured in groups 2, 3, and 4 by RIA at the Syntex Corporation. Seminal fluid was obtained by rectal electroejaculation. Sperm counts were performed in the Seminal Fluid Core Laboratory (C. Alvin Paulsen, Director) of the Population Center for Research in Reproduction.

All animals (n = 22) were studied for an initial 4-month control period during which baseline measurements were obtained. The animals were then divided into four groups: Group 1 (n = 5) received antagonist, 250 µg/kg/day, plus sham implants, for 12 weeks. Group 2 (n = 5) received GnRH antagonist, 250 µg/kg/day plus T via implants for 20 weeks. Group 3 (n = 5) received antagonist, 750 µg/kg/day, plus T via implants for 16 weeks. Group 4 (n = 7) received vehicle alone for 20 weeks. Animals were monitored daily and observed for any physical or behavioral effects of the drug treatment. Throughout the control and experimental periods, seminal fluid, blood samples, and body weights were obtained every 2 weeks.

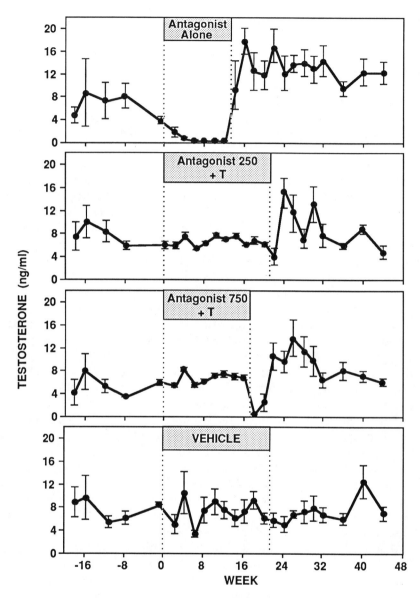

FIGURE 20.1. Mean serum testosterone levels in normal adult male monkeys before, during, and after administration of a GnRH antagonist alone (top panel), or of GnRH antagonist in two dosages plus testosterone (middle panels), or of vehicle alone (bottom panel). Reprinted with permission from Bremner WJ, Bagatell CJ, Steiner RA. Gonadotropin-releasing hormone antagonist plus testosterone: a potential male contraceptive. J Clin Endocrinol Metab, September 1991. © by The Endocrine Society.

Two animals in each treatment group were chosen randomly to undergo testicular biopsy during the treatment period and again following recovery. Open biopsies were performed by sterile technique after the animals had received general anesthesia. Tissue samples were fixed in Cleland's solution, sectioned, and stained with hematoxylin and eosin.

Differences among control, treatment, and recovery period values for sperm counts, body weight, and T levels were determined by analysis of variance with repeated measures and multiple comparison procedures. Differences between groups were determined by analysis of variance. For each group, a chi square test was used to determine diffferences between baseline, treatment, and recovery periods.

Results

In group 1 (antagonist alone) serum T levels decreased significantly, from 21.2 ± 6.6 nmol/L to 1.4 ± 0.4 nmol/L (Fig. 20.1) during 12 weeks of treatment ($P < 0.05$). Within a week after the end of injections, the mean serum T levels had increased to 35.0 ± 14.9 nmol/L, and remained elevated at the end of the recovery period. Serum T levels in group 2 (antagonist 250 µg/kg/day + T) and group 3 (antagonist 750 µg/kg/day + T) did not change significantly during drug administration. After the end of injections and removal of the T implants, serum T levels decreased transiently, but by the end of the recovery period, T levels in both groups were similar to the baseline levels. T levels in group 4 (vehicle) did not change significantly throughout the course of the study.

Sperm counts in the antagonist-treated groups dropped markedly by 8 weeks, and by 12 weeks all the animals in groups 1 and 3 were azoospermic (Fig. 20.2). At 16 and 20 weeks of antagonist administration, only one animal in group 2 failed to become azoospermic, and this animal's sperm counts were very low (50–100,000/ejaculate). At the end of the recovery period, sperm counts in all groups were comparable to pretreatment values. The mean sperm count in the group receiving vehicle alone did not change significantly during the study period.

Representative sections demonstrated normal testicular histology in animals receiving placebo (Fig. 20.3, top) and marked regression of spermatogenesis in animals receiving the antagonist (Fig. 20.3, bottom). Antagonist-treated animals (at both doses and including those animals receiving T) demonstrated a marked decrease in tubular diameter with loss of spermatocytes and spermatids, but with preservation of spermatogonia and Sertoli cells. In the antagonist-treated animals, histology returned to normal during the recovery period.

Animals in group 1 (antagonist alone) lost weight during the treatment period (5.3 ± 0.4 to 4.7 ± 0.3 kg, $P < 0.05$). By the end of the recovery period, the animals had regained the lost weight and had gained some additional weight; mean weight at the end of the recovery period was 5.7

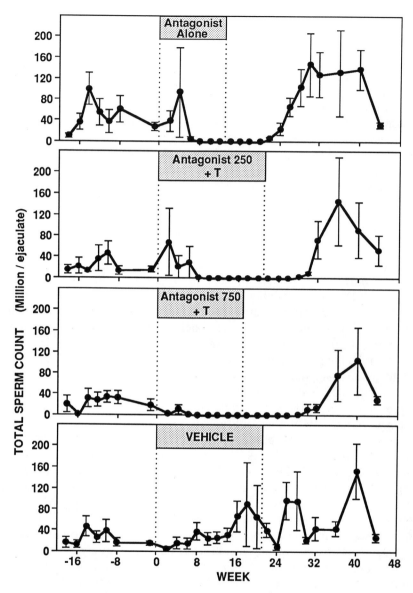

FIGURE 20.2. Mean total sperm counts in normal adult male monkeys before, during, and after administration of a GnRH antagonist alone (top panel), or of a GnRH antagonist in two dosages plus testosterone (middle panels), or of vehicle alone (bottom panel). Reprinted with permission from Bremner WJ, Bagatell CJ, Steiner RA. Gonadotropin-releasing hormone antagonist plus testosterone: a potential male contraceptive. J Clin Endocrinol Metab, September 1991. © by The Endocrine Society.

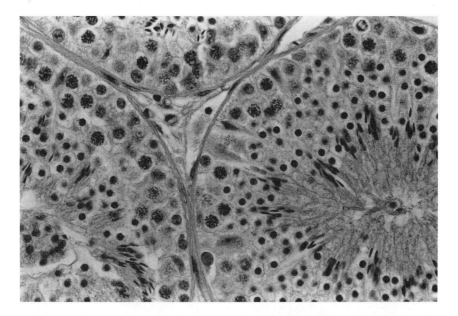

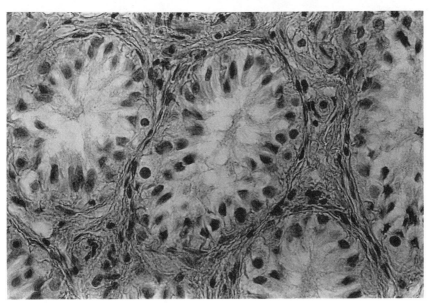

FIGURE 20.3. Testicular histology during administration of vehicle (top) and with GnRH antagonist (750 µg/kg/day) plus T (bottom). During antagonist plus T administration, tubular diameter decreased and spermatids and spermatocytes were absent, leaving only Sertoli cells and spermatogonia in the tubules. Reprinted with permission from Bremner WJ, Bagatell CJ, Steiner RA. Gonadotropin-releasing hormone antagonist plus testosterone: a potential male contraceptive. J Clin Endocrinol Metab, September 1991. © by The Endocrine Society.

TABLE 20.1. GnRH antagonist plasma levels in monkeys receiving daily antagonist injections.

Treatment	GnRH antagonist plasma levels (ng/ml)	
	Before injection	6 h after injection
Group 2 (250 μg/kg/d + T)	59 ± 11	131 ± 20
Group 3 (750 μg/kg/d + T)	228 ± 38	428 ± 69
Group 4 (vehicle)	Undetectable	Undetectable

± 0.3 kg. Animals receiving T replacement (groups 2 and 3) neither lost nor gained a significant amount of weight during the study. In group 4, (vehicle alone), body weights increased slightly during the treatment period, (5.1 ± 0.2 to 5.4 ± 0.2 kg, $P < 0.05$). This increase was maintained to the end of the recovery period.

Mean serum levels of antagonist increased after injections and were maintained at an elevated level until the next injection (Table 20.1). Animals in group 4 had antagonist levels that were undetectable before and 6 h after the injection of vehicle.

Discussion and Conclusions

We administered a GnRH antagonist, with and without testosterone replacement, to sexually mature male monkeys for periods of 12 to 20 weeks. The antagonist alone consistently led to suppression of serum T levels to the castrate range and to azoospermia. When combined with T, the antagonist caused azoospermia in all animals receiving the 750 μg/kg dose and in 4 of the 5 animals receiving the 250 μg/kg dose. These findings were associated with testicular histology showing lack of progression of spermatogenesis beyond spermatogonia in the antagonist-treated animals. These effects were reversible by the end of the recovery period. These results suggest that the combination of a GnRH antagonist plus androgen replacement may be an effective male contraceptive regimen and that the antagonist alone may be an effective treatment for testosterone-dependent neoplasia.

GnRH antagonists without androgen replacement have been shown by others to induce azoospermia in male monkeys (13–15); our work confirms this finding and extends it to include androgen supplementation as part of the experimental design. Since long-term androgen deficiency would have unacceptable behavioral and physiologic sequellae for normal men, androgen replacement would be an important component of a hormonal contraceptive regimen. In contrast to previous studies (15, 16), we found that azoospermia could be induced when a GnRH antagonist and T were administered concomitantly. We used antagonist doses of 250 and 750 μg/kg/day, while Weinbauer et al. (15, 16) used doses of 400 to 460 μg/kg/day. The Nal-Glu analog used by Weinbauer et al. in one of their studies is similar in potency to Detirelix (5), which was used in their other work (16) and in our study reported here. Since 4 of the 5 animals receiving the lower antagonist dose became azoospermic in our study and the fifth was nearly azoospermic, the magnitude of the dose cannot explain the difference in results. We administered the antagonist in daily subcutaneous injections, whereas Weinbauer et al. used osmotic mini-pumps (15). The injections were very effective in maintaining high blood levels of the antagonist (Table 20.1); this is a plausible explanation for the more consistent suppression of spermatogenesis in our animals when compared with those of Weinbauer et al. (15). It is not clear why Weinbauer et al. (16), when using daily injections of a potent antagonist, were unable to induce azoospermia. Their explanation that the con-current administration of testosterone stimulated spermatogenesis directly seems unlikely, since we were able to induce azoospermia using a GnRH antagonist and testosterone in this study.

Azoospermia was achieved within 12 weeks in all animals in groups 1 and 3, while in group 2, azoospermia was reached in 4 animals at 14–16 weeks and the fifth animal became severely oligospermic. Thus, 14 of 15 animals treated with antagonist became azoospermic, including 9 of 10 receiving testosterone replacement. These results suggest that the com-bination of a GnRH antagonist and T may be an effective contraceptive in men, leading to more consistent induction of azoospermia than is true with T-alone regimens (4). We have recently shown that in normal men the combination of the antagonist plus T causes a greater suppression of FSH, LH, and inhibin than does either T alone or antagonist alone (12). Preliminary results suggest that this combination is effective in suppressing sperm production in men (17–19).

As expected, serum T levels in group 1 declined to castrate levels during antagonist administration. During this treatment period, serum T levels in the T-replaced groups were equal to or slightly higher than during the pretreatment period and were in the same range as those of the control group. These T levels are higher than those achieved by Weinbauer et al. in their 1987 study (16) and in the same range or slightly lower than in a later study by these authors (15). These data suggest that the level of T replacement employed is not the most important factor in determining whether or not azoospermia is achieved. On the other hand, determining an optimal level of T replacement will be very important in preventing the adverse effects of either insufficient or excessive androgen levels (e.g., effects on behavior, lipids, and bone mass).

Body weights decreased significantly in animals receiving the antagonist alone and slightly, but not significantly, in animals receiving antagonist plus T. These effects were not accompanied by noticeable decreases in appetite or food intake during the study. The mechanism of this weight loss is unknown, but it could be due in part to antagonist-induced T deficiency. No other physical or behavioral effects of the experimental regimens were noted.

In conclusion, we have shown that the combination of a GnRH antagonist and testosterone can successfully induce azoospermia in a nonhuman primate species. These data suggest that a similar hormonal regimen might be effective as a contraceptive regimen for the human male. The effectiveness of the antagonist alone in achieving prolonged and profound suppression of serum T levels suggests that this peptide could be an effective treatment of androgen-dependent neoplasias, particularly those of the prostate.

Acknowledgments. This chapter was reprinted in large part from Bremner WJ et al., GnRH antagonist plus testosterone: a potential male contraceptive, J Clin Endocrinol Metab, 1991. We thank Ms. Pam Kolb, Ms. Connie Nosbisch, Ms. Connie Pete, Ms. Florida Flor, and Ms. Elaine Rost for their technical assistance. We appreciate the work of Ms. Liza Noonan in the biostatistical analysis and Mr. Larry Mix in manuscript preparation. This work was supported in part by the Contraceptive Development Branch, NIH and by NIH Grants HD-12629, HD-12625, and RR-00166, and by Medical Research funds from the Department of Veterans' Affairs.

References

1. Matsumoto AM, Bremner WJ. Modulation of pulsatile gonadotropin secretion by testosterone in man. J Clin Endocrinol Metab 1984;58:609–14.
2. Sheckter CB, Matsumoto AM, Bremner WJ. Testosterone administration inhibits gonadotropin secretion by an effect directly on the human pituitary. J Clin Endocrinol Metab 1989;68:397–401.
3. Finkelstein J, O'Dea L, Whitcomb R, Schoenfeld D, Crowley W. Testosterone infusion suppresses LH secretion at the pituitary and hypothalamic levels in the human male [Abstract]. In: Proceedings of the 70th meeting of The Endocrine Society, New Orleans, LA, 1988:302.
4. Paulsen CA, Bremner WJ, Leonard JM. Male contraception: clinical trials. In: Mishell DR, ed. Advances in fertility research. New York: Raven Press, 1982:157–70.
5. Karten MJ, Rivier JE. Gonadotropin-releasing hormone analog design: structure-function studies toward the development of agonists and antagonists. Endocr Rev 1986;7:44–66.
6. Bouchard P, Garcia E. Influence of testosterone substitution on sperm suppression by LHRH agonists. Horm Res 1987;28:175–80.
7. Bhasin S, Heber D, Steiner BS, Handelsman DJ, Swerdloff RS. Hormonal effects of gonadotropin-releasing hormone (GnRH) agonist in the human male. III. Effects of long-term combined treatment with GnRH agonist and androgen. J Clin Endocrinol Metab 1985;60:998–1003.
8. Akhtar FB, Marshall GR, Nieschlag E. Testosterone supplementation attenuates the antifertility effects of an LHRH agonist in male rhesus monkeys. Int J Androl 1983;6:461–8.

9. Mann DR, Gould KG, Smith MM, Duffey T, Collins DC. Influence of simultaneous gonadotropin-releasing hormone agonist and testosterone treatment on spermatogenesis and potential fertilizing capacity in male monkeys. J Clin Endocrinol Metab 1987;65:1215–24.

10. Burgo-Briceno LA, Schally AV, Bartke A, Asch RH. Inhibition of serum luteinizing hormone and testosterone with an inhibitory analog of luteinizing-hormone releasing hormone in adult male rhesus monkeys. J Clin Endocrinol Metab 1984;59:601–7.

11. Adams LA, Bremner WJ, Nestor JJ, Vickery BH, Steiner RA. Suppression of plasma gonadotropins and testosterone in adult male monkeys (*Macaca fascicularis*) by a potent inhibitory analog of gonadotropin-releasing hormone. J Clin Endocrinol Metab 1986;62:58–63.

12. Bagatell CJ, McLachlan RI, deKretser DM, et al. A comparison of the suppressive effects of testosterone and a potent new gonadotropin-releasing hormone antagonist on gonadotropin and inhibin levels in normal men. J Clin Endocrinol Metab 1989;69:43–8.

13. Weinbauer GF, Surmann FJ, Akhtar FB, Shah GV, Vickery BH, Nieschlag E. Reversible inhibition of testicular function by a gonadotropin-releasing hormone antagonist in monkeys (*Macaca fascicularis*). Fertil Steril 1984;42:906–14.

14. Bint Akhtar F, Weinbauer GF, Nieschlag E. Acute and chronic effects of a gonadotropin-releasing hormone antagonist on pituitary and testicular function in monkeys. J Endocrinol 1985;104:345–54.

15. Weinbauer GF, Gockeler E, Nieschlag E. Testosterone prevents complete suppression of spermatogenesis in the gonadotropin-releasing hormone antagonist-treated nonhuman primate (*Macaca fascicularis*). J Clin Endocrinol Metab 1988;67:284–90.

16. Weinbauer GF, Surmann FJ, Nieschlag E. Suppression of spermatogenesis in a nonhuman primate (*Macaca fascicularis*) by concomitant gonadotropin-releasing hormone antagonist and testosterone treatment. Acta Endocrinol (Copenh) 1987;114:138–46.

17. Pavlou SN, et al. Complete suppression of spermatogenesis without loss of libido by administering a GnRH antagonist plus testosterone. In: Proceedings of the 72nd annual meeting of The Endocrine Society, 1990:134.

18. Tom L, Bhasin S, Salameh W, Peterson M, Steiner B, Swerdloff RS. Male contraception: combined gonadotropin releasing hormone antagonist and testosterone enanthate. Clin Res 1991;39:91A.

19. Bagatell CJ, Bremner WJ. Unpublished observations.

21

GnRH Antagonists: Primate Models for Clinical Indications

KEITH GORDON, DOUGLAS R. DANFORTH, ROBERT F. WILLIAMS, AND GARY D. HODGEN

The impact of gonadotropin releasing hormone and its analogs on clinical management of infertility and reproductive endocrinology (both realized and anticipated) are far-reaching. The reproductive processes of both males and females are orchestrated by the gonadotropic hormones follicle stimulating hormone and luteinizing hormone, which are in turn largely dependent on the stimulatory effect of GnRH, which is released in a pulsatile manner from the hypothalamus (1). Clinical applications for GnRH and its analogs fall into two broad categories: those dependent upon stimulatory effects on gonadotropin secretion and those dependent upon inhibitory effects on gonadotropin secretion. Applications dependent on stimulatory effects of GnRH on gonadotropins, such as treatment of Kallmann's syndrome (2) and hypothalamic amenorrhea (3), are mostly achieved using the native decapeptide GnRH. Applications dependent on the suppression of gonadotropin concentrations, which constitute the vast majority of applications, are currently fulfilled by GnRH agonists, of which at least half a dozen are commercially available worldwide. It is somewhat of a paradox that compounds originally designed to have more powerful and long-lasting stimulatory actions than the native decapeptide are now used to achieve exactly the opposite end point, inhibition of gonadotropin secretion. Initial efforts at chemically modifying native GnRH were directed at producing both GnRH agonists and antagonists. However, success was much more rapid with GnRH agonists, and product development proceeded rapidly; hence their current prevalence in the market today.

Suppression of gonadotropin secretion, which is after all the end point desired for many of the clinical applications, can be achieved with either GnRH agonists or GnRH antagonists. GnRH agonists accomplish this via the phenomena of down-regulation and desensitization that occur when an overabundance of GnRH is presented to the pituitary receptors. However, the initial response of the pituitary to GnRH agonists is stimulatory: the so-called "flare effect," which can have undesirable clinical consequences. Conversely, GnRH antagonists achieve suppression of gonadotropin concentrations via classical receptor antagonism—i.e., GnRH antagonists monopolize the GnRH receptors to such an extent that native GnRH is unable to bind to sufficient numbers to cause the release of gonadotropins. This difference has some important consequences for potential clinical applications.

Ovulation Induction with Gonadotropins

GnRH agonists are now widely used as part of ovulation induction protocols for various forms of assisted reproductive technologies. The principal objective of such usage is to reduce the incidence of premature LH surges and to provide more precise control over the timing of follicular development, thereby facilitating scheduling of patients for oocyte collection. Combination therapy with GnRH agonist plus gonadotropin rarely shifts a nonresponsive patient into a responsive one. However, avoidance of premature luteinization gets more patients to oocyte collection, increases the yield of high-quality eggs and, in turn, pre-embryos, which is reflected in a higher rate of total take-home babies from the combined transfer of "fresh" and, in subsequent cycles, thawed pre-embryos that were available for and tolerant of cryopreservation (4–12).

GnRH antagonists, when they become clinically available, are likely to offer several advantages over the currently available GnRH agonists for this application. First, GnRH antagonists produce immediate suppression of pituitary gonadotropin secretion without the flare effect, thus avoiding potentially detrimental effects on oocyte quantity and quality. Second, intermediate doses of GnRH antagonists may be employed to allow a balance to be achieved whereby the LH surge is blocked without nullifying tonic FSH/LH secretion, thereby reducing the number of ampules of gonadotropins needed per stimulation. Third, there is the possibility that some women suffering from PCOD who were previously untreatable with standard stimulation protocols may be treatable with a combination therapy of GnRH antagonist plus pulsatile GnRH (see later section).

In early studies (13–15) we have established the feasibility of combining GnRH antagonist-induced inhibition of endogenous gonadotropins with exogenous gonadotropin therapy for ovulation induction. Three intact female cynomolgus monkeys received 6 daily injections of Pergonal (37.5 IU/day) and Antide (1 mg/kg/day), followed by hCG (1000 IU) on day 7. Blood samples were drawn from the day of initiation of treatment until 30 days posttreatment or until the resumption of normal menstrual cycles. Two of the three monkeys displayed a classical endocrine response

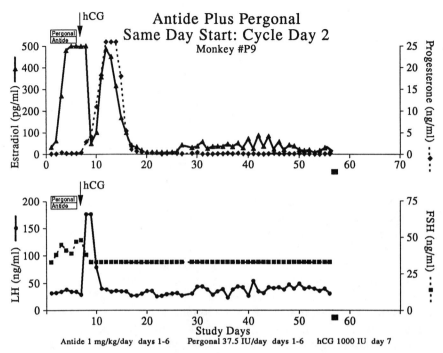

FIGURE 21.1. Serum concentrations of estradiol, progesterone, LH, and FSH in an individual monkey (#P9) undergoing a combination of GnRH antagonist-induced inhibition of endogenous gonadotropins with exogenous gonadotropin therapy for ovulation induction. Treatment involved 6 daily injections of Pergonal (37.5 IU/day) and Antide (1 mg/kg/day), followed by hCG (1000 IU) on day 7.

(Figs. 21.1 and 21.2). Estradiol concentrations rose steadily to reach >500 pg/ml by the day of hCG administration. Administration of hCG induced multiple ovulations accompanied by appropriately elevated progesterone concentrations (>25 ng/ml). The third monkey did not respond well (Fig. 21.3). Although the initial response was promising, with estradiol levels rising from <100 pg/ml to >500 pg/ml on day 5 of treatment, concentrations of estradiol declined prior to hCG injection and there was minimal resultant luteal function. However, note that this was not due to a premature LH surge, since LH concentrations remained basal until after the hCG administration (hCG cross-reacts in the assay used for monkey LH). Also note that the FSH levels in this monkey were elevated (approximately 50 ng/ml) compared to normal (approximately 30 ng/ml), possibly indicating a perimenopausal condition of this monkey. Thus, it appears that Antide, and presumably other GnRH antagonists, are effective as an adjunct to gonadotropin stimulation for ovulation induction. Future studies will be required to evaluate effects on oocyte quality and overall efficiency before clinical trials can be undertaken.

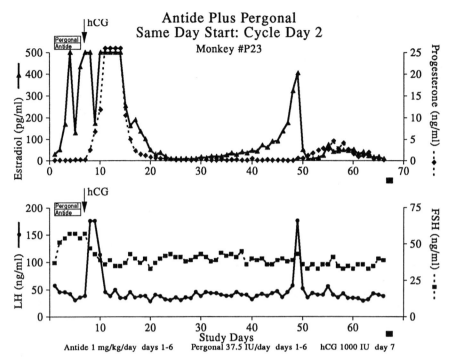

FIGURE 21.2. Serum concentrations of estradiol, progesterone, LH, and FSH in an individual monkey (#P23) undergoing a combination of GnRH antagonist-induced inhibition of endogenous gonadotropins with exogenous gonadotropin therapy for ovulation induction. Treatment involved 6 daily injections of Pergonal (37.5 IU/day) and Antide (1 mg/kg/day), followed by hCG (1000 IU) on day 7.

Ovulation Induction with Pulsatile GnRH

Management of patients with PCOD, or more specifically androgen ovarian dystrophy (16), desiring relief from the sequelae of hyperandrogenism and anovulatory infertility continues to be one of the more challenging clinical presentations (17–21). Prescribed therapies have included the use of glucocorticoids, clomiphene citrate, and pulsatile GnRH for ovulation induction (17, 22, 23). However, there remain a significant number of women for whom these therapies are ineffective. The usage of GnRH analogs to achieve suppression of ovarian androgen secretion has become increasingly common over the past few years (24–32). Large doses of GnRH agonists are used to down-regulate the pituitary ovarian axis, suppressing LH levels and preventing the occurrence of premature LH surges. Ovulations are then induced using exogenous gonadotropins just as in standard ovulation protocols. Since

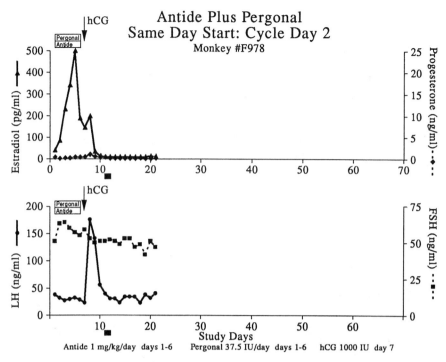

FIGURE 21.3. Serum concentrations of estradiol, progesterone, LH, and FSH in an individual monkey (#PF978) undergoing a combination of GnRH antagonist-induced inhibition of endogenous gonadotropins with exogenous gonadotropin therapy for ovulation induction. Treatment involved 6 daily injections of Pergonal (37.5 IU/day) and Antide (1 mg/kg/day), followed by hCG (1000 IU) on day 7. Notice that this monkey did not respond well (see text for details).

GnRH antagonists, unlike GnRH agonists, do not render the pituitary refractory to administration of exogenous GnRH, this potentially allows for a novel approach to ovulation induction in women with PCOD.

We have recently demonstrated the feasibility of combining GnRH antagonist with pulsatile GnRH therapy for the controlled restoration of gonadotropin secretion and gonadal steroidogenesis, culminating in apparently normal ovulatory menstrual cycles. Four normal intact cynomolgus monkeys having regular menstrual cycles were studied in one of two regimens (33). Regimen A comprised a series of initial large loading doses of Antide (10 mg/kg, sc), with no further Antide administrations. Regimen B comprised an initial 3 mg/kg dose followed by 1 mg/kg administered on alternate days to sustain Antide concentrations at a pharmacoeffective level until ovulation had been successfully induced via the exogenous GnRH pulses. Pulsatile GnRH treatment was initiated 4 days after the first Antide injections at a rate of 5 µg/pulse, with one

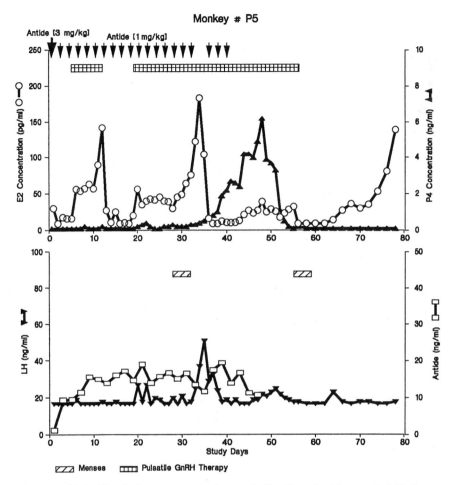

FIGURE 21.4. Circulating concentrations of P, E_2, Antide, and LH in a representative intact monkey treated with Antide plus pulsatile GnRH in a sustaining dose regimen comprised of an initial 3 mg/kg dose of Antide with subsequent 1 mg/kg/doses administered on alternate days to achieve sustained levels of Antide. Pulsatile GnRH was given at a dose of 5 µg pulse (one 1-min pulse/h) from study day 5 until study day 26. Thereafter, pulsatile GnRH was given at a dose of 10 µg/pulse.

1-min pulse/h. The amplitude was subsequently raised to 10 µg/pulse after approximately 21 days.

The results from the two treatment regimens were comparable, thus for brevity we will illustrate the point with data from a representative monkey given treatment B. In monkey P5 (Fig. 21.4), concentrations of Antide rose promptly with initiation of treatment to levels between 10 and 20 ng/ml, and they remained there throughout the course of the study. Notice that the initial pulsatile GnRH treatment resulted in prompt elevations of estradiol. However, the initial cohort of follicles was lost due to technical difficulties, as was evidenced by a precipitous decline in estrogen concentrations without accompanying ovulation. After repair of technical difficulties and on reinitiation of GnRH therapy (5 µg/pulse), E_2 concentrations again rose promptly off the hypoestrogenic baseline caused by Antide. Tonic E_2 concentrations were at 50 to 70 pg/ml for about 10 days. When the GnRH pulse amplitude was increased to 10 µg/pulse, a rapid rise in E_2 concentrations ensued, leading to an apparently normal preovulatory E_2 peak antecedent to ovulation, with subsequent luteal phase length of 19 days and normal P production, despite sustained pharmacoeffective levels of Antide.

The results of this study clearly demonstrated the feasibility of over-riding the Antide-induced suppression of ovulatory menstrual cycles in intact monkeys by providing appropriate GnRH pulse therapy during the continued presence of pharmacoeffective levels of Antide. Our findings from this primate model suggest that a clinical study using Antide to suppress LH excess and/or hyperandrogenism (polycystic ovarian disease) with its sequelae in women while giving pulsatile GnRH to induce folliculogenesis, ovulation, and corpus luteum function may be warranted.

Endometriosis

Endometriosis is the aberrant occurrence of endometrial tissue within the pelvic cavity. It often occurs with adhesive disease in association with dysmenorrhea, dyspareunia, pelvic pain, and infertility. The method of treatment is somewhat dictated by the reason behind the woman's presentation in the clinic. The most common reason for seeking medical help is for alleviation of pelvic pain. A number of therapeutic options are available including surgical intervention (34), treatment with Danazol (a synthetic derivative of 17 ethynyl testosterone) (35), or the use of GnRH agonists (36–39). The use of GnRH agonists given daily (37) or on an individualized approximately weekly basis (38) has been shown to be effective in controlling endometriosis and is becoming more prevalent. However, as is the case for all applications of GnRH agonists for gonadotropin suppression, there is an initial period of enhanced gonadotropin secretion lasting anywhere from 7 to 21 days before down-regulation occurs, which can aggravate pain from the endometriosis condition. It would obviously be desirable to achieve alleviation of pain as quickly as possible, and there is reason to believe that this could be achieved much quicker by using GnRH antagonists than it can by using GnRH agonists. The prospects for long-term control of endometriosis with either the GnRH agonists or the GnRH antagonists is less clear. Both are accompanied by the problems of hypoestrogenism. However, it may be practical to titer the dosage of GnRH antagonists such that control of endometriotic implants is achieved without the need for absolute suppression of estrogen concentrations.

Prostatic Carcinoma

Prostatic carcinoma is the second most common cause of cancer-related deaths among American men over the age of 55 (40). Historically, a variety of treatment regimens have been employed, including orchiectomy, estrogen administration, adrenalectomy, hypophysectomy, corticosteroid therapy, and antiandrogen therapy (41). More recently, GnRH analogs have been utilized as therapeutic agents for patients with androgen-sensitive prostatic adenocarcinoma, which constitutes approximately 70% of all cases of prostatic neoplasms at the time of diagnosis (40). Treatment of patients with GnRH agonists leads to clinical improvement of urinary outflow obstruction and decrease in size of prostate (42) without the adverse side effects of estrogens or the psychological impact of surgical castration (43). However, continued long-term efficacy is not always achieved. There is a tendency for LH and T elevations to reappear after prolonged therapy (44). The principle of GnRH antagonist-induced suppression of the pituitary-testicular axis is already well established (45), and with the increased safety of the newer GnRH antagonists such therapy is likely to become very popular, providing more immediate relief of symptoms and avoiding the adverse consequences of the flare effect common to GnRH agonist regimens (46). In addition, the prolonged duration of action of GnRH anatagonists such as Antide, or galenic formulations, will reduce the need for frequent administrations, thereby improving patient compliance and efficiency, while minimizing adverse side effects. In preliminary studies conducted on adult male cynomolgus monkeys we have been able to demonstrate suppression of serum testosterone levels for up to 60 days in some individuals following a single injection of 10 mg/kg of an experimental formulation of Antide (47).

Contraception

The need for new contraceptive options is great and the desire to have a readily reversible male contraceptive is paramount. A number of clinical trials with both GnRH agonists and antagonists have already been performed (48–54), and the efficacy of these compounds for contraceptive action has been proven. However, the suppressed gonadotropin levels are accompanied by suppressed gonadal steroid secretion, with associated undesirable consequences.

In men, replacement androgens would have to be given to combat the reduced libido that results. This may seem like an awkward compromise; however, since there are currently no practical steroid contraceptives for men, the combination of GnRH analog treatment for gonadotropin suppression, with androgen replacement therapy for alleviation of reduced libido and impotence, may prove successful (53–56).

In women, long-term usage of GnRH analogs would almost certainly be accompanied by the common sequelae of the menopause. Thus, a balance must be achieved between; (1) the need for effective blockade of follicular development, ovulation, and corpus luteum function; and (2) the maintenance of sufficient estrogen production for beneficial effects on CNS, vaginal, bone, and cardiovascular tissues. The feasibility of an intermittent (weekly) administration of GnRH antagonist to achieve such a balance has recently been demonstrated in a nonhuman primate model (57). These limitations notwithstanding, GnRH analogs may be an attractive alternative for women over 35 who wish to reduce the increased risk of cardiovascular problems associated with steroidal contraceptive usage. These analogs may also be ideal for extending the interval of lactational amenorrhea (58), thus avoiding the adverse effects of steroidal combination pills on lactation. Since breastfeeding women are likely to use this method for only relatively short intervals of time and since estrogen production is normally low during this interval anyway, the GnRH analog-associated hypoestrogenism is of lesser concern. Furthermore, since GnRH analogs are only minimally bioavailable when administered orally, there is little concern over passage of bioactive levels to the infant in the milk.

Diagnosis of Osteoporosis Risk

Although many postmenopausal women gain one or more benefits from estrogen replacement therapy (59–61), the question of whether all post-menopausal women should receive estrogen replacement therapy is a matter of balancing potential benefits with the increased risks of undesirable side-effects. Typically, estrogen replacement therapy, even in combination with a progestin, is considered among risk factors in breast and endometrial carcinomas, hypertension, embolytic tendency, and long-term cardiovascular status (62–67). Among the sequelae of severe estrogen deprivation, accelerated bone mineral loss leading to osteoporosis and skeletal fractures remains among the most debilitating. Complications following bone fractures are a leading cause of death in U.S. women over 65; as many as 26,000 die annually soon after hip fractures (68). For some women, evaluation of bone loss by densitometric methods after the menopause may come too late for effective estrogen replacement therapy. One recent study questions the value of bone densitometry in assessing fracture potential (69). Thus, a reliable objective metabolic test for use in conjunction with subjective criteria, including body habitus, diet, exercise, smoking, and other life-style factors, may be useful to physicians considering management for perimenopausal women.

In 1986, we reported that induction of an acute reversible hypo-estrogenic condition mimicking postmenopausal status by acute administration of a GnRH antagonist resulted in elevated urinary calcium excretion in a primate model (70). Importantly, those individuals with the highest calcium:creatinine ratios following GnRH antagonist administration and suppression of ovarian estrogen secretion also demonstrated the greatest increases in urinary calcium excretion following ovariectomy. Thus, these observations left open the possibility that a GnRH antagonist-based diagnostic test given in premenopausal conditions may be indicative of individual risk of osteoporosis in subsequent postmenopausal years. Unfortunately, at that time the studies in laboratory primates could not be extended into the clinic, because the first-generation GNRH antagonists were notoriously high in anaphylactic side-effects (71). However, in a recent study, utilizing the second-generation GNRH antagonist Nal-Glu, we have confirmed that the primate model for a premenopausal GnRH antagonist test has some predictive value for indicating risk of diminished bone density within 1 year after ovariectomy (72), and with the recent advent of GnRH antagonists with further reduced histamine-releasing effects (73–75), cautious initiation of human studies may be warranted.

References

1. Knobil E. The neuroendocrine control of the menstrual cycle. Recent Prog Horm Res 1980;36:53–88.
2. Crowley WF, McArthur JW. Stimulation of the normal menstrual cycle in Kallmann's syndrome by pulsatile administration of luteinizing hormone-releasing homone (LHRH). J Clin Endocrinol Metab 1980;51:173–5.
3. Leyendecker G, Wildt L, Hansmann M. Pregnancies following chronic intermittent (pulsatile) administration of GnRH by means of a portable pump ("Zyklomat")—a new approach to the treatment of infertility in hypo-thalamic amenorrhea. J Clin Endocrinol Metab 1980;51:1214–6.
4. Palermo R, Amodeo G, Navot D, Rozenwaks Z, Cittadini E. Concomitant gonadotropin-releasing hormone agonist and menotropin treatment for the synchronized induction of multiple follicles. Fertil Steril 1988;49:290–5.
5. Meldrum DR, Wisot A, Hamilton F, Gutlay AL, Huynh D, Kempton W. Timing of initiation and dose schedule of leuprolide influence the time course of ovarian suppression. Fertil Steril 1988;50:400–2.
6. Katayama KP, Roesler M, Gunnarson C, Stehlik E, Jagusch S. Short-term use of gonadotropin-releasing hormone agonist (leuprolide) for *in vitro* fertilization. J *In Vitro* Fertil Embryo Transf 1988;5:332–4.
7. Caspi E, Ron-El R, Golan A, et al. Results of *in vitro* fertilization and embryo transfer by combined long-acting gonadotropin-releasing hormone

analog D-Trp-6-luteinizing hormone-releasing hormone and gonadotropins. Fertil Steril 1989;51:95–9.

8. Droesch K, Muasher SJ, Brzyski RG, et al. Value of suppression with a gonadotropin-releasing hormone agonist prior to gonadotropin stimulation for *in vitro* fertilization. Fertil Steril 1989;51:292–7.

9. Sathanandan M, Warnes GM, Kirby CA, Petrucco OM, Mathews CD. Adjuvant leuprolide in normal, abnormal, and poor responders to controlled ovarian hyperstimulation for *in vitro* fertilization/gamete intrafallopian transfer. Fertil Steril 1989;51:998–1006.

10. Ashkenazi J, Dicker D, Feldberg D, Goldman GA, Yeshaya A, Goldman JA. The value of GnRH analogue therapy in IVF in women with unexplained infertility. Hum Reprod 1989;6:667–9.

11. Cheskowski RJ, Kruse LR, Nass TE. Improved pregnancy outcome with the addition of leuprolide acetate to gonadotropins for *in vitro* fertilization. Fertil Steril 1989;52:250–5.

12. Hodgen GD. Uses of GnRH analogs in IVF/Gift. Contemp Obstet Gynecol 1990;35:10–24.

13. Kenigsberg D, Littman BA, Williams RF, Hodgen GD. Medical hypophysectomy: II. Variability of ovarian response to gonadotropin therapy. Fertil Steril 1984;42:116–26.

14. Simon JA, Danforth DR, Hutchison JS, Hodgen GD. Characterization of recombinant DNA-derived human luteinizing hormone *in vitro* and *in vivo*: efficiency in ovulation induction and corpus luteum support. JAMA 1988; 259:3290–5.

15. Gordon K, Williams RF, Danforth DR, Hodgen GD. The use of a GnRH antagonist (antide) as adjunctive therapy with gonadotropins for ovulation induction in cynomolgus monkeys [Abstract]. Presented at the Canadian Fertility and Andrology Society annual meeting, Esterel, Quebec, 1990.

16. Netter A. Polycystic ovary syndrome. Fertil Steril 1990;54:182–3.

17. McKenna TJ. Pathogenesis and treatment of polycystic ovary syndrome. N Engl J Med 1988;318:558–62.

18. Franks S, Mason HD, Polson DW, Winston RML, Margara R, Reed MJ. Mechanism and management of ovulatory failure in women with polycystic ovary syndrome. Hum Reprod 1988;3:531–4.

19. Franks S. Polycystic ovary syndrome: a changing perspective. Clin Endocrinol 1989;31:87–120.

20. Salat-Baroux J, Alvarez S, Antoine JM, et al. Results of IVF in the treatment of polycystic ovary disease. Hum Reprod 1988;3:331–5.

21. Salat-Baroux J, Alvarez S, Antoine JM, et al. Comparison between long and short protocols of LHRH agonists in the treatment of polycystic ovary disease by in-vitro fertilization. Hum Reprod 1988;3:535–9.

22. Coney P. Polycystic ovarian disease: current concepts of pathophysiology and therapy. Fertil Steril 1984;42:667–82.

23. Barnes R, Rosenfield RL. The polycystic ovary syndrome: pathogenesis and treatment. Ann Intern Med 1989;110:386–99.

24. Fleming R, Haxton MJ, Hamilton MPR, et al. Successful treatment of infertile women with oligomenorrhea using a combination of an LHRH agonist and exogenous gonadotropins. Br J Obstet Gynaecol 1985;92:369–73.

25. Chang RJ, Laufer LR, Meldrum DR, et al. Steroidal secretion in polycystic ovarian disease after ovarian suppression by a long-acting gonadotropin-releasing hormone agonist. J Clin Endocrinol Metab 1983;56:897–903.
26. Andreyko JL, Monroe SE, Jaffe RB. Treatment of hirsutism with a gonadotropin-releasing hormone agonist (nafarelin). J Clin Endocrinol Metab 1986;63:854–9.
27. Couzinet B, Le Strat N, Brially S, Schaison G. Comparative effects of cyproterone acetate or a long-acting gonadotropin-releasing hormone agonist in polycystic ovarian disease. J Clin Endocrinol Metab 1986;63:1031–5.
28. Mongioi A, Maugeri G, Macchi M, et al. Effect of gonadotropin-releasing hormone analogue (GnRH-A) administration on serum gonadotropin and steroid levels in patients with polycystic ovarian disease. Acta Endocrinol (Copenh) 1986;111:228–34.
29. Calogero AE, Macchi M, Montanini V, et al. Dynamics of plasma gonadotropin and sex steroid release in polycystic ovarian disease after pituitary-ovarian inhibition with an analog of gonadotropin-releasing hormone. J Clin Endocrinol Metab 1987;64:980–5.
30. Steingold K, De Zeigler D, Cedars M, et al. Clinical and hormonal effects of chronic gonadotropin-releasing hormone agonist treatment in polycystic ovarian disease. J Clin Endocrinol Metab 1987;65:773–8.
31. Faure N, Lemay A. Ovarian suppression in polycystic ovarian disease during 6 month administration of luteinizing hormone-releasing hormone (LH-RH) agonist. Clin Endocrinol 1987;27:703–13.
32. Adashi EY. Potential utility of gonadotropin-releasing hormone agonists in the management of ovarian hyperandrogenism. Fertil Steril 1990;53:765–79.
33. Gordon K, Williams RF, Danforth DR, Hodgen GD. A novel regimen of GnRH antagonist plus pulsatile GnRH: controlled restoration of gonadotropin secretion and ovulation induction. Fertil Steril 1990;54:1140–5.
34. Buttram VC. Surgical treatment of endometriosis in the infertile female: a modified approach. Fertil Steril 1979;32:635–9.
35. Buttram VC, Belue JB, Reiter R. Interim report of a study of Danazol for the treatment of endometriosis. Fertil Steril 1982;37:478–83.
36. Schriock E, Monroe SE, Henzl M, Jaffe RB. Treatment of endometriosis with a potent agonist of gonadotropin-releasing hormone (nafarelin). Fertil Steril 1985;44:583–8.
37. Meldrum DR, Chang RJ, Lu J, Vale W, Rivier J, Judd HL. "Medical oophorectomy" using a long-acting GnRH agonist—a possible new approach to the treatment of endometriosis. J Clin Endocrinol Metab 1982;54:1081–3.
38. Werlin LB, Hodgen GD. Gonadotropin-releasing hormone agonist suppresses ovulation, menses, and endometriosis in monkeys: an individualized, intermittent regimen. J Clin Endocrinol Metab 1983;56:844–8.
39. Meldrum DR. Management of endometriosis with gonadotropin-releasing hormone agonists. Fertil Steril 1985;44:581–2.
40. Schally AV, Comaru-Schally A-M, Redding TW. Antitumor effects of analogs of hypothalamic hormones in endocrine-dependent cancers. Proc Soc Exp Biol Med 1984;174:259–81.
41. Walsh PC. Physiological basis for hormonal therapy in carcinoma of the prostate. Urol Clin North Am 1975;2:125–40.

42. Tolis G, Ackman D, Stellos A, et al. Tumor growth inhibition in patients with prostatic carcinoma treated with luteinizing hormone-releasing agonists. Proc Natl Acad Sci USA 1982;79:1658–62.

43. Schally AV, Redding TW, Comaru-Schally A-M. Potential use of analogs of luteinizing hormone-releasing hormone in the treatment of hormone-sensitive neoplasms. Cancer Treat Rep 1984;68:281–9.

44. Kerle D, Williams G, Ware H, Bloom SR. Failure of long term luteinizing hormone releasing hormone treatment for prostate cancer to suppress serum luteinizing hormone and testosterone. Br Med J 1984;289:468–9.

45. Tenover JS, Dahl KD, Vale WW, Rivier JE, Bremner WJ. Hormonal responses to a potent gonadotropin hormone-releasing hormone antagonist in normal elderly men. J Clin Endocrinol Metab 1990;71:881–8.

46. Kahan A, Delrieu F, Amor B, Chiche R, Steg A. Disease flare induced by D-Trp[6]-LHRH analogue in patients with prostatic cancer. Lancet 1984;1: 971–2.

47. Edelstein MJ, Gordon K, Williams RF, Danforth DR, Hodgen GD. Single dose long-term suppression of testosterone secretion by a gonadotropin-releasing hormone antagonist (antide) in male monkeys. Contraception 1990;42:209–16.

48. Bergquist C, Nillius SJ, Wide L. Intranasal gonadotropin-releasing hormone-releasing hormone agonist as a contraceptive agent. Lancet 1979;2:215–6.

49. Bergquist C, Nillius SJ, Wide L. Long-term intranasal luteinizing hormone-releasing hormone agonist treatment for contraception in women. Fertil Steril 1982;38:190–3.

50. Nillius SJ, Bergquist C, Wide L. Inhibition of ovulation in women by chronic treatment with a stimulatory LRH analogue—a new approach to birth control? Contraception 1978;17:537–45.

51. Lemay A, Faure N, Labrie F, Fazekas ATA. Inhibition of ovulation during discontinuous intranasal luteinizing hormone-releasing hormone agonist dosing in combination with gestagen-induced bleeding. Fertil Steril 1985;43: 868–77.

52. Linde R, Doelle GC, Alexander AN, et al. Reversible inhibition of testicular steroidogenesis and spermatogenesis by a potent gonadotropin releasing hormone agonist in normal men. N Engl J Med 1981;305:663–7.

53. Heber D, Swerdloff RS. Gonadotropin-releasing hormone analog and testosterone synergistically inhibit spermatogenesis. Endocrinology 1981;108: 2019–21.

54. Bhasin S, Yuan QX, Steiner BS, Swerdloff RS. Hormonal effects of gonadotropin-releasing hormone (GnRH) agonist in men: effects of long-term treatment with GnRH agonist infusion and androgen. J Clin Endocrinol Metab 1987;65:586–74.

55. Evans RM, Doelle GC, Alexander AN, Uderman HD, Rabin D. Gonadotropin and steroid secretory patterns during chronic treatment with a luteinizing hormone-releasing hormone agonist analog in men. J Clin Endocrinol Metab 1984;58:862–7.

56. Bagatell CJ, McLachlan RI, de Kretser DM, et al. A comparison of the suppressive effects of testosterone and a potent new gonadotropin-releasing hormone antagonist on gonadotropins and inhibin levels in normal men. J Clin Endocrinol Metab 1989;69:43–8.

57. Danforth DR, Williams RF, Hsiu JG, et al. Intermittent GnRH antagonist plus progestin contraception conserving tonic ovarian estrogen secretion and reducing progestin exposure. Contraception 1990;41:623–31.
58. Fraser HM, Dewart PJ, Smith SK, Cowen SK, Sandow J, McNeilly AS. Luteinizing hormone releasing hormone agonist for contraception in breast feeding women. J Clin Endocrinol Metab 1989;69:996–1002.
59. Nordon BEC, Horsman A, Grilly RG, Marshall DH, Simpson M. Treatment of spinal osteoporosis in postmenopausal women. Br Med J 1980;280:451–4.
60. Horsman A, Nordon BEC, Gallagher JC, Kirby PA, Milner RM, Simpson M. Observations of sequential changes in bone mass in postmenopausal women: a controlled trial of estrogen and calcium therapy. Calcif Tissue Res 1977;22(suppl):217–24.
61. Campbell S, Whitehead M. Estrogen therapy and the postmenopausal syndrome. Clin Obstet Gynecol 1977;4:1–30.
62. Mandel FP, Geola FL, Lu JKH, et al. Biological effects of various doses of equine estradiol in postmenopausal women. Obstet Gynecol 1982;59:673–9.
63. Stern MP, Brown BW, Haskell WL, Farquhar JW, Wehrle CL, Wood PDS. Cardiovascular risk and use of estrogens or estrogen-progestogen combinations. JAMA 1976;235:811–5.
64. Bradley DD, Wingard J, Petitti DB, Krauss RM, Ramcharan S. Serum high-density-lipoprotein cholesterol in women using oral contraceptives, estrogens and progestins. N Engl J Med 1978;299:17–20.
65. Nachtigall LE, Nachtigall RH, Nachtigall RD, Bechman EM. Estrogen replacement therapy: I. A 10-year prospective study in the relationship to osteoporosis. Obstet Gynecol 1979;53:277–81.
66. Hirvonen E, Malkonen M, Manninen V. Effects of different progestogens on lipoproteins during postmenopausal replacement therapy. N Engl J Med 1981;305:560–3.
67. Paffenberger RS Jr, Kampert JB, Chang H-G. Characteristics that predict risk of breast cancer before and after the menopause. Am J Epidemiol 1980;112:258–63.
68. Reese WD. A better way to screen for osteoporosis. Contemp Obstet Gynecol 1983;22:116–32.
69. Ott Sn, Kilcoyne RF, Chesnut CH III. Comparisons among methods of measuring bone mass and relationship to severity of vertebral fractures in osteoporosis. J Clin Endoocrinol Metab 1988;65:501–7.
70. Abbasi R, Hodgen GD. Predicting the predisposition to osteoporosis: gonadotropin-releasing hormone antagonist for acute estrogen deficiency test. JAMA 1986;255:1600–4.
71. Schmidt F, Sundaram K, Thau RB, Bardin CW. [Ac-D-Nal(2)^1,4FD-Phe^2, D-Trp^3,D-Arg^6]-LHRH, a potent antagonist of LHRH, produces transient edema and behavioral changes in rats. Contraception 1984;29:283–9.
72. Danforth DR, Itskovitz J, Chillik C, Hahn DW, McGuire JL, Hodgen GD. Test for risk of osteoporosis: one-year follow-up data on bone densitometry and second-generation gonadotropin releasing hormone (GnRH) antagonist. In: Koreman SG, ed. Menopause: biological and clinical consequences of ovarian failure—evaluation and management: proceedings of the Serono Symposium for Menopause, Napa, CA, March 5–8, 1989. New York: Plenum Press: 17–24.

73. Ljungqvist A, Feng D-M, Tang P-FL, et al. Design, synthesis and bioassays of antagonists of LHRH which have high antiovulatory activity and release negligible histamine. Biochem Biophys Res Commun 1987;148:849–56.
74. Ljungqvist A, Feng D-M, Hook WA, Shen Z-X, Bowers C, Folkers K. Antide and related antagonists of luteinizing hormone release with long action and oral activity. Proc Natl Acad Sci USA 1988;85:8236–40.
75. Ljungqvist A, Feng D-M, Bowers C, Hook WA, Folkers K. Antagonists of LHRH superior to antide: effective sequence/activity relationships. Tetrahedron 1990;46:3297–304.

22

Use of Gonadotropin Releasing Hormone Analogs to Influence Sexual and Behavioral Development

David R. Mann, Kenneth G. Gould, and Kim Wallen

GnRH analogs have been valuable experimental and clinical tools in studies of sexual and behavioral development. In this report, we will review recent work using GnRH antagonism to assess the importance of activation of the hypothalamic-pituitary-gonadal axis for normal sexual and behavioral development, and examine the impact of GnRH agonist treatment on reproductive development, secondary sex characteristics, and the growth velocity and skeletal maturation of children with true precocious puberty (TPP).

Use of GnRH Antagonism to Alter Sexual and Behavioral Development in Male Primates

The perinatal and early postnatal periods of primates are characterized by an activation of the hypothalamic-pituitary-testicular axis. Toward the end of gestation, LH levels in the umbilical cord blood are low and indistinguishable between human males and females (1, 2); but when measured in the peripheral blood at the time of birth, LH concentrations are significantly higher than in cord blood and 10-fold greater in male than in female infants (3). Serum LH concentrations begin to decline by 1 h after birth, and by 6 h there is no difference in levels between males and females. A secondary increase in LH secretion begins during week 2 in both sexes (4), but it appears earlier (5) and is of greater magnitude in boys than in girls (6–8). In infants, plasma FSH levels rise more rapidly and reach higher levels in girls than they do in boys (4). Plasma LH and FSH secretion reach maximum values (comparable to those in adults) in both sexes between 2 and 4 months of postnatal life and decline thereafter, approaching prepubertal levels by 1 year of age (4, 5, 7, 9). The neonatal pattern of gonadotropin secretion in a variety of other primate species is similar to that reported in humans (10–13).

The elevated levels of circulating LH in newborn boys increase production of testicular testosterone (3). Serum T doubles over the first 3 h and continues to increase over the next 9 h after birth in boys, whereas in girls serum T is low at birth and remains low over the next 21 h. Cord blood T levels in boys are low, but significantly higher than in newborn girls (14, 15). During this period, peripheral serum T levels are 3 to 4 times greater in boys than in girls (16). This rise of serum T in boys is short-lived, and within 2 to 4 days levels fall below values obtained shortly after birth (17, 18). A second rise in serum T begins during the second week of life in male infants, reaching peak levels between weeks 3 and 12 (4). The magnitude of this rise is 50 to 60% of adult levels (4, 7, 15, 16). Levels of serum T then fall gradually to low juvenile values by 6 to 8 months of life. In contrast, T values in female infants decline over the first month of life, and overall values average between 5 and 10% of levels in infant males during this period (4). Between 7 months and 2 years of age, there are no differences in serum T between males and females.

There is controversy as to the physiological significance of the neonatal increase in T secretion in male primates. While total serum T levels in male infants rise to values that approach the low normal range in adult men, apparently free T levels do not show a similar magnitude of change (19, 20). Salivary T concentration, which serves as an index of the free fraction of serum steroid (21), actually declines from the day of birth through 6 months of age in male infants (19, 20). Moreover, sex hormone binding globulin (SHBG) in the serum increases in boys and to a greater extent in girls in early infancy; and the free androgen index (ratio of T to SHBG) in infant boys is relatively low, being comparable to that in women (22). We have also observed a more than 4-fold increase in SHBG in male rhesus monkeys during the first 2 to 3 weeks of postnatal life (unpublished data). Thus, it has been postulated that the secondary peak in total serum T observed in infant boys between 1 month and 3 months of age may lack biological significance (20, 22).

On the other hand, the free androgen index in infant boys is 10-fold higher than that observed in infant girls (22); and the degree of which salivary T correlates with serum T in infants is not known (19). The changes in salivary T with age in infants are also at variance with data on levels of unbound T in infants (4, 7, 9). These investigators showed that the amount of bound T in the peripheral blood at birth was low, but increased rapidly over the first 2 weeks of life and then more gradually over the next 2 months to values comparable to those in the prepubertal child. The pattern of unbound T levels in the male infant paralleled that of total T, except that the unbound T peak between 1 month and 3 months of age did not reach adult male levels as it did on the day of birth. It is, therefore, premature to conclude that neonatal T is not physiologically important.

While it is well established that neonatal T contributes substantially to sexual differentiation in short-gestation rodents, such as rats and hamsters, it has generally been accepted that T exerts its influences on sexual differentiation prenatally in primates. However, there is some evidence that neonatal T may play a role in testicular descent, sexual differentiation of the central nervous system, and behavioral differentiation and development (23–31). Of particular interest is the demonstration of sexual dimorphism in the preoptic area (POA) and corpus callosum of the human brain (24, 29, 30). Histologic examination of the brains of men and women (10 to 93 years of age) revealed that in men the sexually dimorphic cell group (SDN) of the POA is 2.5-fold larger in size and contains 2.2 times more cells than in women, and that the volume and number of cells in the SDN decrease with age in both sexes (29). Sexual dimorphism of this nucleus, however, does not develop during gestation, but is only present after 4 years of postnatal life (30). It was postulated that T secretion in the male facilitates later cell survival by interfering with programmed cell death that occurs in the female SDN (30). The volume and number of cells in the SDN appear independent of the adult hormonal environment, since measurements of the POA of a 46-year-old woman with a virilizing tumor in the adrenal cortex did not differ from other female values. These data are similar to those reports indicating that the size of the SDN of POA of the rat is independent of adult sex hormone treatment (31). The POA is involved in the regulation of gonadotropin secretion and sexual behavior in a number of mammalian species (32–35). The function of the SDN in rats and humans has yet to be clarified (29), but it may inhibit female sexual behavior in males. Although lesions encompassing the SDN failed to influence sexual behavior of male rats (35), animals with these lesions show excellent female sexual behavior in response to estrogen treatment and show a progesterone facilitation of female sexual behavior not seen in neurologically intact males (36, 37). In this regard, it is intriguing that the size of the SDN in three male transsexuals was outside the range of normal males and comparable to that of female SDNs (30).

A sex difference has also been reported in the shape and size of the corpus callosum of the human brain (24). The caudal part of the corpus callosum is larger and more bulbous in the female than in the male. This area is of special interest because of its possible importance in determining sex differences in the degree of cerebral lateralization for visuospatial function, which may be related to the ability of men to perform better on spatial measures (27, 38). Moreover, men with idiopathic hypogonadotropic hypogonadism and resulting androgen deficiency have impaired spatial ability compared with controls or with men who developed hypogonadism after the onset of puberty (26). Androgen therapy does not correct the behavioral deficit. These data suggest that the presence of androgen before (such as during the neonatal period) or at the time of puberty has an important organizational effect on the CNS that results in the sex difference in spatial ability of adults. Of particular importance is that patients with idiopathic hypogonadotropic hypogonadism possess a normal 46, XY genotype and that the level of prenatal masculinization is nearly normal, suggesting that sex differences in spatial ability develop postnatally (26).

Despite these clinical data suggesting a permanent organization effect of postnatal T on CNS, it has generally been accepted that neonatal T secretion is of little consequence in the normal process of sexual and behavioral development in male primates. However, to the best of our knowledge, we are the first group to assess directly the possible importance of neonatal activation of the pituitary-testicular axis on developmental processes in primates (39, 40).

During the birth seasons of 1983 and 1984, we treated eight male infant rhesus monkeys with a GnRH agonist (10 µg/day of D-Trp^6-N-α-Me-Leu^7-des-Gly^{10}-Pro^9-NHEt-GnRH; Wyeth-Ayerst Laboratories), using osmotic minipumps beginning at 10 to 13 days of age for 112 days. These infants were part of a large (79 subjects) heterosexual group of animals maintained in a 30×30-m outdoor compound with an indoor housing and capture area. Animals were maintained with their mother in this group throughout the first 3 years of life. Serum LH (bioactive) and T concentrations in control infants were elevated to the low normal range of adult males during the period from 10 to 60 days of age before gradually declining to low prepubertal values by 120 to 130 days of age (Fig. 22.1). In contrast, GnRH agonist infusion caused a precipitous fall of LH and T levels to prepubertal values during the first 2 weeks of treatment, where they remained throughout the first 6 months of postnatal life. It is likely that the GnRH agonist reduced basal LH secretion in neonates by down-regulating pituitary GnRH receptors, as has been reported in adult rats (41), since the LH response to a large bolus of GnRH (5 µg/kg BW) was abolished during GnRH infusion (39). The results suggested that the pituitary of neonates is functional, similar to the adult pituitary (42, 43), in its response to the inhibitory actions of chronically administered GnRH agonists.

It appears that the neonatal surge of T secretion does not have an effect on somatic growth in male infants. Crown-rump length and body weight over the first 20 weeks of postnatal life did not differ between control and GnRH agonist-treated infants (39, 40). This is in contrast to the peripubertal monkey, in which the surge of T is of primary importance for the pubertal growth spurt (44).

The juvenile (6 months to 3 years of age) pattern of basal LH and T secretion did not differ between control monkeys and those treated neonatally with a GnRH agonist (40). Serum LH and T levels during this period were low, and the pituitary and testicular response to exogenous GnRH was minimal (40). Apparently the GnRH pulse generator that becomes functional in the fetus and continues to function in the neonate

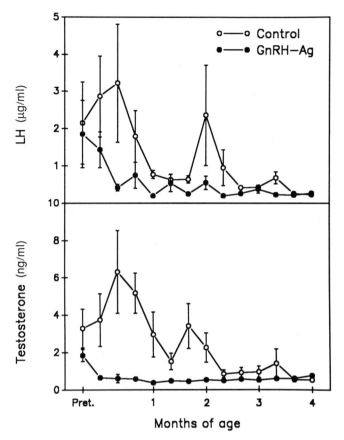

FIGURE 22.1. Mean (±SEM) levels of serum LH (top) and testosterone (bottom) in control (n = 10) and GnRH agonist-treated (n = 8) infant male monkeys. Treatment was initiated between 10 and 13 days of age and was continued for 112 days. These graphs represent the combined data from Refs. 39 and 40.

shuts down and remains quiescent during the juvenile period (45–47). Neonatal T does not appear to play a role in the shutdown of the GnRH pulse generator, since the decline in LH secretion occurs at approximately the same time in intact male monkeys and in animals orchidectomized at 1 week of age (46, 47).

Male monkeys raised in large heterosexual groups in outdoor compounds at the Yerkes Regional Primate Research Center begin to show signs of increased gonadal function during the early portion of the breeding season (September–January) during their fourth year of life (approximately 3.5 years of age) (48). The peripubertal period is characterized by a rapid increase in testicular volume (40), an increase in the pituitary and testicular response to GnRH (40), a seasonal rise in

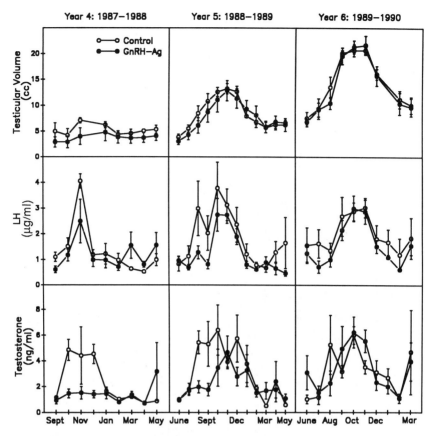

FIGURE 22.2. Seasonal changes (mean ± SEM) in testicular volume (top), serum LH (middle), and testosterone (bottom) during years 4, 5, and 6 in control (n = 4) and GnRH agonist-treated (n = 6) monkeys. The data in this figure are from animals born in 1984.

serum T (40, 48), an increase in the frequency of sexual behavior over year 3 (48), and a decline in play behavior (48). During year 4, all four control males showed seasonal rises in serum LH and T, and testicular volume, whereas the six treated males showed either blunted or no peripubertal changes in these parameters (Fig. 22.2). The treated males fell into two distinct groups: Three had a subnormal, but significant rise in serum T and showed responses to electroejaculation (40). The other three treated males showed a significant rise neither in serum T nor in ejaculatory response (Fig. 22.3A). Thus, GnRH agonist treatment during the neonatal period resulted in a hypogonadotropic-hypogonadal condition that persisted through the expected peripubertal period (40). In addition, those treated males that did not show a peripubertal rise in serum T during year 4 were found to have mounted (P < 0.05) and

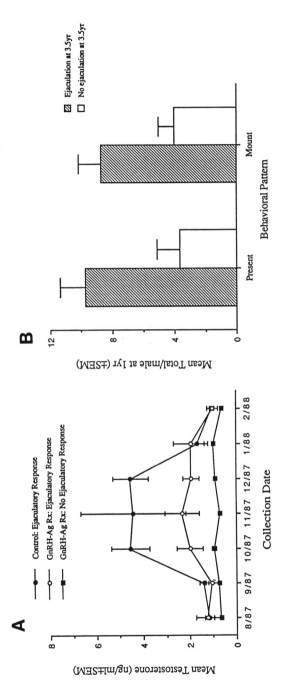

FIGURE 22.3. (A) Peripubertal changes in serum testosterone concentrations (mean ± SEM) in control and GnRH agonist-treated monkeys born in 1984. The treated animals fell into two distinct groups: three animals exhibited a subnormal, but significant, rise in testosterone and responses to electroejaculation; the other three showed a significant rise neither in serum testosterone nor in ejaculatory response. (B) Mean (±SEM) total presents and mounts in their social group during year 1 of treated monkeys that did or did not exhibit a peripubertal rise in serum testosterone during year 4.

presented (P < 0.06) less in their social group at 1 year of age than did males showing a rise in serum T at 4 years of age (Fig. 22.3B). These results suggest that neonatal T suppression not only delays the pubertal onset of testicular function, but also produces differences in juvenile sexual behavior exhibited before the onset of pubertal activation of testes and after the cessation of neonatal testicular activity. This is the first evidence in rhesus monkeys that the organizing influence of T on male sexual behavior is not limited to prenatal development but continues into the neonatal period.

We have continued to closely monitor hypothalamic-pituitary-testicular function of these 6 treated and 4 control males. During years 5 and 6, seasonal changes in testicular volumes, serum LH, and T between treated monkeys and controls no longer differed statistically (Fig. 22.2); but a close examination of the data suggests a mild, but persistent, hypo-gonadotropic hypogonadal condition in the treated animals.

We have been attempting recently to determine the site(s) of the lesion responsible for the hypogonadotropic-hypogonadal state. Neither pituitary nor testicular function appears to be abnormal in these animals, since the pituitary and testicular responses to two physiological boli of GnRH (separated by 1 h) during year 6 did not differ between control and GnRH agonist-treated monkeys (Fig. 22.4A).

When N-methyl-D-aspartate, an analogue of aspartate, is administered peripherally to rhesus monkeys it stimulates GnRH discharge into the hypophyseal portal vessels and induces LH secretion. This NMDA-stimulated LH secretion is blocked by pretreatment of prepubertal rhesus monkeys with a GnRH receptor or NMDA receptor antagonist (49). It has been postulated that NMDA receptors may play a role in triggering the onset of puberty in primates, since intermittent NMDA adminis-tration to juvenile male monkeys induces precocious puberty (50). Because of the possible importance of the NMDA receptor in mediating reactivation of GnRH secretion at the time of puberty, we evaluated the response to NMDA of control monkeys and animals treated neonatally with a GnRH agonist.

During the nonbreeding season of the sixth year, control and treated monkeys were given a single IV pulse of 5 mg/kg BW of NMDA. Control monkeys showed a significant increment of serum LH (P < 0.05) and a 2-to 4-fold rise in serum T (P < 0.05) in response to NMDA (Fig. 22.4B). In contrast, basal LH and T levels were lower, and there was no sig-nificant LH and T response to NMDA in treated monkeys. These preliminary data need to be repeated using multiple doses of NMDA in a larger number of animals. However, if confirmed, they would suggest that the persistent hypogonadotropic hypogonadism in adult male monkeys treated neonatally with a GnRH agonist may result from a subnormal sensitivity of the CNS to one or more of its excitatory neurotransmitters (e.g., aspartate or glutamate). Thus, abolishing the neonatal surge of

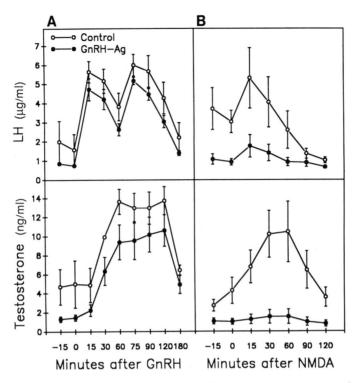

FIGURE 22.4. Mean (±SEM) serum LH (top) and testosterone (bottom) responses to GnRH (A, 50 ng/kg BW at 0 and 60 min) and NMDA (B, 5 mg/kg BW at 0 min) in control and GnRH agonist-treated monkeys during year 6.

T with a GnRH agonist may permanently alter development and differentiation of CNS centers that either are involved in episodic GnRH secretion or govern this process.

There was evidence that the GnRH agonist treatment may have influenced fertility potential during years 4, 5, and 6. Treated monkeys responded to electroejaculation during year 4 less frequently (21.4% of attempts) than did controls (62.5% of attempts), most likely reflecting the subnormal peripubertal rise in serum T in these animals. During years 5 and 6, the frequency of ejaculation did not differ between controls and treated monkeys. Sperm count was highly variable and not different between the groups at any age; however, counts tended to be higher during years 4 ($323 \pm 273 \times 10^6$ versus $131 \pm 80 \times 10^6$/ml) and 5 ($260 \pm 83 \times 10^6$ versus $95 \pm 50 \times 10^6$/ml) in the treated animals, possibly as a result of retarded sexual accessory gland development.

At 6 years of age, adult sexual behavior was tested with six estrogen-treated, ovariectomized females. Sexual behavior was assessed during 2-h tests given 3 days per week for 4 weeks in the spring and 4 weeks in the summer. During behavioral tests, all 10 males were observed with the six females as a group. This testing procedure provided opportunities for competition between the males that might reveal differences in sexual initiative between the GnRH agonist-treated males and the controls. Measures of initiation of proximity as well as traditional copulatory measures of mounts, intromissions, and ejaculations were recorded. In addition, agnostic interactions between males and between females and males were recorded. In this preliminary analysis, we report primarily on the measures of copulatory behavior. The females either received daily injections of 6 µg/kg BW estradiol-17β or received two 4-cm silastic implants containing crystalline estradiol. This was designed to maximize the availability of sexually responsive females, since it was not known which estradiol treatment would be most effective in group-housed animals where the influence of the female's hormonal condition is quite different than that traditionally seen in laboratory pair-tests (51). Behavioral tests were given at two different times to test for seasonal variation in sexual behavior. The observations reported here represent the end of the breeding season (March and April) and the middle of the nonbreeding season (June and July). A third set of tests is currently in progress during the peak of the breeding season. Complete assessment of the behavioral characteristics of these males will have to await the data from the peak of the breeding season; however, there are indications that neonatal treatment with a GnRH agonist may have influenced the adult sexual behavior of these males.

Three of four control males ejaculated at least once during the spring or summer behavioral tests, as opposed to four of the six experimental males. Across all tests, treated males displayed lower frequencies of mounts, intromissions, and ejaculations than the control males, although none of these differences reached statistical significance. For example, treated males averaged 2.24 ± 1.60 mounts per test in the spring and 2.51 ± 1.42 mounts in the summer, the control males averaged 10.13 ± 6.61 mounts per test in the spring and 4.73 ± 2.80 mounts per test in the summer ($f1,8 = 2.44$, $P = 0.15$). Unfortunately, the small numbers of animals and the relatively low levels of sexual behavior by both groups of males produced high variability in the study, even though the control males typically displayed 2 to 3 times the frequencies of mounts and intromissions of treated males. The mounting behavior of the controls, but not the treated males, seemed to vary with the season. The results of the fall breeding season should allow us to determine whether these males differ in sensitivity to seasonal cues as well as in their sexual competency.

Somatic growth has been retarded in monkeys that were not exposed to elevated neonatal levels of T. While body weight has not differed significantly between treated and control monkeys over the first six years of their lives, crown-rump ($P < 0.025$) and tibia ($P < 0.025$) lengths and bone mineral density ($P < 0.025$) of the lumbar spine were subnormal in

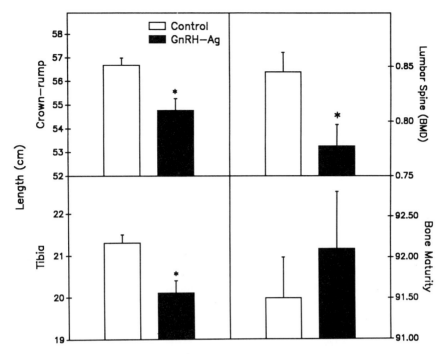

FIGURE 22.5. Mean (±SEM) crown-rump (top left) and tibia (bottom left) length, bone mineral density of lumbar spine (top right), and bone maturity scores (bottom right) in control and GnRH agonist-treated monkeys during year 6. * = Significantly different from the control at P < 0.05 or better.

treated monkeys at 6 years of age (Fig. 22.5). Conversely, bone maturity scores, based on a modified Tanner-Whitehouse system for humans (52) and evaluated by J.M. Tanner, did not differ between controls and treated monkeys (Fig. 22.5). In fact, two of the treated animals, but none of the controls, had achieved full adult bone maturity by 6 years of age, suggesting that the retarded skeletal development in treated monkeys may be permanent. The causes of this effect on the skeletal system remain to be determined. However, peripubertal and seasonal changes in serum insulin-like growth factor-1 (IGF-1) and growth hormone (GH) did not differ between treated monkeys and controls during years 4, 5, or 6 (unpublished data), suggesting that differences in the secretion of these important metabolic hormones do not account for the observed differences in skeletal development. On the other hand, the IGF-1 and GH data are based on monthly morning blood samples. More frequent sampling, including nocturnal, may have detected less obvious differences in GH and IGF-1 between the treated group and controls.

We are uncertain whether neonatal T has direct permanent organizational effect on regulatory systems governing reproduction and skeletal development or whether the disruption of neonatal T secretion retards development of the hypothalamic-pituitary-testicular axis and this in turn impacts on skeletal maturation and sexual behavior. However, we envision neonatal activation of the pituitary-testicular axis of male monkeys as one important event in a continuum of in utero and postnatal events that are needed to ensure normal sexual and behavioral differentiation. The data suggest that the disruption of neonatal T secretion in primates impairs normal development of CNS centers regulating peripubertal reactivation of pulsatile GnRH secretion and the timing of the onset of puberty. Thus, important peripubertal events, such as testicular enlargement and the peripubertal LH and T surge, are subnormal or delayed, and a mild hypogonadotropic-hypogonadal condition persists in these animals as adults. There are some clinical data to suggest that postnatal androgen can alter development of central nervous centers regulating the onset of puberty. Young children (boys and girls less than 8 years old) with congenital adrenal hyperplasia that were diagnosed after 4 years of age experienced the onset of true puberty shortly after the initiation of treatment to suppress adrenal function (53). This suggests that the elevated levels of androgens seen in these patients may have hastened the reawakening of the GnRH pulse generator, resulting in premature onset of puberty.

Neonatal T may also have an organizing influence on male sexual behavior. These data need to be confirmed in a larger group of monkeys, and such efforts are currently underway; however, if confirmed, it would suggest that T's organizing influence is not limited to the prenatal period in primates. The recent finding that the behavior of female rhesus monkeys can be masculinized by androgen treatment late in gestation without masculinizing the female's genitalia (54) supports the idea that there may be several "critical" periods (63) of sensitivity to the organizing actions of androgens for different developmental systems. Our results suggest an early neonatal period of organization in the developing monkey. One might also postulate that conditions (e.g., premature delivery, stress; 55) that significantly alter neonatal T secretion may affect later development.

Other investigators are in the process of examining the importance of gonadotropin and T secretion on sexual maturation in primates (56, 57). Male monkey fetuses were injected with a long-acting GnRH agonist depot at 75 days of gestation and at day 1 and 3 months of neonatal life. Plasma LH, FSH, and T levels were subnormal in treated animals during the first 3 postnatal months, and treated monkeys exhibited microphallus and reduced testicular size at 6 months of age. GnRH agonist treatment did not alter bone density in these animals. It was concluded that prenatal and neonatal gonadotropin and T secretions are essential for normal virilization, but not for normal skeletal maturation in neonates. The effects of this treatment on subsequent sexual development have not yet been reported, but a comparison between the data from this study and our own should establish the relative importance of the late gestational and early neonatal periods of gonadal function to subsequent sexual maturation.

Use of GnRH Antagonism to Alter Sexual and Behavioral Development in Rats

Rats are less well developed at birth than are primates, with the early neonatal period of the rat being equivalent to the midgestational period of human development (58). GnRH antagonists have been utilized to examine the potential role of neonatal activity of the pituitary-testicular axis of the rat on sexual and behavioral differentiation (58–62).

GnRH antagonists were administered to male rats to suppress pituitary gonadotropin secretion at intervals during the first 3 weeks of life, and parameters of sexual maturation and function were monitored through 160 days of age (58–60). Administration of a GnRH antagonist (twice daily) to male rats on days 1 through 15 of age was associated with a delayed onset of puberty (balano-preputial separation) and reduced fertility (59). Although there was an initial delay in pubertal activation of Leydig cell function and, therefore, the peripubertal rise in serum T, by 90 days Leydig cell function had fully recovered and serum T levels were actually supranormal. Despite the elevated levels of serum T, serum LH concentrations were also elevated, suggesting that a resetting of the hypothalamic set-point of the negative feedback system for testicular T secretion had occurred. Moreover, elevated serum FSH levels, reduced numbers of Sertoli cells, and subnormal testes weights in adult animals suggested that postnatal GnRH antagonist suppression of FSH secretion had permanently damaged tubular function (59, 61). Elevated FSH secretion in these animals may be caused by reduced inhibin secretion (61). It appears that the first 2 to 3 weeks of life in the male rat may be a critical period for development of the hypothalamic negative feedback systems regulating LH and FSH secretion and for maturation of testicular tubular function.

Experiments have also been performed to determine whether specific periods of sensitivity exist in the early postnatal period of male rats that are responsible for changes in hypothalamic-pituitary-testicular function that occur during sexual maturation (60). Induction of a gonadotropin deficiency for varying 5-day periods between days 1 and 15 delayed the onset of puberty and reduced adult testes weight and fertility (by as much as 88%). The pronounced impaired fertility was not the result of gross abnormality of spermatogenesis, since motile sperm were present in the epididymis and produced a 100% pregnancy rate when used for artificial insemination (59–61). Certain of the effects (e.g., reduced adult testes weight and testicular FSH receptors) of the GnRH antagonist were independent of the timing of the treatment period. However, reduced numbers of testicular LH receptors only occurred in animals treated between days 1 and 5, and fertility effects were most pronounced in, but not entirely confined to, the youngest treatment group.

The disruption of gonadotropin secretion during the first 2 weeks of life in the male rats appears to alter differentiation of brain centers important to male sexual behavior, resulting in infertility (58, 62). Treated animals had elevated male sexual interest (anogenital inspection) in females, but exhibited an inability to ejaculate (62). The development of the sexual dimorphic nucleus of the spinal cord of rats appears dependent on neonatal secretion of androgens, and this motor nucleus may be necessary for penile reflexes in adults (63). Deficient secretion of androgen during postnatal life may, therefore, impair the ability of the male to perform sexually, resulting in reduced fertility (60). Alternatively, GnRH antagonist treatment initiated after the early period (postnatal day 6) of brain sensitivity to steroids also altered adult male sexual behavior, suggesting a possible direct central organizing effect of the antagonist on sexual behavior (62). The central processing of external sexual stimuli may be impaired, or the peripheral sensitivity to these stimuli is attenuated by early postnatal administration (before 3 weeks of age) of a GnRH antagonist (62).

Neonatal activation of the pituitary-testicular axis may also be important for programming CNS centers that subsequently regulate the pubertal secretion of IGF-1 (64). GnRH antagonist treatment of neonatal rats (days 1 to 6), but not prepubertal castration, reduced the magnitude of the pubertal surge of IGF-1 (64). These data support the contention that activation of the pituitary-gonadal axis is involved in programming the pubertal surge in IGF-1, but this surge of IGF-1 occurs independently of a functional peripubertal gonad.

In females, the effects of postnatal GnRH antagonist treatment on reproductive function are transient and far less pronounced (65). Administration of a GnRH antagonist at 6, 9, 12, and 15 days of age attenuated the normal gonadotropin surge of prepubertal rats and reduced ovarian weights at first estrus, although other parameters of sexual maturation (e.g., age at first estrus and number of eggs shed at first ovulation) and fertility at 4 months were normal. This study suggested that GnRH antagonist administration did not have organizational effects on CNS centers regulating gonadotropin secretion or sexual behavior in the female rats, and that postnatal differentiation of these centers in the female proceed independently of the influence of GnRH and ovarian steroids.

GnRH antagonists have also been used to establish the importance of the prepubertal elevation of serum FSH and LH on the recruitment of primordial follicles into the pool of growing follicles (66, 67). A GnRH antagonist administered on days 6, 9, 12, and 15 of age reduced the number of growing follicles and increased the number of primordial follicles at 15 and 28 days of age; but on the day of first estrus and at 90 and 300 days of age, there was no difference in the two follicle pools between control and treated rats. Thus, the prepubertal gonadotropin surge in rats is important for recruitment of follicles into the growing pool, but is not a prerequisite for sexual maturation or later female cyclicity. At the time of first estrus, a control of follicular dynamics is established, that is for the most part independent of prepubertal gonadotropin secretion and follicle dynamics.

Use of GnRH Antagonism to Treat True Precocious Puberty

TPP results when there is premature (approximately 50% before the age of 6 years) activation of the GnRH pulse generator resulting in physical, behavioral, and hormonal changes that are characteristic of normal puberty. The elevated circulating levels of gonadotropin cause premature maturation of the gonads and increased sex steroid secretion, leading to the development of secondary sexual characteristics, an acceleration of linear growth, and skeletal maturation. TPP occurs more frequently in girls than in boys.

TPP has been managed and treated with medroxyprogesterone, cyproterone acetate, and a variety of potent GnRH agonists (68, 69). Until 1980, medroxyprogesterone and cyproterone acetate were used exclusively to treat TPP and were effective in slowing the rate of sexual development and blunting sexual behavior (70–74), but were not fully effective in suppressing gonadotropin secretion or decelerating the rate of bone maturation (71, 72, 75–77). These drugs also had significant side-effects related to their inherent progestational and glucocorticoid activity (72, 78, 79).

GnRH agonists have a paradoxical inhibitory action on reproductive function when administered chronically (43, 80). The earlier studies utilizing GnRH agonists to treat TPP employed the D-Trp^6,Pro^9 ethylamide analog administered by daily subcutaneous injection (81–83). More recent studies have used the intranasal or intramuscular (depot preparations; monthly) modes of administration (84–88). Although there have been differences in the effectiveness of the analogs related to their potency and bioavailability, overall GnRH agonists have been an effective and efficacious method of treating TPP for prolonged intervals of time (6–7 years).

Chronic GnRH agonist therapy (after a latency period of 2 to 4 weeks) reduces the secretion of gonadotropin and sex steroids to prepubertal levels, causes regression of the physical signs of puberty (e.g. in girls, cessation of menses, reduced ovarian size, and breast fullness; in boys, reduced testes size and pubic hair), reduces sexual behavior, decreases the growth velocity and the rate of skeletal maturation, and improves the predicted final height of children with TPP (68, 81–85). Following the termination of treatment, sexual maturation resumes promptly with onset of menses in girls within a year and presence of pubertal levels of T in boys within 6 months (68, 87–89). Only one group has reported on the actual height obtained in TPP patients after the termination of treatment with GnRH agonists (87). Of eight girls treated for TPP that have achieved their final height, four reached a final height that was above, three reached a final height equal to, and one reached a final height below posttreatment prediction. All girls were above or equal to pretreatment height predictions. The number of subjects was very limited and the period of time on treatment was highly variable (1 year, 3 months to 5 years, 2 months), but these very preliminary data on final height in TPP patients treated with a GnRH agonist are at least promising.

Few adverse effects have resulted from GnRH agonist treatment of TPP children. A few patients showed a local hypersensitivity response, and one exhibited an analphylactic reaction to the $D\text{-Trp}^6,\text{Pro}^9$ ethylamide analog (68). Three of 14 girls experienced frequent hot flushes. Allergic reactions were also reported in 2 of 20 girls treated with Naferelin (68). During the initial phase of treatment with another analog (Buserelin; intranasal administration), there was an increased frequency of aggressive behavior and masturbation in one of three boys and an increased incidence of vaginal bleeding in girls (86). It was recommended that simultaneous cyproterone acetate administration during the first month of treatment might minimize the side-effects associated with the initial stimulation of gonadotropin and sex steroids by GnRH agonists. The determination of whether or not the administration of GnRH agonists to children for as long as 6 to 8 years will have any significant effects on adult reproductive potential and behavioral processes will have to await the full assessment of these patients after they reach adulthood.

Treatment of TPP children with GnRH agonists provides an opportunity to examine the importance of gonadal and adrenal sex steroids, IGF-1, and GH on skeletal development and maturation, and to assess the involvement of sex steroids in driving the pubertal rise in IGF-1 and GH secretion (68, 90). The decline in the linear growth velocity in young TPP children (all were preadrenarchal and less than 5 years of age) treated for 2 years with a GnRH agonist to suppress ovarian steroidogenesis was associated with a reduction in the nocturnal surges of serum GH and plasma IGF-1 (90). These data also suggested that the pubertal rise in the growth velocity is mediated in part by gonadal hormone-stimulated GH secretion. Interestingly, the growth velocity of TPP patients treated with GnRH agonists does not correlate with IGF-1 levels (68, 90–92). Circulating IGF-1 levels decline in these patients to levels that are appropriate for bone age, not chronological age, suggesting that the onset of puberty causes changes in IGF-1 secretion that are not reversed when gonadal sex steroid secretion is suppressed with GnRH agonists (90).

Important information on the sex steroid regulation of GH-independent growth has been provided by a subset of TPP patients that are also GH-deficient (68). Before treatment with a GnRH agonist, height was appropriate for chronological age in this group but was less than in TPP patients with normal GH levels. Bone age was less advanced in the GH-deficient group, but the growth velocities were elevated and similar in the two groups. After 1 year of treatment with a GnRH agonist, the growth velocity was reduced in both groups, but was less in the group that was GH-deficient. Administration of GH eliminated this difference in growth rate. The data suggested that sex steroids were of greater importance to the pubertal growth spurt than is GH.

Summary

We have briefly reviewed contributions made using GnRH antagonism toward our understanding of developmental processes. The contributions have been substantial and significant, and with the continued future development and availability of more potent GnRH analogs, should continue to add to our knowledge in this area.

Acknowledgments. This work was supported by NIH Grants HD-26423, RR-08248 (via cofunding from the NIMH), and RR-00165. We thank Wyeth-Ayerst Laboratories for providing the GnRH agonist used in our studies, the NIDDK and Drs. Gordon Niswender and Leo Reichert, Jr., for providing bioassay and radioimmunoassay reagents, and Dr. J.M. Tanner for determining bone maturity scores.

References

1. Crosignani PG, Nencioni T, Brambati B. Concentration of chorionic gonadotropin and chorionic somatomammotrophin in maternal serum, amniotic fluid and cord serum at term. J Obstet Gynaecol 1972;79:122–6.
2. Penny R, Olambiwonnu O, Frasier D. Follicle stimulating hormone (FSH) and luteinizing hormone-human chorionic gonadotropin (LH-HCG) concentrations in paired maternal and cord sera. Pediatrics 1974;53:41–7.
3. Corbier P, Dehennin L, Castanier M, Mebazaa A, Edwards DA, Roffi J. Sex differences in serum luteinizing hormone and testosterone in the human neonate during the first few hours after birth. J Clin Endocrinol Metab 1990;71:1344–8.
4. Forest MG. Pituitary gonadotropin and sex steroid secretion during the first two years of life. In: Grumbach MM, Sizonenko PC, Auberrt ML, eds.

Control of the onset of puberty. Baltimore: Williams & Wilkins, 1990: 451–77.

5. Winter JSD, Faiman C, Hobson WC, Prasad AV, Reyes FI. Pituitary-gonadal relations in infancy: I. Patterns of serum gonadotropin concentrations from birth to four years of age in man and chimpanzee. J Clin Endocrinol Metab 1975;40:545–51.

6. Faiman C, Winter JSD. Sex differences in gonadotrophin concentrations in infancy. Nature 1971;232:130–1.

7. Forest MG, Sizonenko PC, Cathiard AM, Bertrand J. Hypophysogonadal function in infants during the first year of life: I. Evidence for testicular activity in early infancy. J Clin Invest 1974;53:819–28.

8. Ryle M, Stephenson J, Williams J, Stuart J. Serum gonadotrophins in young children. Clin Endocrinol 1975;4:413–9.

9. Penny R, Olambiwonnu N, Frasier SD. Serum gonadotrophin concentrations during the first four years of life. J Clin Endocrinol Metab 1974;38:320–1.

10. Mann DR, Castracane VD, McLaughlin F, Gould KG, Collins DC. Developmental patterns of serum luteinizing hormone, gonadal and adrenal steroids in the sooty mangabey (*Cercocebus atys*). Biol Reprod 1983;28:279–84.

11. Frawley LS, Neill JD. Age related changes in serum levels of gonadotropins and testosterone in infantile male rhesus monkeys. Biol Reprod 1979;20: 1147–51.

12. Fuller GB, Faiman C, Winter JSD, Reyes FI, Hobson WC. Sex-dependent gonadotropin concentrations in intact chimpanzees and rhesus monkeys. Proc Soc Exp Biol Med 1982;169:494–500.

13. Steiner R, Bremner WJ. Endocrine correlates of sexual development in the male monkey, *Macaca fascicularis*. Endocrinology 1981;109:914–9.

14. Forest MG, Cathiard AM, Bertrand J. Total and unbound testosterone levels in the newborn and in normal and hypogonadal children: use of a sensitive radioimmunoassay for testosterone. J Clin Endocrinol Metab 1973;36: 1132–42.

15. Pang S, Levine LS, Chow D, Sagiani F, Saenger P, New MI. Dihydrotestosterone and its relationship to testosterone in infancy and childhood. J Clin Endocrinol Metab 1979;48:821–6.

16. Forest MG, Cathiard AM. Pattern of plasma testosterone and ⁴androstenedione in normal newborns: evidence for testicular activity at birth. J Clin Endocrinol Metab 1975;41:977–80.

17. Stahl F, Götz F, Poppe I, Amendt P, Dörner G. Pre- and early postnatal testosterone levels in rat and human. In: Dörner G, Kawakami M, eds. Hormones and brain development. Amsterdam: Elsevier, 1978:99–109.

18. Tapanainen J. Hormonal changes during the perinatal period: serum testosterone, some of its precursors, and FSH and prolactin in preterm and fullterm male infant cord blood and during the first week of life. J Steroid Biochem 1983;18:13–8.

19. Huhtaniemi I, Dunkel L, Perheentupa J. Transient increase in postnatal testicular activity is not revealed by longitudinal measurements of salivary testosterone. Pediatr Res 1986;20:1324–7.

20. Huhtaniemi IT, Warren DW. Ontogeny of pituitary-gonadal interactions: current advances and controversies. Trends Endocrinol Metab 1990;1: 356–62.

21. Riad-Fahmy D, Read GF, Walker RF, Griffiths K. Steroids in saliva for assessing endocrine function. Endocrinol Rev 1982;3:367–95.
22. Bolton NJ, Tapanainen J, Koivisto M, Vihko R. Circulating sex hormone-binding globulin and testosterone in newborns and infants. Clin Endocrinol 1989;31:201–7.
23. Hadziselimovic F. Pathogenesis and treatment of undescended testes. Eur J Pediatr 1982;139:255–65.
24. de Lacoste-Utamsing C, Holloway RL. Sexual dimorphism in the human corpus callosum. Science 1982;216:1431–2.
25. MacLuskey NJ, Naftolin F. Sexual differentiation of the central nervous system. Science 1981;211:1294–303.
26. Hier DB, Crowley WF Jr. Spatial ability in androgen-deficient men. N Engl J Med 1982;306:1202–5.
27. Gur RC, Gur RE, Obrist WD, et al. Sex and handedness differences in cerebral blood flow during rest and cognitive activity. Science 1982;217:659–61.
28. Money J, Schwartz M, Lewis VG. Adult erotosexual status and fetal hormonal masculinization and demasculinization: 46,XX congenital virilizing adrenal hyperplasia and 46,XY androgen-insensitivity syndrome compared. Psychoneuroendocrinology 1984;9:405–14.
29. Swaab DF, Fliers E. A sexually dimorphic nucleus in the human brain. Science 1985;228:1112–5.
30. Swaab DF, Hofman MA. Sexual differentiation of the human hypothalamus: ontogeny of the sexually dimorphic nucleus of the preoptic area. Dev Brain Res 1988;44:314–8.
31. Gorski RA. Critical role for the medial preoptic area in the sexual differentiation of the brain. Prog Brain Res 1984;61:129–46.
32. Oomura Y, Yoshimatsu H, Aou S. Medial preoptic and hypothalamic neuronal activity during sexual behavior of the male monkey. Brain Res 1983;266:340–3.
33. Hart BL. Medial preoptic-anterior hypothalamic area and sociosexual behavior of male dogs: a comparative neuropsychological analysis. J Comp Physiol Psychol 1974;86:328–49.
34. Rodriguez-Sierra JF, Terasawa E. Lesions of the preoptic area facilitate lordosis behavior in male and female guinea pigs. Brain Res Bull 1979;4:513–7.
35. Arendash GW, Gorski RA. Effects of discrete lesions of the sexually dimorphic nucleus of the preoptic area or other medial preoptic regions on sexual behavior of male rats. Brain Res Bull 1983;10:147–54.
36. Hennessey AC, Wallen K, Edwards DA. Preoptic lesions increase the display of lordosis by male rats. Brain Res 1986;370:21–8.
37. Cherry JA, Baum MJ. Effects of lesions of a sexually dimorphic nucleus in the preoptic/anterior hypothalamic area on the expression of androgen- and estrogen-dependent sexual behaviors in male ferrets. Brain Res 1990;522:191–203.
38. Harris LJ. Sex differences in spatial ability: possible environmental, genetic, and neurologic factors. In: Kinsbourne M, ed. Asymmetrical function of the brain. Cambridge: Cambridge University Press, 1978:405–522.
39. Mann DR, Davis-DaSilva M, Wallen K, Coan P, Evans DE, Collins DC. Blockade of neonatal activation of the pituitary-testicular axis with con-

tinuous administration of a gonadotropin-releasing hormone agonist in male rhesus monkeys. J Clin Endocrinol Metab 1984;59:207–11.

40. Mann DR, Gould KG, Collins DC, Wallen K. Blockade of neonatal activation of the pituitary-testicular axis: effect on peripubertal luteinizing hormone and testosterone secretion and on testicular development in male monkeys. J Clin Endocrinol Metab 1989;68:600–7.

41. Heber D, Dodson R, Stoskopf C, Peterson M, Swerdloff RS. Pituitary desensitization and the regulation of pituitary gonadotropin-releasing hormone (GnRH) receptors following chronic administration of a superactive GnRH analog and testosterone. Life Sci 1982;30:3201–8.

42. Mann DR, Gould KG, Collins DC. Influence of continuous gonadotropin-releasing hormone (GnRH) agonist treatment on luteinizing hormone and testosterone secretion, the response to GnRH, and the testicular response to human chorionic gonadotropin in male rhesus monkeys. J Clin Endocrinol Metab 1984;58:262–7.

43. Mann DR, Gould KG, Smith MM, Duffey T, Collins DC. Influence of simultaneous gonadotropin releasing hormone agonist and testosterone treatment on spermatogenesis and potential fertilizing capacity in male monkeys. J Clin Endocrinol Metab 1987;65:1215–24.

44. Catchpole HR, van Wagenen G. Reproduction in the rhesus monkey, *Macaca mulatta*. In Bourne GH, ed. The rhesus monkey: management, reproduction, and pathology. Volume II. New York: Academic Press, 1975:117–40.

45. Plant TM. Pulsatile luteinizing hormone secretion in the neonatal male rhesus monkey (*Macaca mulatta*). J Endocrinol 1982;93:71–4.

46. Plant T. Puberty in primates. In: Knobil E, Neill J, eds. The physiology of reproduction. New York: Raven Press, 1988:1763–88.

47. Plant TM. The effects of neonatal orchidectomy on the developmental pattern of gonadotropin secretion in the male rhesus monkey (*Macaca mulatta*). Endocrinology 1980;106:1451–4.

48. Rose RM, Bernstein IS, Gordon TP, Lindsley JG. Changes in testosterone and behavior during adolescence in the male rhesus monkey. Psychosom Med 1978;40:61–70.

49. Gay VL, Plant TM. N-methyl-D,L-aspartate elicits hypothalamic gonadotropin-releasing hormone release in prepubertal male rhesus monkeys (*Macaca mulatta*). Endocrinology 1987;120:2289–95.

50. Plant TM, Gay VL, Marshall GR, Arslan M. Puberty in monkeys is triggered by chemical stimulation of the hypothalamus. Proc Natl Acad Sci USA 1989;86:2506–10.

51. Wallen K. Desire and ability: hormones and the regulation of female sexual behavior. Neurosci Biobehav Rev 1990;14:233–41.

52. Tanner JM, Whitehouse RH, Cameron N, Marshall WA, Healy MJR, Goldstein H. Assessment of skeletal maturity and prediction of adult height (TW2 method). New York: Academic Press, 1983:50–103.

53. Pang S, Levine LS, New MI. Puberty in congenital adrenal hyperplasia. In: Grumbach MM, Sizonenko PC, Aubert ML, eds. Control of the onset of puberty. Baltimore: Williams & Wilkins, 1990:669–89.

54. Goy RW, Bercovitch FB, McBrair MC. Behavioral masculinization is independent of genital masculinization in prenatally androgenized female rhesus macaques. Horm Behav 1988;22:552–71.

55. Tapanainen J, Koivisto M, Vihko R, Huhtaniemi I. Enhanced activity of the pituitary-gonadal axis in premature human infants. J Clin Endocrinol Metab 1981;52:235–7.

56. Liu L, Cristiano AM, Southers JL, et al. Effects of pituitary-testicular axis suppression *in utero* and during the early neonatal period with a long-acting LHRH analog on the development of secondary sexual characteristics and growth of male cynomolgus monkeys [Abstract]. In: The Endocrine Society 71st annual meeting, 1989:27A.

57. Liu L, Reynolds JC, Banks SM, et al. Effect of pituitary-testicular axis suppression *in utero* and during early neonatal period with a long-acting LHRH analog on bone density of the left radius and femur in male cynomolgus monkeys [Abstract]. In: The Endocrine Society 72nd annual meeting, 1990:395A.

58. Huhtaniemi I, Pakarinen P, Sokka T, Kolho K-L. Pituitary-gonadal function in the fetus and neonate. In: Delemarre van de Waal HA, Plant TM, van Rees GP, Schoemaker J, eds. Control of the onset of puberty, III. Amsterdam: Excerpta Medica 1989:101–9.

59. Huhtaniemi IT, Nevo N, Amsterdam A, Naor Z. Effect of postnatal treatment with a gonadotropin-releasing hormone antagonist on sexual maturation of male rats. Biol Reprod 1986;35:501–7.

60. Kolho K-L, Nikula H, Huhtaniemi I. Sexual maturation of male rats treated postnatally with a gonadotrophin-releasing hormone antagonist. J Endocrinol 1988;116:241–6.

61. van den Dungen HM, van Disten JAMJ, van Rees GP, Schoemaker J. Testicular weight, tubular diameter and number of sertoli cells in rats are decreased after early prepubertal administration of an LHRH-antagonist; the quality of spermatozoa is not impaired. Life Sci 1990;46:1081–9.

62. van den Dungen HM, Dijkstra H, Hiehle MAH, van Rees GP, Schoemaker J. Effects of LHRH antagonist administration to immature male rats on sexual development. Physiol Behav 1989;46:779–85.

63. Breedlove SM, Arnold AP. Hormone accumulation in a sexual dimorphic motor nucleus of the rat spinal cord. Science 1980;21:564–6.

64. Handelsman DJ, Spaliviero JA, Scott CD, Baxter RC. Hormonal regulation of the peripubertal surge of insulin-like growth factor-I in the rat. Endocrinology 1987;120:491–6.

65. van den Dungen HM, van Dieten JAMJ, Tilders FJH, van Rees GP, Schoemaker J. Administration of a GnRH-antagonist to immature rats affects subsequent female and male pubertal development differently. Acta Endocrinol 1989;120:778–84.

66. van Cappellen WA, Meijs-Roelofs HMA, Kramer P, van den Dungen HM. Ovarian follicle dynamics in immature rats treated with a luteinizing hormone-releasing hormone antagonist (org. 30276). Biol Reprod 1989; 40:1247–56.

67. Meijs-Roelofs HMA, van Cappellen WA, van Leeuwen ECM, Kramer P. Short- and long-term effects of an LHRH antagonist given during the prepubertal period on follicle dynamics in the rat. J Endocrinol 1990;124:247–53.

68. Kaplan SL, Grumbach MM. True precocious puberty: treatment with GnRH-agonists. In: Delemarre van de Waal HA, Plant TM, van Rees GP,

Schoemaker J, eds. Control of the onset of puberty, III. Amsterdam: Excerpta Medica, 1989:357–73.

69. Kaplan SL, Grumbach MM. Pathogenesis of sexual precocity. In: Grumbach MM, Sizonenko PC, Auberrt ML eds. Control of the onset of puberty. Baltimore: Williams & Wilkins, 1990:620–68.

70. Styne DM, Grumbach MM. Puberty in the male and female: its physiology and disorders. In: Yen SSC, Jaffee RB, eds. Reproductive endocrinology. Philadelphia: W.B. Saunders, 1978:189–240.

71. Lee PA. Medroxyprogesterone therapy for sexual precocity in girls. Am J Dis Child 1981;135:443–5.

72. Kaplan SA, Ling SM, Irani NG. Idiopathic isosexual precocity. Am J Dis Child 1968;116:591–8.

73. Schoen EJ. Treatment of idiopathic precocious puberty in boys. J Clin Endocrinol Metab 1966;26:363–70.

74. Rager K, Huenges R, Gupta D, Bierich JR. The treatment of precocious puberty with cyproterone acetate. Acta Endocrinol 1973;74:399–408.

75. Kauli R, Prager-Lewin R, Keret R, Laron Z. The LH response to LH-releasing hormone in children with true isosexual precocious puberty treated with cyproterone acetate. Clin Endocrinol 1975;4:305–11.

76. Werder EA, Muret G, Zachmann M, Brook CGD, Prader A. Treatment of precocious puberty with cyproterone acetate. Pediatr Res 1974;8:248–56.

77. Sorgo W, Kiraly E, Homoki J, et al. The effects of cyproterone acetate on statural growth in children with precocious puberty. Acta Endocrinol (Copenh) 1987;115:44–56.

78. Sadeghi-Nejad A, Kaplan SL, Grumbach MM. The effect of medroxy-progesterone acetate on adrenocortical function in children with precocious puberty. J Pediatr 1971;78:616–24.

79. Savage DCL, Swift TGF. Effect of cyproterone acetate on adrenocortical function in children with precocious puberty. Arch Dis Child 1981;56:218–22.

80. Rivier C, Rivier J, Vale W. Chronic effects of [D-Trp^6,Pro^9-NEt]-LHRH on reproductive functions in the male rat. Endocrinology 1979;105:1191–201.

81. Crowley WF Jr, Comite F, Vale W, et al. Therapeutic use of pituitary desensitization with a long-acting LHRH agonist: a potential new treatment for idiopathic precocious puberty. J Clin Endocrinol Metab 1981;52:370–2.

82. Comite F, Cutler GB, Rivier J, et al. Short-term treatment of idiopathic precocious puberty with a long-acting analogue of luteinizing hormone-releasing hormone. N Engl J Med 1981;305:1546–50.

83. Styne DM, Harris DA, Egli CA, et al. Treatment of true precocious puberty with a potent luteinizing hormone-releasing factor agonist: effect on growth, sexual maturation, pelvic sonography, and the hypothalamic-pituitary-gonadal axis. J Clin Endocrinol Metab 1985;61:142–51.

84. Oostdjk W, Hummedlink K, Odink RJH. Treatment of children with central precocious puberty by a slow-release gonadotropin-releasing hormone agonist. Eur J Pediatr 1990;149:308–13.

85. Kreiter M, Burstein S, Rosenfield RL, et al. Preserving adult height potential in girls with idiopathic true precocious puberty. J Pediatr 1990;117:364–70.

86. Werther GA, Warne GL, Ennis G, et al. Luteinizing hormone-releasing hormone analogue (Buserelin) treatment for central precocious puberty: a multi-centre trial. J Pediatr Child Health 1990;26:4–8.

87. Kauli R, Kornreich L, Laron Z. Pubertal development, growth and final height in girls with sexual precocity after therapy with the GnRH analogue D-Trp-6-LHRH: a report on 15 girls, followed after cessation of gonadotrophin suppressive therapy. Horm Res 1990;33:11–7.
88. Ward PS, Ward I, McNinch AW, Savage DCL. Reversible inhibition of central precocious puberty with a long-acting GnRH analogue. Arch Dis Child 1985;60:872–4.
89. Manasco PK, Pescovitz OH, Feuillan PP, et al. Resumption of puberty after long-term luteinizing hormone-releasing hormone agonist treatment of central precocious puberty. J Clin Endocrinol Metab 1988;67:368–72.
90. Mansfield MJ, Rudlin CR, Crigler JF, et al. Changes in growth and serum growth hormone and plasma somatomedin-C levels during suppression of gonadal sex steroid secretion in girls with central precocious puberty. J Clin Endocrinol Metab 1988;66:3–8.
91. Harris DA, Van Vliet G, Egli CA, et al. Somatomedin-C in normal puberty and in true precocious puberty before and after treatment with a potent luteinizing hormone-releasing hormone agonist. J Clin Endocrinol Metab 1985;61:152–9.
92. Pescovitz OH, Rosenfeld RG, Hintz RL, et al. Somatomedin-C in accelerated growth of children with precocious puberty. J Pediatr 1985;107:20–5.

Author Index

Subject Index